WN 180 KES

D1323083
369 0291525

## INTE
## RADIO

## DATE DUE

| 25 8 15 | |
|---|---|
| 24 10 16 | |
| | |
| | |
| | |
| | |
| | |
| | |
| | |
| | |
| | |
| | |
| | |
| | |
| | |
| | |
| | |
| | |

GAYLORD                    PRINTED IN U.S.A.

NHS Ayrshire & Arran
Libraries
Crosshouse Hospital

*Commissioning Editor*: Michael Houston
*Development Editor*: Sharon Nash
*Project Manager*: Srikumar Narayanan
*Design*: Charles Gray
*Illustration Manager*: Bruce Hogarth
*Marketing Managers (UK/USA)*: Richard Jones/Cara Jespersen

# INTERVENTIONAL RADIOLOGY

## A SURVIVAL GUIDE

### THIRD EDITION

**David Kessel** MB BS MA MRCP FRCR

Consultant Radiologist
St. James's University Hospital
Leeds, UK

**Iain Robertson** MB ChB MRCP FRCR

Consultant Radiologist
Gartnavel General Hospital
Glasgow, UK

With a contribution by:
Tarun Sabharwal FRCSI FRCR
Consultant Lead Interventional Radiologist
Honorary Senior Lecturer
Guy's and St Thomas' Hospital
London, UK

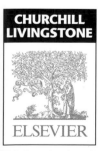

CHURCHILL LIVINGSTONE

ELSEVIER

Edinburgh   London   New York   Oxford   Philadelphia   St Louis   Sydney   Toronto   2011

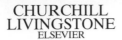

# CHURCHILL LIVINGSTONE
### ELSEVIER

CHURCHILL LIVINGSTONE an imprint of Elsevier Limited,

© 2011, Elsevier Limited. All rights reserved.

First edition 2000
Second edition 2005
Third edition 2011
    Reprinted 2011, 2012, 2013

No part of this publication may be reproduced or transmitted in any form or by any means, electronic or mechanical, including photocopying, recording, or any information storage and retrieval system, without permission in writing from the publisher. Details on how to seek permission, further information about the Publisher's permissions policies and our arrangements with organizations such as the Copyright Clearance Center and the Copyright Licensing Agency, can be found at our website: **www.elsevier.com/ permissions**.

This book and the individual contributions contained in it are protected under copyright by the Publisher (other than as may be noted herein).

**Notices**
Knowledge and best practice in this field are constantly changing. As new research and experience broaden our understanding, changes in research methods, professional practices, or medical treatment may become necessary. Practitioners and researchers must always rely on their own experience and knowledge in evaluating and using any information, methods, compounds, or experiments described herein. In using such information or methods they should be mindful of their own safety and the safety of others, including parties for whom they have a professional responsibility.

With respect to any drug or pharmaceutical products identified, readers are advised to check the most current information provided (i) on procedures featured or (ii) by the manufacturer of each product to be administered, to verify the recommended dose or formula, the method and duration of administration, and contraindications. It is the responsibility of practitioners, relying on their own experience and knowledge of their patients, to make diagnoses, to determine dosages and the best treatment for each individual patient, and to take all appropriate safety precautions.

To the fullest extent of the law, neither the Publisher nor the authors, contributors, or editors, assume any liability for any injury and/or damage to persons or property as a matter of products liability, negligence or otherwise, or from any use or operation of any methods, products, instructions, or ideas contained in the material herein.

ISBN: 978-0-7020-3389-6

1. **British Library Cataloguing in Publication Data**
Interventional radiology : a survival guide. – 3rd ed.
    1. Interventional radiology.    2. Interventional radiology–Equipment and supplies.
    I. Kessel, David.   II. Robertson, Iain, 1962-
    617'.0757–dc22

2. **Library of Congress Cataloging in Publication Data**
A catalog record for this book is available from the Library of Congress

 **ELSEVIER**   your source for books, journals and multimedia in the health sciences
**www.elsevierhealth.com**

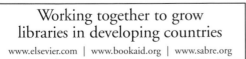

Working together to grow libraries in developing countries

www.elsevier.com | www.bookaid.org | www.sabre.org

ELSEVIER    BOOK AID International    Sabre Foundation

The publisher's policy is to use paper manufactured from sustainable forests

Printed in China

# Contents

# Section 3: Non-vascular intervention

# Preface

*"Hey, did you really write that survival book?" says trainee with opposable thumbs.*
*"Well ... yes, but there were two of us," replies modest author.*
*Yawn ... scratch ... trainee replies, "It's not bad, you know."**

Well, there you go. It makes the several hundred hours spent writing this third edition seem a fantastic investment. The life of an author, it's not all flashbulbs and glamour, you know.

So what's changed for edition number three? The major changes include a rewrite to incorporate non-invasive imaging as the predominant method of diagnostic investigation. It's truly remarkable to think that in the first edition in 2000 non-invasive imaging barely featured and we now rarely start an intervention without a previous CT or MR angiogram. We have also expanded the focus on Interventional Oncology and are extremely grateful to Tarun Sabharwal for agreeing to contribute the chapter on tumour ablation. We certainly learnt a lot about tumour ablation and extend our thanks to Tarun for dealing with our 'shock and awe' editing style with diplomacy and tact.

As the book, and we, get older it's been harder and harder to stop the mid-life bulge appearing. We've done our best to keep the weight down and maintain an easy-to-read style that many, well at least several, readers have kindly complimented us on.

We do hope you enjoy this new edition and hope you agree it's even better than *"not bad."*

*Trainee with opposable thumbs™ assures us that "not bad" in the North of the UK is fairly close to Nobel prize winning; they're not big on compliments (Northerners and trainees).

# Acknowledgements

We are both greatly indebted to the many people who have contributed to the delivery of this text.

Thanks to everyone who told us that they appreciated the first edition and motivated us to get typing again. We must mention the many patients who have endured and frequently entertained us during procedures and who have allowed us to use their images in the book. We are grateful to representatives from industry for providing some of the equipment that we have used to illustrate the manuscript. Our thanks to Sharon Nash for her timely and tenacious encouragement. Lastly, there are radiologists, surgeons, nurses and radiographers who have helped us practically, and willingly shared their knowledge, skill and wisdom with us.

Special thanks to our families: Ben, Holly, Jamie, Ross and Anna, children who have not questioned what their dads were up to. Carrie and Debbie, our much better halves, who supported us throughout the writing and editing.

# Abbreviations

| | | | |
|---|---|---|---|
| **AAA** | abdominal aortic aneurysm | **MRA** | magnetic resonance angiography |
| **AV** | atrioventricular | | |
| **CCA** | common carotid artery | **MRI** | magnetic resonance imaging |
| **CCF** | congestive cardiac failure | **NSAID** | non-steroidal anti-inflammatory drug |
| **CE-MRA** | contrast-enhanced MRA | | |
| **CFA** | common femoral artery | **PA** | popliteal artery |
| **CFV** | common femoral vein | **PE** | pulmonary embolism |
| **CIA** | common iliac artery | **PFA** | profunda femoris artery |
| **CTA** | computed tomography angiography | **PIG** | peroral image-guided gastrostomy |
| **CVA** | cerebrovascular accident | **PTC** | percutaneous transhepatic cholangiography |
| **DSA** | digital subtraction angiography | **PV** | popliteal vein |
| **DVT** | deep vein thrombosis | **PVA** | polyvinyl alcohol |
| **EIA** | external iliac artery | **RAO** | right anterior oblique |
| **ERCP** | endoscopic retrograde cholangiopancreatography | **RAS** | renal artery stenosis |
| | | **RHV** | right hepatic vein |
| **FBC** | full blood count | **RIG** | radiologically inserted gastrostomy |
| **FFP** | fresh frozen plasma | | |
| **FNA** | fine-needle aspiration | **RIJV** | right internal jugular vein |
| **FNAC** | fine-needle aspiration cytology | **RPV** | right portal vein |
| **fps** | frames per second | **rt-PA** | recombinant tissue plasminogen activator |
| **GTN** | glyceryl trinitrate | | |
| **IADSA** | intra-arterial digital subtraction angiography | **RVEDP** | right ventricular end-diastolic pressure |
| **IJV** | internal jugular vein | **SFA** | superficial femoral artery |
| **IM** | intramuscular | **STD** | sodium tetradecyl sulphate |
| **IMA** | inferior mesenteric artery | **SVCO** | superior vena cava obstruction |
| **IV** | intravenous | **SVT** | supraventricular tachycardia |
| **IVC** | inferior vena cava | **TIPS** | transjugular intrahepatic portosystemic shunting |
| **LAO** | left anterior oblique | | |
| **LGA** | left gastric artery | **TJB** | transjugular liver biopsy |
| **MIP** | maximum intensity projection | **TN** | tibial nerve |
| **MPDSA** | multiposition DSA | **TOS** | thoracic outlet syndrome |

# Section One

# General principles of angiography and intervention

# Preparing for successful and safe procedures

This chapter covers the cornerstones of good practice. You may be tempted to skip past to get to the action and give this section little more than a perfunctory glance. Do so at your own peril! Stop and think before rushing off, needle in hand; maximize your chances of a positive outcome by ensuring that the procedure is appropriate to the clinical situation. In particular, you should identify risk factors in individual patients and take steps to minimize them. The remainder of this chapter focuses on steps you should take to optimize patient safety.

## Patient preparation

The key elements to ensure that patients are properly prepared for a procedure are **evaluation** and **information**. Each assumes that you understand the procedure yourself.

### Evaluation

The focus of evaluation is identifying factors that may increase the risk of the procedure. Complex procedures should be discussed at multidisciplinary team meetings where all the different therapeutic options can be considered.

**Screening tests** Routine investigation (blood testing and electrocardiogram [ECG]) of all patients is unnecessary and merely increases the cost of patient care. In deciding whom to screen, consider the 'invasiveness' of the planned procedure and the likelihood of detecting an abnormality which would affect patient management. There is little evidence on which to base management except in the case of prevention of contrast-induced nephropathy. The guidelines below are suggestions for screening and are not absolute; if in doubt, it is better to perform a non-invasive test.

    **Evaluation of renal function is indicated when the patient**:

- Has a history of renal dysfunction
- Has a disease likely to impair renal function, e.g. hypertension, especially with peripheral vascular disease
- Is diabetic and has not had recent evaluation of renal function
- Has heart failure
- Is receiving nephrotoxic drugs.

    **Clotting studies are indicated when the patient**:

- Has clinical evidence of a coagulopathy
- Has a disease likely to affect clotting, e.g. liver disease; therefore, it is unwise to perform a liver biopsy without knowing the coagulation status
- Is receiving medication that affects coagulation, e.g. heparin or warfarin.

**Full blood count (FBC) is seldom indicated, but platelet count is often useful** in conditions that affect blood cell production or consumption, e.g. leukaemia, hypersplenism and cancer chemotherapy.

- FBC is obtained in the context of bleeding but is less important than physiological status.

**Alarm:** Remember numbers may be misleading, e.g.:

- Haemoglobin can be normal for several hours after acute haemorrhage.
- Platelet number may be normal but function may be abnormal, particularly in patients on dual antiplatelet agents.

**ECG is indicated when the patient:**

- Has a history of cardiac disease
- Is to undergo a procedure likely to affect cardiac output or cause arrhythmia, e.g. cardiac catheterization.

## Information

In order to decide whether to have treatment, patients need a basic understanding of their condition and its prognosis. Expect them to have researched their condition on the internet; your job is to help them to make sense of the bewildering mixture of fact and fiction they have found. For all but the most basic procedures it is best to see the patient in advance either on the ward or in an outpatient clinic. Be straightforward and honest about your ability and expertise and don't be afraid to allow a patient the opportunity to seek a second opinion. Patients will respect this and it is the least you would expect from someone treating you.

**Things a sensible patient might want to know**

- Are there alternative therapeutic options?
- The experience of the operator?
- What are the risks of the procedures?
- What is the likelihood of the procedure being a technical success?
- Will this have the clinically desired effect?
- Is the treatment a cure?
- What is the likelihood of recurrence?
- Will this treatment strategy impact on their future management?

In practical terms, a patient can only make a choice when they are empowered with sufficient knowledge.

**Informed consent**  Patients have a right to be given sufficient information to make informed decisions about the investigation/treatment (these terms will be used synonymously) options available to them. Your role is to provide relevant information in a way that they can comprehend. The laws regarding informed consent vary from country to country; these guidelines are based on the current situation in England but the ethos is broadly applicable. The following summary outlines the key issues relating to informed consent, which are applicable in most instances.

**Consent issues**  A qualified doctor who understands the risks and side effects of the procedure should be responsible for obtaining consent for treatment. Usually the doctor performing the treatment is in the best position to provide this information. If this is not practicable, the doctor may delegate to an appropriately experienced colleague. You must provide a balanced explanation of the treatment and management options along with the risks and benefits of each. Include:

- The general nature and purpose of the proposed treatment, including analgesia, sedation and aftercare
- Realistic expectations of the outcomes of the procedure
- Details of common and serious side effects (and their management) of the proposed intervention, particularly where these may have special significance for the patient
- The name of the doctor with overall responsibility for the patient and relevant members of the doctor's team
- The fact that they can change their mind or seek a second opinion at any time without prejudicing the care.

The form of the explanation and the amount of information provided vary depending on the patient's wishes, their capacity to understand, and the nature and complexity of the treatment. The patient should be allowed time to consider the information and must not be pressurized to make a decision.

 **Alarm:** It is unsatisfactory to mention only those complications that occur in at least 1% of patients! You should comment when the treatment is complex or involves significant risk for the patient's health, employment, or social or personal life. Document the key elements of any explanation and record any other wishes that the patient has in relation to the proposed treatment.

Review the patient's decision close to the time of treatment. This is mandatory when:

- Significant time has elapsed since consent was obtained. Many consent forms have a section to allow reaffirmation of consent
- There have been changes that may affect the treatment
- Someone else has obtained consent.

 **Alarm:** Compliance is not the same as consent! The patient's presence in the angiography suite does not indicate that the patient knows what the treatment entails. Checking the consent will avoid the possibility of misunderstanding later.

**Special circumstances** There are instances in which it is difficult or impossible to obtain informed consent. There are some general guidelines for what is acceptable procedure. If there is any doubt, legal advice should be obtained either from the hospital administration department, or your medical protection society or union.

*Emergencies* When consent cannot be obtained, you may only provide whatever medical treatment is necessary to save life or prevent significant deterioration in the patient's condition.

**Competence to make decisions** This is the ability to understand and retain information for long enough to evaluate it and make a decision.

*Inability to comprehend* Seemingly irrational decisions and refusal of treatment are not evidence of a lack of competence. Take time and review whether the patient has been provided with sufficient information or has not fully understood any of the explanation. Where doubt exists, seek advice; there is guidance for the formal assessment of competence.

*Fluctuating capacity* When the patient's mental state varies, consent should be obtained during periods of lucidity. This should be reviewed at intervals and recorded in the patient's notes.

No one can give or withhold consent of treatment on behalf of a mentally incapacitated patient. Try to establish whether the patient has previously indicated a preference, e.g. in a 'living will'. If the patient complies, you may carry out any treatment that is judged to be in the patient's best interest.

*Children* At the age of 16, the patient should be treated as an adult. Children below the age of 16 who are able to understand the nature, purpose and consequence of the procedure or its refusal have the capacity to make decisions regarding their treatment. In England, if a competent child refuses treatment, a person with parental authority or a court may give consent for any treatment in the child's best interest. Seek legal advice when doubt exists. A person with parental authority may authorize or refuse treatment for a child who is not competent to give consent. You are not bound by parental refusal; seek legal advice. In an emergency, proceed as above.

# Managing high-risk patients

The role of interventional therapy is extending to some of the highest-risk patients such as those with major bleeding from the gastrointestinal tract and secondary to trauma. Having identified patients who are at increased risk, it is necessary to have strategies to manage them. Consider the risk in the context of the patient's condition. While the risks of the procedure should be minimized, a life-saving procedure should not be delayed. From time to time you will be told that 'the patient is too unstable to bring to radiology' but remember there is no logic saying that the patient is too ill to have a potentially life-saving procedure! This section aims to help you keep the risk to yourself and the patient as small as possible.

This list is not comprehensive, so pause to consider before every case and never hesitate to seek advice.

 **Tip:** In many cases the simplest, safest strategy is to perform a non-invasive investigation. If you don't do this routinely, now is the time to start!

# The patient's general condition

## American Society of Anesthesiologists (ASA) status classification system

Anaesthetists will often quote ASA scores to you. The grading allows a common understanding of a patient's pre-procedure physical condition. The ASA score should not be used for prognostic indication as actual risk will be affected by other factors such as age, body mass index, type of procedure, anaesthetic technique and operator experience.

**In practice you need assistance with PS4 patients, and PS5 patients require immediate attention!**

**The patient has a history of anaphylactic reaction to intravascular contrast** This is fully discussed in Chapter 2, Interventional Pause. Consider alternative imaging strategies such as duplex ultrasound and magnetic resonance angiography (MRA), or another contrast agent such as gadolinium or carbon dioxide ($CO_2$).

**The patient is anticoagulated or has a severe bleeding diathesis** Correction of coagulopathy is discussed in Chapter 5, Drugs Used in Interventional Radiology. The risk relates to the nature of the procedure; simple drainage and venous puncture are safer than arterial puncture or core biopsy. The risk of haematoma following angiography increases when the platelet count is $100 \times 10^9/L$. For surgery and invasive procedures the platelet count should be $\geq 50 \times 10^9/L$.

Evaluate each case on its own clinical merit, consider postponing elective procedures to allow investigation and correction of the coagulopathy. Only intervene to correct the clotting if the procedure is urgent.

**Tip:** Abnormal clotting is relevant mainly when the time comes to obtain haemostasis. Consider using a closure device (Chapter 12, Haemostasis). Alternatively, leave a sheath in the artery until the clotting is corrected. An arterial line may be helpful for patients in the intensive therapy unit.

**Diabetes**  Diabetic patients are at particular risk because of:
- The protean manifestations of diabetes, especially cardiovascular and renal disease
- Potential problems with diabetic control in the peri-procedural period.

*Non-insulin-dependent diabetic patients*  The current UK recommendation is that patients with non-insulin-dependent diabetes should stop metformin at the time of any procedure involving intravascular iodinated contrast and should not restart until renal function has been checked 48 hours after the procedure. **The risk of lactic acidosis is vanishingly small unless there is prior renal dysfunction**. Some patients will need to take insulin to control their diabetes over this period.

*Insulin-dependent diabetic patients*  Should avoid prolonged fasting; they should be scheduled to have their procedure early in the morning. In this case they should take their long-acting insulin as usual but omit the short-acting insulin. If the procedure is later in the day, leave out the short-acting insulin and halve the dose of the long-acting insulin. A 5% dextrose solution should be infused to provide 5–10 g/h of glucose; this will usually maintain the blood glucose in the range 6–11 mmol/L.

**Alarm:** Hypoglycaemia is more important than transient hyperglycaemia. It is seldom unsafe to give the patient dextrose!

**Renal impairment**  Chronic renal impairment is common in very sick patients and those with peripheral vascular disease and may be exacerbated by contrast. The aetiology of contrast-induced nephropathy (a rise in creatinine of 0.5–1 mg/dL or 44–88 µmol/L) is complex. Although few patients will require dialysis, prevention is better than cure. **The most important factor in protecting renal function is ensuring adequate hydration**. If iodinated contrast is essential then non-ionic isosmolar agents probably minimize the risk. The evidence for other regimens such as N-acetylcysteine is weak but this regimen is relatively innocuous and can be administered as 600 mg PO pre and post procedure.

**Alarm:** Roughly 50% of renal function has been lost by the time the creatinine rises above the normal limit. Many labs now supply the estimated glomerular filtration rate (eGFR) calculated from age, race and sex of the patient. If your lab doesn't supply it, you can use calculators available online.

1. **Is this the most appropriate investigation?** Consider using alternative tests (MRA, Doppler, $CO_2$). Remember that there is a risk of nephrogenic systemic sclerosis in patients given gadolinium-based contrast for magnetic resonance imaging (MRI).

2. **Review medication. If possible stop:**
   - Non-steroidal anti-inflammatory drugs (NSAIDs)
   - Angiotensin-converting enzyme inhibitors (ACE-Is) unless there is severe heart failure
   - METFORMIN (stop for 48 hours and restart if creatinine stable).

   Avoid loop diuretics if possible.
3. Act according to the creatinine clearance (serum creatinine if you don't have a calculator):
   - **Minimal risk CrCl >60 or Cr <120**
     **Ensure hydration** Oral fluids 1 L pre and post procedure
   - **Low risk CrCl 30–60 or Cr 120–180**
     **Inpatient**: Non-ionic contrast, IV normal saline 1 mL/kg/h 12 hours pre and post procedure
     **Outpatient**: Iso-osmolar contrast (iodixanol). Encourage oral fluids 1 L pre and post
       procedure, if possible IV normal saline started on arrival 1 L over 4 hours.
   - **Intermediate risk CrCl <30, Cr >180 or renal transplant**
     **If possible admit for procedure**: iso-osmolar contrast IV normal saline 1 mL/kg/h
       (caution if congestive cardiac failure [CCF]) 12 hours pre and post procedure
       N-acetylcysteine 600 mg PO (two doses pre and post procedure).
   - **High risk CrCl <20 mL/min**
     **Admit for procedure**; as above. Repeat Cr at 7 days.
   - **Avoid further contrast exposure for 72 hours if possible**.
4. Other risk factors, e.g. diabetes mellitus, multiple myeloma, CCF, cirrhosis: consider
   promoting to the next level of CrCl.

 **Tip:** Hydration – in the presence of CCF or cirrhosis with ascites use 5% dextrose instead of saline.

**Hypertension** Hypertension is common and is exacerbated by anxiety and pain. Hypertension increases the risk of haematoma. Review the ward charts to check the normal baseline blood pressure (BP). The Society of Cardiovascular and Interventional Radiology (SCVIR) standards define uncontrolled hypertension as a diastolic pressure >100 mmHg. Systolic hypertension is present when the systolic pressure is >180 mmHg.

Controlling high blood pressure starts on the ward. The patient should take any antihypertensive medication (except diuretics) as normal. If they remain hypertensive in the angiography suite, they can be given 10 mg of nifedipine. Sedation and analgesia may also help blood pressure control. Aim to reduce the mean blood pressure by no more than 25%.

 **Tip:** If the blood pressure cannot be controlled by these simple measures, postpone elective cases until the patient is appropriately medicated on the ward.

**Heart failure** The patient's condition should be optimized before angiography. Diuretics should be avoided if possible to minimize the risk of nephrotoxicity. Limit the study to the essential details. If necessary, breathless patients can sit up slightly; this can be compensated for by craniocaudal angulation of the C-arm. Give oxygen as necessary.

**Gastric contents** It is normal to fast patients before invasive procedures but the risk of aspiration of gastric contents is very small except in sedated patients. General guidelines are shown in Table 1.1. These are mandatory before conscious sedation or anaesthesia and advisable before other cases.

In urgent cases, seek anaesthetic advice, avoid sedation and consider metoclopramide to promote gastric emptying, H2 antagonists or proton pump inhibitors to increase gastric pH and antiemetics to minimize the risk of vomiting.

**Table 1.1** General guidelines for fasting time before invasive procedures

| Oral intake | Fasting time |
| --- | --- |
| Solids and non-clear liquids | 6–8 h |
| Clear liquids | 2–3 h |

 **Tip:** Diabetic patients and those at the extremes of age should be given maintenance IV fluids to cover the peri-procedural period.

**Demented, anxious and agitated patients** These patients may require sedation or general anaesthesia for invasive procedures. General anaesthesia is often the safest option for both the patient and staff, and maximizes the chance of performing the procedure successfully. Consent issues are also relevant in this group of patients (see above).

# Suggestions for further reading

### Patient information sheets

British Society of Interventional Radiology (BSIR). Available at: www.bsir.org/.

Cardiovascular and Interventional Radiology Society of Europe (CIRSE). General information for patients available at www.cirse.org; information on specific procedures available at www.cirse.org.

Society of Interventional Radiology (SIR). Available at: www.sirweb.org/; www.sirweb.org/medical-professionals.

### Screening tests

Payne CS. A primer on patient management problems in interventional radiology. AJR Am J Roentgenol 1998;170:1169–1176. Available at www.ajronline.org/cgi/reprint/170/5/1169.

A useful overview of screening for and managing high-risk patients.

Standards of Practice Committee of the American Society for Gastrointestinal Endoscopy. Position statement on routine laboratory testing before endoscopic procedures. Gastrointest Endosc 2008;68:no 5.

Although this issue is about endoscopy, it is also pragmatic about levels of evidence and when a test might be useful.

### High-risk patients

ASA available at: http://my.clevelandclinic.org/services/Anesthesia/hic_ASA_Physical_Classification_System.aspx

Gives examples of how to assign scores.

Aspelin P, Aubry P, Fransson S-G, et al. Nephrotoxic effects in high risk patients undergoing angiography. N Engl J Med 2003;348:491–499.

General Medical Council. Good medical practice. 2006. London: GMC Publications, 178 Great Portland Street, London W1N 6JE. Available at: www.gmc-uk.org/guidance/good_medical_practice/GMC_GMP.pdf.

Up-to-date and informative booklet outlining reasonable practice in the UK. Mandatory reading. There are also interactive case studies on the GMC website: www.gmc-uk.org/guidance/case_studies/index.asp.

General Medical Council. 0–18 years: Guidance for all doctors. 2007. London: GMC Publications, 178 Great Portland Street, London W1N 6JE. Available at: www.gmc-uk.org/guidance/ethical_guidance/children_guidance/index.asp; download from www.gmc-uk.org/guidance/archive/GMC_0-18.pdf

Up-to-date and informative booklet outlining how to deal with children and those under 18 years of age (and their carers) in the UK. Mandatory reading.

General Medical Council. Consent: patients and doctors making decisions together. 2008. London: GMC Publications, 178 Great Portland Street, London W1N 6JE. Available at: www.gmc-uk.org/guidance/ethical_guidance/consent_guidance/Consent_guidance.pdf

Up-to-date and informative booklet describing all issues regarding consent in the UK. Mandatory reading.

Mental Capacity Act. Guidance for health professionals. Succinct explanations of the principles of patients' rights and ability to make informed decisions. 2005. Available at: www.bma.org.uk/health_promotion_ethics/consent_and_capacity/mencapact05.jsp; download from www.bma.org.uk/images/mentalcapacityact_tcm41-146891.pdf.

Mueller C, Buerkel G, Buettner H, et al. Prevention of contrast media associated nephropathy. Randomized comparison of 2 hydration

regimens in 1620 patients undergoing coronary angioplasty. Arch Intern Med 2002;162:329–336.
Level 1 evidence why to use normal saline.
Rihal C, Textor S, Grill D, et al. Level 1 evidence the advantage of iodixanol (Visipaque) over non-ionic contrast media. Incidence and prognostic importance of acute renal failure after percutaneous coronary intervention. Circulation 2002;105:2259–2264.

The true incidence of ARF and its significance in a real population, sobering reading!
Waksman R, King SB, Douglas JS, et al. Predictors of groin complications after balloon and new device coronary intervention. Am J Cardiol 1995;75:886–889.
Big holes, big patients and deranged clotting. Platelets less than 200 and dual antiplatelet = false aneurysm.

# Interventional pause

The World Health Organization (WHO) is actively promoting adoption of a strategy to reduce predictable and preventable errors during procedures. It has been clearly demonstrated that stopping to consider each individual case at three separate stages helps prevent significant patient morbidity. This ethos can simply be applied to interventional radiology.

## Advance planning

It is always worth mentally rehearsing the procedure and trying to anticipate any difficulties you may encounter.

- Reflect on what you are aiming to achieve and think about what you will do if there is a problem and you are not successful? You should always have a 'Plan B' and if necessary little plans C, D and E. Might you stop before your objective is reached; is it better to 'live to fight another day'? Would it help to have assistance from a colleague?
- What might go wrong during the procedure and are you equipped to manage complications? Are there predictable difficulties or aspects of the case that might affect outcome? Have you discussed this with the patient and your colleagues?

## On the day: staff, equipment and room preparation

*Before starting* Liaise with a named individual who is responsible for working on the case. Make sure that they know the plan for the procedure, its steps and any anticipated difficult elements. Ensure that they have checked that all the kit is available and in the room and that they will inform you if anything in missing or in short supply (e.g. embolization coils).

*Introductions* Ensure that everyone knows each other. This is particularly important when working in an unfamiliar environment and with staff you don't know.

*Explanations* If the case is complex, who will ensure that everyone knows their roles and responsibilities, e.g. patient monitoring, running nurse, scrub nurse. Pick your strongest team and ensure that the most appropriate individual is in each role.

**Table 2.1** Checklist for typical interventional cases

| Task | Person responsible | Elements |
|------|--------------------|----------|
| Pre-procedure case review | Doctor | Review intended procedure: site, side, approach, etc. |
| | Nurse | Need for sedation, analgesia, anaesthesia |
| | Radiographer | Monitoring |
| | | Anticipated equipment including patient-specific items, e.g. stent graft, chemoembolization |
| | | Emergency equipment |
| | | Potential difficulties |
| | | Additional equipment, e.g. ultrasound machine |
| | | Important elements of procedure |
| | | Set of room: C-arm position, trolleys, etc. |
| Pre-procedure checklist | Nurse | Patient ID |
| | | Patient notes |
| | | Allergies/drug reactions |
| | | Pre-procedure test results normal or inform doctor |
| | | Intravenous access |
| | | Hydration |
| | | Premedication |
| | | Antibiotic prophylaxis within previous 60 minutes |
| | | Analgesia/sedation |
| | | Check correct equipment available |
| | | Bail out kit (covered stents, etc.) |
| | Doctor | Consent |
| | | Medication required is prescribed |
| | Radiographer | Request available |
| | | Imaging available |
| Post-procedure check | Doctor | Operative sheet completed showing procedure, outcomes, complications, aftercare |
| | | Communication with patient, relatives and other carers |
| | | Planned review stated |
| | Nurse | Sharps disposed safely |
| | | Patient charts completed including prescribed drugs, monitoring |
| | | Specimens labelled and handled correctly |
| | | Handover to ward staff including instructions for aftercare/analgesia |
| | | Patient given information sheets/instructions for care/contact numbers |
| | Radiographer | Images reviewed with doctor |
| | | Images archived |

# Post-procedure care

- Will the patient require any special care or analgesia after the procedure?
- Have you handed over care to an appropriate colleague?
- Do the ward nurses require special orders for observations and patient monitoring?
- Do drains or lines need particular care or management?
- If there are potentially predictable problems what precautions are necessary and what actions should be taken if they occur?
- Who should be notified if there is a problem and how are they to be contacted?
- Will you be visiting to review the patient?
- When can the patient be discharged, has a discharge letter been provided and any medications prescribed?
- Is an outpatient appointment necessary, when and with whom?

Table 2.1 indicates the typical elements that should be considered for almost every procedure.

 **Tip:** This all seems too obvious but it has been shown that planning prevents significant errors, in particular wrong operation, wrong patient, wrong site. Planning doesn't only help patients, it also helps you and your staff to ensure procedures are performed smoothly with the minimum of stress and interruption for all concerned! It will also help you if there is a complication or, worse still, an adverse outcome/litigation. A checklist for typical interventional cases is shown in Table 2.1.

# Suggestions for further reading

Angle JF, Nemcek AA, Cohen AM, et al. Quality improvement guidelines for preventing wrong site, wrong procedure, and wrong person errors: application of the Joint Commission 'Universal Protocol for Preventing Wrong Site, Wrong Procedure, Wrong Person Surgery' to the practice of interventional radiology. J Vasc Interv Radiol 2008;19:1145–1151. Available at: www.jvir.org/article/S1051-0443(08)00473-9/abstract.

Joint Commission on Accreditation of Healthcare Organizations. Healthcare at the crossroads strategies for improving the medical liability system and preventing patient injury. 2005.

Available at: www.jointcommission.org/NR/rdonlyres/167DD821-A395-48FD-87F9-6AB12BCACB0F/0/Medical_Liability.pdf.

Strategies to minimize preventable patient injuries – daft not to think about this really.

WHO Surgical Safety Checklist. 2009. Available at: www.npsa.nhs.uk/nrls/alerts-and-directives/alerts/safer-surgery-alert/.

The size of the problem – 'In industrialized countries major complications are reported to occur in 3–16% of inpatient surgical procedures, with permanent disability or death rates of approximately 0.4–0.8%' – and simple pragmatic solutions.

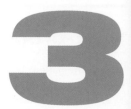

# Contrast

Most vascular computed tomography (CT) and MRI, the vast majority of angiographic procedures, and many non-vascular interventions rely on contrast media to reveal the anatomy. Contrast media can be broadly classified by their use and by their chemical structure. X-ray contrast affects tissue X-ray attenuation, ultrasound contrast affects tissue and blood reflectivity and MRI contrast affects tissue relaxation times. Discussion in this section is confined to contrast media used for angiography and vascular diagnosis.

## Intravascular X-ray contrast agents

The two principal categories of X-ray contrast both affect X-ray attenuation. Details of the chemical and physical properties of these agents are extensively discussed in many texts, and it is important that you are familiar with the different options and their indications.

**Positive contrast agents** are liquids that have greater attenuation than the patient's soft tissues, due either to the presence of iodine or gadolinium.

**Negative contrast** has lower attenuation than the patient's tissues; at present, carbon dioxide gas is the only available option.

## Iodinated contrast media

These are the most frequently used agents. Non-ionic contrast media are recommended in high-risk patients (see below) and have largely replaced ionic contrast agents for intravascular use.

Optimal demonstration of anatomy and pathology requires the correct strength and volume of contrast delivered in the right place. Appropriate catheter positions, contrast volumes and flow rates are indicated throughout the diagnostic angiography chapters.

Most diagnostic and therapeutic intervention is performed using '300 strength' contrast (300 mg/mL iodine). This density of contrast is fine for pump injections into large vessels where the contrast is diluted by rapid blood flow. For selective hand injections in the vascular system and for non-vascular examinations, 300 strength contrast is diluted with saline to two-thirds or half strength. The aim is to adequately opacify the vessel but allow a level of grey scale that allows branches/filling defects to be seen through the contrast. Avoid high-density contrast examinations as lesions can be readily obscured.

As a general principle, the contrast column should opacify the entire vessel segment. To achieve this, the total contrast dose and the duration of the bolus must be correct. When the blood flow is slow, it takes several seconds for the opacified blood to pass through the vessel. Hence, a long contrast bolus is necessary. This is one of the reasons for increasing the volume of contrast to image the more distal vessels. Modern angiography equipment allows integration of multiple images, which has the same effect as increasing the length of the bolus, but it can reduce image quality due to minor degrees of patient movement between frames.

## Contrast reactions with iodinated contrast media

There are two forms of contrast reaction: direct effects and idiosyncratic responses. Up to 2% of patients require treatment for adverse reactions to intravascular iodinated contrast agents. In the majority of cases, only observation and minor supportive treatment are necessary but severe reactions require prompt recognition and immediate treatment.

**Direct effects** Direct effects are secondary to the osmolality and direct chemotoxicity of the contrast, and they include heat, nausea and pain. More important are the effects on organ systems.

*Renal* Chronic renal impairment is relatively common in patients with peripheral vascular disease and is exacerbated by contrast. Contrast-induced nephrotoxicity (a rise in creatinine of 0.5–1 mg/dL or 44–88 µmol/L) is common; the effect is usually transient but may be irreversible. Patients with pre-existing renal impairment, particularly diabetic patients, have the greatest risk, and increasingly eGFR is used to stratify patients into risk groups. No single protocol is available but if eGFR is below 45 consider using alternative tests, iso-osmolar contrast agents (e.g. iodixanol) and non-iodinated contrast agents, such as carbon dioxide.

The most important factor in protecting renal function is **actively promoting hydration**. Normal saline provides the optimal protection and can be used in patients who are nil by mouth. *N*-acetylcysteine may confer additional benefit (see Chapter 1, Preparing for Successful and Safe Procedures). Diabetic patients treated with metformin have a risk of developing lactic acidosis if they experience renal failure. The current UK guidelines are that metformin should be discontinued on the day of the examination and for 48 hours afterwards until the creatinine has returned to the pre-examination normal level.

*Cardiac* Cardiac problems are most likely to occur during coronary angiography and are usually manifest as arrhythmias or ischaemia. It is prudent to use non-ionic contrast in patients with ischaemic heart disease or heart failure.

*Haematological* Significant haematological interactions are uncommon. Non-ionic iodinated contrast can induce clotting if mixed with blood; hence, scrupulous attention to catheter flushing and avoidance of contaminating syringes with blood are essential.

*Neurological* Most neurological sequelae occur during carotid angiography and are related to angiographic technique. Genuine contrast-related problems are rare and are usually seen in patients with abnormalities in the blood–brain barrier.

**Idiosyncratic reactions** The mechanism of these reactions is uncertain; vasoactive agents such as histamine, serotonin, bradykinin and complement have been implicated but a causal role has not been established.

Idiosyncratic reactions are classified according to severity.

**Minor**: Common, ~1:30, e.g. metallic taste, sensation of heat, mild nausea, sneezing; these do not require treatment.

**Intermediate**: Common, ~1:100, e.g. urticaria; not life-threatening; respond quickly to treatment.

**Severe**: Rare, ~1:3000, e.g. circulatory collapse, arrhythmia, bronchospasm, dyspnoea; may be life-threatening, require prompt therapy. Remember the A, B, C, D approach and don't hesitate to call for help.

**Death**: Rare, ~1:40 000, mostly caused by cardiac arrhythmia, pulmonary oedema, respiratory arrest or convulsions.

**Assessing the risk** The risk of a contrast reaction varies depending on the circumstances of individual patients; however, the following are associated with an increased risk of a severe idiosyncratic reaction:

- Previous allergic reaction to iodine-containing contrast and shellfish allergy: 10×
- Cardiac disease: 5×
- Asthma: 5×
- General allergic responses: 3×
- Drugs: β-blockers, interleukin-2 3×
- Age >50 years: 2× risk of death.

Remember that these factors increase the relative risk; the absolute risk remains very low!

**Reducing the risk** The vast majority of severe and fatal contrast reactions occur within 20 minutes of administration and therefore it is vital that patients are kept under constant supervision during this period. There have been a few isolated reports of delayed hypotensive reactions hours after contrast injection.

The ideal method of reducing risk is to avoid iodine-containing contrast examinations by using other imaging modalities such as ultrasound or MRI. When this is not possible:

- **Prepare for reaction**. Ensure that resuscitation equipment and drugs are immediately available every time contrast is injected. Make sure that you are familiar with the management of the reaction; most catheter laboratories have charts on the wall to remind you in times of need (it is much less stressful to check it out in advance).
- **Use non-ionic contrast agents**. Non-ionic contrast agents certainly reduce the risk of minor reactions and may reduce the risk of more significant reactions.
- **Reassure the patient**. Explain that contrast reactions are unlikely and that the situation is under control. In severe anxiety, short-acting anxiolytic agents may be warranted.
- **Consider steroid pre-medication**. There is some evidence that oral steroid premedication may reduce the risk of moderate–severe reactions, though this is hotly contested. Treatment has to be started 24 hours before contrast administration and therefore this is only suitable for elective examinations. Intravenous hydrocortisone 200 mg has been given prior to urgent examinations, although this is of questionable value. Many departments have local guidelines on steroid administration.

In the rare patient with a previously documented severe reaction:

1. Avoid iodinated contrast; use $CO_2$ or gadolinium or another imaging modality.
2. If this is impossible and the examination is essential, monitor the patient carefully.
3. Ensure resuscitation personnel, equipment and drugs are immediately available. You may need expert assistance maintaining the airway – consider enrolling anaesthetic assistance.
4. Obtain secure IV access before contrast administration.
5. Use non-ionic contrast.
6. Consider steroid premedication; consult local guidelines.
7. Reassure the patient.

## Treatment of contrast reactions

Warn patients that a sense of warmth, a metallic taste and transient nausea are all common after rapid IV injection of contrast and these effects wear off after a few minutes.

## Minor reactions

- **Nausea and vomiting.** Active treatment rarely required. Reassure and monitor patient.
- **Urticaria.** One of the commonest contrast reactions. Localized patches of urticaria do not require treatment. Simply observe and monitor the patient (pulse, BP). Generalized urticaria or localized urticaria in sensitive areas, e.g. periorbital, should be treated by chlorphenamine 20 mg given slowly by IV injection.
- **Vasovagal syncope.** Monitor the patient's pulse, BP, oxygen saturation and ECG. Elevate the legs. Establish IV access. Give atropine 0.6–1.2 mg by IV injection for bradycardia. Volume expansion with IV fluids for persistent hypotension.

## Intermediate–severe reactions

- **Bronchospasm.** Monitor the patient's pulse, BP, oxygen saturation and ECG. Give 100% $O_2$. Treat initially with β-agonist inhaler, e.g. salbutamol. If continuing bronchospasm, administer adrenaline (epinephrine) subcutaneously: 0.3–0.5 mL of 1 : 1000 solution. If severely shocked, then administer adrenaline 1 mL (0.1 mg) 1:10000 by slow IV injection. IV steroids are also usually given and in acute reactions, steroids may work surprisingly quickly, although it can take a few hours for them to achieve full effect.
- **Laryngeal oedema/angioneurotic oedema.** Monitor the patient's pulse, BP, oxygen saturation and ECG. Give 100% $O_2$ and watch the oxygen saturation closely. Administer adrenaline subcutaneously 0.3–0.5 mL of 1 : 1000 solution. Chlorphenamine 20 mg by slow intravenous injection should also be given. Get an anaesthetist to assess the airway. Tracheostomy may be required in severe cases.
- **Severe hypotension.** Hypotension accompanied by tachycardia may indicate vasodilation and increased capillary permeability. Monitor the patient's pulse, BP, oxygen saturation and ECG. Rapid infusion of IV fluids is essential and several litres of fluid replacement may be necessary. Adrenaline is often of value.
- **Cimetidine**, the H2 receptor antagonist, has been effective in severe reactions resistant to conventional therapy. The drug is given by slow intravenous infusion (cimetidine 300 mg in 20 mL saline). An H1 receptor blocker, such as chlorphenamine, should be given first.

# MRI contrast agents

## Gadolinium

Gadolinium works well as an MRI contrast agent. Its use has been described in X-ray angiography but it is a poor X-ray contrast agent and is often difficult to see on fluoroscopy. Gadolinium is handled in the same way as conventional contrast agents and can be injected by hand or with an injection pump.

There is increasing interest in the use of 'blood pool agents' for MRA. These have a longer dwell time in the circulation and this improves imaging in the venous phase.

Gadolinium-based agents are much more expensive than iodinated contrast, therefore their use is almost exclusively reserved for MRI and the occasional patient who needs a limited volume of contrast and has a genuine reason to avoid iodinated contrast, e.g. severe contrast reaction.

It is now recognized that gadolinium poses particular risks in patients with renal impairment. Gadolinium-based agents are nephrotoxic in their own right especially when doses greater than 40 mL are used in MRA.

## Nephrogenic systemic fibrosis (NSF)

Risk factors for NSF are still being established; NSF has not been described in patients with GFR >60 mL/min/1.7 m$^2$. This limits the utility of gadolinium-based agents for MRA and conventional angiography in patients with renal impairment. Some agents appear to have increased risk but the list is changing and you should refer to contemporary local and national guidelines. Macrocyclic agents such as gadoterate meglumine (Dotarem) may also reduce the incidence of NSF in high-risk patients.

 **Alarm:** Pay particular attention in the following groups:

- GFR <30 mL/min/1.7 m$^2$ including patients on dialysis and children aged <1 year.
- Patients with renal dysfunction who have had or are awaiting liver transplantation.

The prevalence in patients on dialysis or with hepatorenal syndrome is 4%.

# Negative contrast agents – CO$_2$

Carbon dioxide is most commonly used for the following reasons:
- History of severe reaction to iodinated contrast
- Renoprotection
- Where there is another advantage such as the use of CO$_2$ for wedged hepatic venography.

CO$_2$ is only effective with digital subtraction angiography (DSA) and additional software is necessary to optimize the image. CO$_2$ dissolves rapidly in blood and is excreted through the lungs. Consider using CO$_2$ when there is a contraindication to conventional iodinated contrast and to opacify the portal vein during wedged hepatic venography.

 **Alarm:** There is a risk of cerebral toxicity with CO$_2$ and for this reason it should never be used intra-arterially above the diaphragm or intravenously in patients with right-to-left shunts.

## Equipment

- Basic angiography set
- Medical grade CO$_2$ from a disposable* cylinder
- Standard bacterial filter (from a blood-giving set)
- High-pressure connector
- 3-way tap
- Lockable stopcock for each syringe
- 60-mL Luer lock syringes.

The circuit is set up as shown in Figure 3.1.

 **Alarm:** The pressurized CO$_2$ must never be connected directly to the patient as this risks inadvertent injection of a large volume of gas that may cause a 'vapour lock'.

---

*Reusable cylinders may be contaminated with water or rust particles; hence the need for a disposable system. The bacterial filter is a further safeguard. In an ideal world one would use disposable stainless steel cylinders. These are more expensive but cause less patient discomfort.

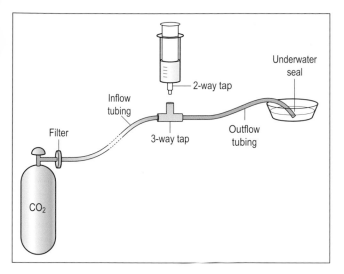

**Fig. 3.1** ■ Preparation of $CO_2$ for hand injection.

# Injecting $CO_2$

You can inject by hand or via a dedicated pump. $CO_2$ gas has very low viscosity and so is very readily injected even through small catheters. Injecting a colourless, odourless and invisible gas is disconcerting at first. It is essential to have a foolproof system for filling the syringes to prevent inadvertent air embolization.

### Filling syringes with $CO_2$

1. Fill a 10-mL syringe from the system; this flushes the system and purges any air from the connecting tube. Repeat this each time that the gas is turned off.
2. Angiography requires a volume of around 50 mL, therefore use a 50-mL Leur lock syringe and allow the syringe to fill 'passively' from the cylinder; this ensures that it is filling with $CO_2$.
3. Use the 3-way tap to discard the contents three times to flush out any residual air in the syringe before finally filling.
4. Shut the lockable stopcock and disconnect the syringe from the 3-way tap.
5. The syringe will now contain $CO_2$ at slightly above atmospheric pressure.

   **Alarm:** The $CO_2$ in an open syringe will be replaced with air in about an hour! Always prepare $CO_2$ syringes just before use and keep the stopcock closed.

The catheter is flushed with saline as normal. As the filled syringe is connected to the catheter, the stopcock is opened; this has two functions:

- Air is flushed from the catheter hub
- The $CO_2$ in the syringe falls to atmospheric pressure and so the true volume of the gas is known.

The catheter is now gently flushed with $CO_2$; this expels the saline from the lumen. You will know when the catheter is flushed as there is a marked fall in resistance. Close the tap and disconnect this syringe and discard its contents. Connect a fresh syringe of $CO_2$ and you are ready to inject. The volume and rate of injection are adjusted according to the size of the vessel. There is no dose limit as long as injections are restricted to 100 mL every 2 minutes.

If performing venography, always fluoroscope over the pulmonary artery to look for gas trapping.

## Troubleshooting

**Dependent vessels are not seen**. Intravascular $CO_2$ displaces blood rather than mixing with it like a liquid contrast. The $CO_2$ is buoyant and floats over the blood column, dependent branches tend not to fill and in general there is an underestimate of vessel size. If necessary, the patient can be turned to elevate the vessel of interest, e.g. side of interest up for renal angiography. C-arm angulation must be adjusted accordingly.

**There is gas trapping**. The $CO_2$ collects above the blood and forms a 'vapour lock'. This reduces the surface area for the gas to dissolve. Potentially, this can lead to ischaemia or thrombosis. This is most likely to happen with large (>100 mL) injections of $CO_2$ or in capacious vessels with anterior branches, e.g. in an aortic aneurysm. If gas trapping occurs, simply turn or tilt the patient head down so that the gas can disperse. If necessary, the gas can be aspirated via a catheter. **Do not elevate the patient's head!**

**The gas column fragments**. This happens particularly in the distal vessels (Fig. 3.2). Use image summation techniques to integrate several frames onto the same image. Consider raising the leg as this improves filling of the distal vessels.

**The distal vessels cannot be seen**. $CO_2$ is a 'negative contrast' and not as good as conventional contrast media (otherwise we would use it all the time!). Sometimes bolus fragmentation and poor opacification require the use of a liquid contrast agent.

The patient experiences pain during injection. Try a slower injection rate.

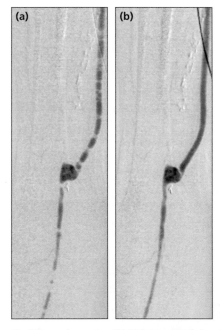

**Fig. 3.2** ■ Gas fragmentation with $CO_2$ angiography: (A) before multiple image summation; (B) after image summation.

# Suggestions for further reading

Ansell G. Complications of intravascular iodinated contrast media. In: Ansell G, et al. eds. Complications in diagnostic imaging and interventional radiology, 3rd edn. Oxford: Blackwell Science, 1996;245–300.
An excellent summary with everything that you might ever wish to know about iodinated contrast and more besides.
Bettmann MA, Heeren T, Greenfield A, et al. Adverse events with radiographic contrast agents: Results of the SCVIR contrast registry. Radiology 1997;203:611–620.
A prospective review of adverse outcomes in over 60 000 patients. There is some study bias but unless you are dealing with a high-risk patient, ionic contrast agents are safe.

### Alternatives to iodinated contrast media

Caridi JG, Hawkins IF. $CO_2$ digital subtraction angiography: Potential complications and their prevention. J Vasc Interv Radiol 1997;8:383–891.
How to work with $CO_2$. A useful starter.
Bettmann M. Frequently asked questions: iodinated contrast agents. Radiographics 2004;24:S3–S10.
Kessel DO, Peters K, Robertson I, et al. Carbon dioxide guided vascular interventions: technique and pitfalls. CVIR 2002;25:476-483.
Massicotte A. Contrast medium-induced nephropathy: strategies for prevention. Pharmacotherapy 2008;28:1140–1150.
Rao QA, Newhouse JH. Risk of nephropathy after intravenous administration of contrast material: a critical literature analysis. Radiology 2006;239:392-397.

# 4

# Sedation

Radiologists frequently administer sedation to patients undergoing prolonged interventional procedures. Sedation can also be useful in anxious or hypertensive patients. Remember that sedation may result in respiratory depression and aspiration of gastric contents; in addition, there is a small but significant mortality. Children are at particular risk. Unfortunately most of us have not been trained in anaesthesia and may lack the ability to maintain a patient's airway in an emergency.

This chapter defines conscious sedation and outlines patient selection and management within the radiology department. If you have any doubts about your ability to manage a particular patient, seek advice from an anaesthetist.

## Conscious sedation

This refers to a controlled state of reduced consciousness throughout which the patient retains the ability to make purposeful, verbal responses. Protective reflexes are preserved and the airway is maintained. Drugs used in conscious sedation should have a sufficient margin of safety to make unintended loss of consciousness unlikely.

 **Alarm:** If verbal responsiveness is lost the patient requires a level of care identical to that needed for general anaesthesia.

**Deep sedation and anaesthesia** Involve a further reduction in conscious level from which the patient is not readily roused and during which protective reflexes and the ability to maintain the airway may be lost along with the ability to respond to physical and verbal stimulation. In terms of patient management, deep sedation should be regarded as a form of general anaesthesia.

 **Alarm:** Clinical observation is vital during conscious sedation; machines do not detect responsiveness. Someone must maintain verbal and tactile contact with the patient and assess the patient's mental state and alertness.

## To sedate or not to sedate, that is the question

Practices differ widely between countries and cultures. Patient tolerance varies enormously; it is unnecessary to use sedation routinely. Try to establish whether sedation is likely to be required before starting the procedure. In this way, the patient can be properly assessed and risk minimized.

Take time to talk to the patient before, during and after the procedure and you will find that the majority of patients are not distressed if they are actively reassured and not in pain. Remind them that if they become distressed, sedation can be administered during the procedure. Consider sedation in the following circumstances:

- Prolonged procedures where the patient is likely to become uncomfortable.
- Patients who remain very anxious despite explanation.
- Painful procedures, It is important not to equate sedation with analgesia, and if performing a painful procedure, give adequate analgesia. Remember that sedation and analgesia are synergistic and take care.
- Patients who are unlikely to cooperate, e.g. children. Now you have considered it, dismiss the idea – agitated or confused patients often become unmanageable following even light sedation. In these circumstances you need anaesthetic support and general anaesthesia may be the safest option!

## Sedation guidelines

- Assess the requirements and risks for each patient.
- Make sure the patient has IV access and pulse, BP and $O_2$ monitoring.
- Remember, benzodiazepines are more potent in patients >60 years: the dose should be reduced accordingly. Diazepam dosage is more predictable in patients >70 years.
- Start with a small dose and increase it as necessary. A large bolus is more likely to result in hypoxia (oxygen saturation <90%) and apnoea, e.g. use 1–2-mg aliquots of midazolam.
- Designated personnel should be responsible for monitoring the patient and maintaining records.
- Resuscitation equipment must be readily available and staff should be familiar with its use. It helps to have a designated staff member to respond in case of emergency.

 **Alarm:** Do not hesitate to seek anaesthetic assistance if you have any doubts about sedation; it is much better than having to deal with a problem during a case.

## Patient selection

Most serious adverse events are not predictable and can occur in 'healthy' patients. Extremes of age and pre-existing cardiorespiratory disease and severe illness contribute to increased risk of sedation. Ask an anaesthetist to assess high-risk patients; a general anaesthetic may be safer for them than sedation. Do not forget that aspiration of gastric contents is associated with significant morbidity in patients who are not fasted.

## Care and monitoring of sedated patients

**Care** It is essential that there are adequate numbers of trained staff and appropriate facilities to allow constant monitoring of the patient's condition. Radiologists often take responsibility for sedation; this is unsatisfactory during interventional procedures when your attention is focused elsewhere.

**Monitoring** A named member of staff is responsible for monitoring each patient. They must be capable of recognizing and managing important changes in the sedated patient's condition. Many of the complications caused by sedation can be avoided if the patient is closely and responsively observed during the procedure and in the recovery period. The following parameters should be monitored:

*Pulse oximetry and respiratory rate* Allows prompt recognition of hypoxia long before it is clinically obvious. Prompt action should be taken when the oxygen saturation falls below 95%. The patient should be encouraged to take some deep breaths and oxygen should be administered by mask or nasal cannulae. If this fails, try to establish an airway using the jaw thrust manoeuvre or a plastic airway. Seek assistance sooner rather than later.

 **Tip:** Give oxygen routinely to sedated patients; this saves an unseemly scuffle when the pulse oximeter alarm starts to ring.

*ECG* The ECG demonstrates heart rate and cardiac rhythms and detects signs of myocardial ischaemia. It is invaluable in the management of cardiac arrest and arrhythmia. It is not uncommon for you to hear a change in rate and rhythm before anyone else notices. **N.B. Most cardiac events are late manifestations of hypoxia.**

*Pulse and blood pressure* These are best monitored by an automatic device. Warn the patient that this is:

- Uncomfortable
- Normal practice and not a sign of impending problems.

Most machines have alarms that can be set to respond to significant increases or falls in blood pressure. Record the pressure every 5 minutes and make additional recordings during procedures likely to affect the blood pressure. **N.B. Tachycardia and hypertension are usually the response to pain but may also reflect hypercapnoea.**

 **Alarm:** Make sure that your staff notify you of any upward or downward trends in the record and warn them if you are going to do something likely to affect the values, e.g. give hyoscine butylbromide (Buscopan) or a vasodilator.

## Aftercare

Remember that sedated patients require close observation until they are alert and oriented and able to drink. Inpatients may return to the ward as soon as they are stable enough to be cared for on the ward, but this varies considerably with the type of ward. Baseline observations should be stable for at least 1 hour before discharge. Outpatients should not drive or operate machinery for 24 hours and must be accompanied by a responsible adult. Clear instructions should be provided for the carer, detailing what to expect in the postprocedural period. State clearly who should be contacted (and how to contact them) in case of problems.

## Suggestions for further reading

Practice guidelines for sedation and analgesia by non-anesthesiologists. Anesthesiology 2002;96:1004–1017.

Royal College of Radiologists and the Royal College of Anaesthetists. Sedation and anaesthesia in radiology: report of a joint working party. 1992. Available at; www.rcr.ac.uk/publications.aspx?PageID=310&PublicationID=186. A good overview compiled jointly by anaesthetists and radiologists.

Safe sedation, analgesia and anaesthesia within the radiology department. Ref No: BFCR(03)4 ISBN 1872599 91 5. BFCR(03)4.

Shabanie A. Conscious sedation for interventional procedures: a practical guide. Tech Vasc Interv Radiol 2006;9:84–88.

# Pain control and analgesia

Many interventional radiology procedures do not require any analgesia; some procedures are intrinsically painful, especially if they are prolonged, and others are unpredictably uncomfortable. The procedure will be simpler and the patient less distressed if pain can be kept to a minimum. Preventing severe pain is likely to increase everyone's confidence in you! Remember pain and anxiety affect the patient pre, peri and post procedure to a varying degree so there is no 'one size fits all' solution. As always, forward planning is the key to success: recognize which procedures and which particular stages are likely to require analgesia.

**If a procedure is predicted to be painful** e.g. some embolization procedures:
- Explain this to the patient in advance and reassure them that this is normal and that effective pain control will be provided.
- Prophylactic analgesia should be given to minimize/prevent it. Combinations of non-steroidal and opiate analgesics are often used.
- Prescribe appropriate medication before starting (e.g. analgesic, antiemetic, sedative).
- Have someone check regularly whether the pain control is effective. Give additional analgesia and pain control as necessary. Patient-controlled analgesia (PCA) is useful here.
- Suitable analgesia should be prescribed for the post-procedural period.

 **Tip:** If you anticipate giving drugs on several occasions during a procedure, attach a low pressure connector to the venous access and locate it in an easily accessible position. This means you will not have to interrupt the procedure while someone rummages around under the drapes trying to find a cannula each time a drug is given.

**If a patient experiences unexpected pain during or after a procedure**
- Establish what is causing the pain and what can be done to resolve it, e.g. stress-related angina may respond to the usual glyceryl trinitrate spray.
- Treat pain swiftly and effectively. This is not the time for oral paracetamol (acetaminophen); **intravenous opiate analgesics** are the order of the day, so remember to ensure that venous access is obtained in advance.

**If a procedure is likely to have painful consequences**
- Plan for this in advance by prescribing a suitable analgesic regimen. This is particularly important following embolization.
- Review the patient to ensure that clinical evolution is satisfactory.

You should become familiar with the regimens and preparations in use at your institution. Remember that the actions of sedatives and analgesics are often synergistic (antidotes to reverse the effects of both are available). Anaesthetists are expert at managing pain and should be consulted if there is any doubt regarding appropriate medication or the need for adjunctive procedures such as epidural or spinal anaesthesia.

## Some typical regimens

Pre-procedure medication for painful procedures, especially those likely to induce inflammation, e.g. embolization of solid organs.

**Non-steroidal anti-inflammatory drugs** e.g.:
- Intravenous (IV) paracetamol 1 g
- Per rectum (PR) diclofenac 25–50 mg
  Single dose pre procedure.

**Opiate analgesics** e.g.:
- Morphine 1–5 mg estimated according to patient size (little old lady 1 mg)
- Fentanyl (Sublimaze) usually given in 20–40-μg aliquots. Fentanyl has faster onset and shorter duration of action and is almost 100 × more potent than morphine.

Give a loading dose before starting the procedure and then further top up doses as required during the procedure.

**Alarm:** When using opiate analgesics:
- Cautions. Start with a low dose and increase as necessary. Elderly patients are often very sensitive. Opiates and sedatives have a synergistic effect.
- Consider concomitant antiemetic therapy. Cyclizine (50 mg), ondansetron (4 mg), metoclopramide 10 mg are all effective.
- Monitor. Pulse, BP and oxygen saturation.
- Reversal. Naloxone 100–200 mg (1.5–3 mg/kg) by IV injection. If response inadequate, give increments of 100 mg every 2 minutes. Repeat as necessary.

## Patient-controlled analgesia

PCA is an important weapon in your armamentarium; in essence, following an initial loading dose, the patient self-medicates whenever they feel pain. To prevent overdose there is typically a 'lockout period' of 5–10 minutes during which the patient cannot administer further drug.

PCA can be set up simply to give dosage on demand or to give a background infusion dose which can be supplemented on demand; this is very useful following the procedure (Table 5.1).

**During a procedure** a suitably trained member of staff should regularly assess the patient to gauge the effectiveness of pain control and to administer further analgesia in accordance with your local protocol.

**After a procedure** there is a tendency for interventional radiologists to forget this component of patient care or to devolve it to others who may not be familiar with the needs of patients post intervention. Post-procedure pain control is essential. Make sure that the

**Table 5.1** Patient controlled analgesia (PCA) dosage table

| Drug | Loading dose | Background infusion dose / hour | Patient administered dose | Lock-out time |
|------|------|------|------|------|
| Fentanyl | 10–50 μg | 0–10 μg | 5–20 μg | 3–10 minutes |
| Morphine | 1.0–2.5 mg | 0.2–0.4 mg | 0.2–0.4 mg | 5–15 minutes |

patient will be cared for on a ward that is appropriately staffed and equipped to monitor and manage the patient. If there is a high level of support then analgesia can be prescribed as required; if there is a lower level of care, then regular dosage is advisable in the first instance.

## Suggestions for further reading

Keyoung JA, Levy EB, Roth ER, et al. Intraarterial lidocaine for pain control after uterine artery embolization for leiomyomata. J Vasc Interv Radiol 2001;12:1065–1073.

Lang EV, Berbaum KS, Pauker SG, et al. Beneficial effects of hypnosis and adverse effects of empathic attention during percutaneous tumor treatment: when being nice does not suffice. J Vasc Interv Radiol 2008;19: 897–905.

Lee SH, Hahn ST, Park SH. Intraarterial lidocaine administration for relief of pain resulting from transarterial chemoembolization of hepatocellular carcinoma: Its effectiveness and optimal timing of administration. Cardiovasc Intervent Radiol 2001;24:368–371.

# Drugs used in interventional radiology

This chapter provides a brief guide to the use of some of the drugs frequently used and encountered in the practice of interventional radiology. The drugs are broadly grouped according to their actions, with an additional section on prescribing in patients with atherosclerosis. Familiar drugs in common general usage will not be discussed in detail. The list is not comprehensive and we do not address pharmacological interactions. For other drugs and paediatric dose schedules, consult drug formularies, conventional texts and local guidelines.

## Antidotes

This seems like an unusual and cautious place to start but antidotes are often needed more urgently than treatments. You should be familiar with reversal of central/respiratory depression due to benzodiazepine sedation and opiate analgesia and also correction of anticoagulation.

### Benzodiazepine reversal

#### Flumazenil (Anexate)

- **Action**: short-acting benzodiazepine antagonist.
- **Dose**: IV 200 µg over 15 seconds. Repeated doses may be necessary; maximum total dose is 3 mg.

### Opiate reversal

#### Naloxone

- **Action**: short-acting opiate antagonist.
- **Dose**: IV 0.1–0.2 mg at 2–3-minute intervals until desired degree of reversal is achieved. Try to titrate the dose, as rapid reversal may result in complete reversal of analgesia and elevation of blood pressure.

 **Alarm:** If a patient requires treatment to reverse the effects of benzodiazepine or opiate drugs they must be cared for in an environment in which they can safely be monitored in case central/respiratory depression reoccurs!

# Abnormal clotting and anticoagulation reversal

The risk of bleeding relates to the procedure; clearly, simple drainage and venous puncture are safer than arterial puncture or core biopsy.

 **Alarm:** Routine reversal of anticoagulation is often unnecessary and can be hazardous for the patient, e.g. metallic heart valves. Consider the balance of risks.

## Correcting coagulopathy – when and how

This is a frequent issue in interventional radiology, especially for urgent cases. The golden rule is to postpone the examination if the clinical scenario allows. **Only intervene to correct the clotting if the procedure is urgent**.

### Abnormal INR

Patients with liver disease frequently have deranged clotting; they should be given vitamin K1 unless the procedure is urgent, in which case proceed as for reversal of warfarin.

### Vitamin K1

- **Indication**: correction of the international normalized ratio (INR) in patients with liver synthetic dysfunction. Vitamin K1 takes at least 12 hours to normalize the INR.
- **Dose**: slow IV injection (1 mg/min). The dose depends on the INR and the condition of the patient (see Table 6.1).

 **Alarm:** Following vitamin K1, it may take 2–3 weeks to re-establish anticoagulation with warfarin. Do not use vitamin K1 when continued anticoagulation is desired!

## Reversal of warfarin

Warfarin affects vitamin K1 metabolism. For elective cases warfarin should be stopped for 3 days before intervention and INR checked on the day of the procedure.

### Rapid reversal of warfarin

It is prudent to consult a haematologist, especially if anticoagulation will need to be restarted.

**Table 6.1** Dose of Vitamin K1

| INR | Dose of Vitamin K1 |
| --- | --- |
| 6–10 | 0.5–1 mg |
| 10–20 | 3–5 mg |
| >20 | 10 mg |

**Table 6.2** Dried prothrombin complex dosage

| Initial INR | 2–3.9 | 4–5.9 | >6 |
|---|---|---|---|
| Dose mg/kg | 1 | 1.4 | 2 |
| Dose factor IX IU/kg | 25 | 35 | 50 |

**Table 6.3** Reversal of unfractionated heparin with protamine

| Time since heparin administration | Protamine dose | Protamine dose for 5000 units of heparin | Protamine dose for 3000 units of heparin |
|---|---|---|---|
| <15 minutes | 10 mg/1000 units | 50 mg | 30 mg |
| 30 minutes | 5 mg /1000 units | 25 mg | 15 mg |
| 60 minutes | 2.5 mg /1000 units | 12.5 mg | 7.5 mg |
| 90 minutes | 1.25 mg/1000 units | 6.25 mg | 3.75 mg |

# Fresh frozen plasma (FFP)

- **Indication**: transient reversal of warfarin. FFP is effective for approximately 6 hours.
- **Action**: replacement of clotting factors.
- **Dose**: at least 2 units are usually required. Each unit of FFP has clotting factors equivalent to 1 unit of fresh blood. At least 1 unit of FFP is usually given before starting the procedure.

# Dried prothrombin complex (Beriplex)

- **Indication**: immediate reversal of warfarin.
- **Action**: a combination of human clotting factor IX with factors II, VII and X.
- **Dose**: IV no more than 3 units/kg /mL based on the INR (see Table 6.2). Maximum dose 210 units. The maximum dose should not exceed 5000 IU of factor IX. 5–10 mg of vitamin K is usually given with dried prothrombin complex.
- **Cautions**: can cause severe thrombosis, hypersensitivity, anaphylaxis.

 **Tip:** Beriplex and FFP are used when rapid correction of coagulopathy or temporary reversal of anticoagulation is necessary.

# Reversal of heparin

## Protamine sulphate

- **Action**: binds strongly to unfractionated heparin (UFH).
- **Alarm**: protamine binding to low molecular weight heparin (LMWH) is incomplete and normalizes activated partial thromboplastin time (APTT) but does not reverse antifactor Xa completely, hence anticoagulant activity persists.
- **Indication**: rapid correction of APTT.
- **Dose**: Slow IV injection no more than 1 mg/minute. Maximum 50 mg. Dosage depends on heparin dose and time since administration (see Table 6.3).
- **Cautions**: Risk of allergic reaction increased if previous exposure.

 **Tip:** As a general rule, 10 mg of protamine will neutralize 1000 units of heparin; the dose should be halved every 30 minutes after heparin administration.

## Reversal of low molecular weight heparin

Seek haematological advice. Within 8 hours of administering LMWH, the dose of protamine is 1 mg/100 anti-Xa units for enoxaparin. Smaller doses are needed beyond 8 hours after LMWH administration.

# Prevention of crises

## Antihypertensive agents

True hypertensive crisis with immediate life-threatening consequences such as pulmonary oedema and stroke is sometimes seen in patients with phaeochromocytoma. Severe hypertension with a diastolic blood pressure in excess of 120 mmHg is not uncommon in patients undergoing intervention.

Hypertension is a common problem and is exacerbated by anxiety and pain. Hypertension increases the risk of haematoma. When faced with a hypertensive patient, review the ward charts to check the normal baseline blood pressure and to ensure that the patient has taken any antihypertensive medication as normal. Blood pressure reduction is indicated if the diastolic pressure rises above 100 mmHg before or during an interventional procedure. Sedation and analgesia may also help blood pressure control. If the patient remains hypertensive in the angiography suite, aim to reduce the mean blood pressure by no more than 25%.

### Nifedipine

- **Action**: calcium channel blocker.
- **Dose**: 10 mg oral; this dose can be repeated at 20-minute intervals up to a dose of 30 mg.
- **Monitor**: Pulse, BP and ECG.

**Tip:** To speed up the effect, the capsule should be chewed and the contents swallowed. The effect begins in 5–10 minutes, peaks at 40 minutes and lasts 6 hours.

### Labetalol

- **Action**: Mixed α- and β-adrenoreceptor blockade.
- **Indication**: Patients with phaeochromocytoma, hypertensive crisis.
- **Dose**: Usually oral 100 mg twice daily. In emergency, slow IV injection of 50 mg repeated at 2-minute intervals up to a maximum of 200 mg.
- **Cautions**: Asthma and heart block. Postural hypotension for up to 3 hours.
- **Monitor**: Pulse, BP and ECG.

### Carcinoid crisis

Carcinoid crisis is the sudden onset of the manifestations of carcinoid syndrome: cutaneous flushing, severe dyspnoea, peripheral cyanosis, tachycardia and diarrhoea. Patients may be haemodynamically unstable. Crisis can be precipitated by embolization of carcinoid metastases.

## Octreotide

- **Action**: octreotide is a synthetic somatostatin analogue that binds receptors in carcinoid tumours and reduces the release of 5-hydroxytryptamine (5-HT) and other vasoactive chemicals.
- **Indication**: prevention and treatment of carcinoid crisis. Patients undergoing embolotherapy for carcinoid syndrome should be premedicated with octreotide.
- **Dose**: 100 µg IV over 5 minutes.

# Anaesthetics, analgesics and sedatives

## Local anaesthetics

Local anaesthesia is the first stage in almost every interventional procedure. Warn the patient that the injection may sting for a few seconds before the anaesthetic takes effect; remember to pause a few seconds before making that first incision! Local anaesthetics are remarkably free from adverse reactions. The majority of 'reactions' are psychogenic or the result of systemic toxicity usually owing to inadvertent intravascular injection, overdose or rapid absorption. True anaphylactoid and anaphylactic reactions to lidocaine occur very rarely (about one per year in the UK) and represent only 1% of reported adverse reactions. Skin testing may be useful to establish cases of true type I hypersensitivity. In true allergy, prilocaine should be used. Systemic effects on the central nervous system include dizziness, confusion, paraesthesia and convulsions with bradycardia, and cardiovascular effects (e.g. arrhythmia and hypotension).

### Lidocaine hydrochloride (Xylocaine)

- **Action**: stabilizes nerve membrane, preventing generation and transmission of impulses.
- **Indication**: local anaesthesia.
- **Dose**: 1% lidocaine (10 mg/mL) is sufficient for local anaesthesia; the total dose should not usually exceed 20 mL (200 mg).
- **Cautions**: allergic reactions.
- **Monitor**: pulse, BP and oxygen saturation.
- **Reversal**: none. Oxygen helps prevent and treat systemic effects; give circulatory support and maintain airway.

### Prilocaine hydrochloride

- **Indication**: allergy to lidocaine; adverse reactions are commoner with prilocaine but there is little cross-reactivity.
- **Dose**: 1% prilocaine (10 mg/mL). Maximum dose 400 mg.

### Bupivacaine hydrochloride (Marcain)

Bupivacaine is a long-acting local anaesthetic and is sometimes useful for prolonged procedures or when a device is left in situ. It is not used to induce anaesthesia as it takes up to 30 minutes to reach full effect.

- **Indication**: prolonged local anaesthesia.
- **Dose**: 0.25% bupivacaine (2.5 mg/mL). Maximum dose 150 mg (60 mL).

# Analgesics (see Chapter 5, Pain control and analgesia)

Non-opioid agents: used to control mild to moderate pain. NSAIDs also have anti-inflammatory action.

## Paracetamol (acetaminophen)

- **Action**: cyclo-oxygenase inhibitor.
- **Indications**: analgesia.
- **Dose**:
  - Oral 500–1000 mg 4–6-hourly, maximum 4 g/day
  - IV 1 mg infused over 15 minutes, child 10–50 kg, 15 mg/kg 6-hourly
- **Cautions**: liver dysfunction.

## Diclofenac

- **Actions**: NSAID cyclo-oxygenase inhibitor analgesic (equivalent to paracetamol).
- **Indications**: pain control and prevention/reduction in inflammation.
- **Dose**:
  - 25–50 mg tds (oral or rectal). Maximum 150 mg in 24 hours.
  - IV: infusion over 30 minutes, dilute according to instructions.
- **Cautions**: hypersensitivity to aspirin or NSAIDs, severe heart failure, arterial disease.

## Opiates

- **Indication**: moderate to severe pain.
- **Side effects**: nausea (give prophylactic antiemetic) and respiratory depression.
- **Monitoring**: verbal assessment of pain control, pulse, BP, oxygen saturation for cardiorespiratory depression. Give prophylactic oxygen.

## Morphine

Still the most commonly used analgesic.

- **Actions**: maximum effect reached after 10 minutes, lasts 4–6 hours.
- **Indications**: Moderate to severe pain.
- **Dose**: Titrate according to response, start with a low dose, e.g. 1 mg in elderly, 2.5 mg in normal adult.

## Fentanyl

- **Actions**: rapid-acting short half-life synthetic opioid 100× more powerful than morphine. A dose of 0.1 mg of fentanyl is equivalent to 10 mg of morphine. Maximum effect if injected IV reached after 2–5 minutes, lasts 45–90 minutes.
- **Indications**: pre procedural pain control IV bolus or infusion. Post procedural pain transdermal.
- **Dose**:
  - IV 0.1 mg slow injection.
  - Transdermal patch: slow release patches that last 72 hours, nomenclature fentanyl '12' patch gives approximately 12 µg/h. Start at 12–25 µg/h.
- **Cautions**: peak respiratory depressant effect of a single dose of fentanyl is not seen until 5–15 minutes after injection.

# Sedatives (see Chapter 4, Sedation)

Benzodiazepines are the most commonly used sedatives; their dose requirement decreases with increasing age.

- **Monitor**: pulse, BP and oxygen saturation. Give oxygen by nasal prongs or by mask.

## Midazolam

- **Action**: short-acting benzodiazepine with a half-life of 2 hours.
- **Indication**: conscious sedation.
- **Dose**: 2.5–10 mg, IV or IM; IM injection gives slower absorption in elderly patients. The potency of midazolam increases in patients over 60 years and for this reason diazepam is recommended in elderly patients, especially over 70 years old.
- **Cautions**: reduce dose in elderly patients, respiratory depression and aspiration.

## Diazepam

- **Action**: benzodiazepine with a long half-life and active metabolites.
- **Indication**: sedation of elderly patients. Compared with midazolam, the relative potency of diazepam changes little with age, giving it a wider margin of safety.
- **Dose**: 2–10 mg by slow IV injection into a large vein.
- **Cautions**: thrombophlebitis common.

# Vasoactive drugs

## Vasodilators

Vasodilator drugs are used in angiography to prevent and relieve vascular spasm (prevention, as always, is better than cure) and to augment flow during measurement of intra-arterial pressure gradients. Several drugs are in common usage and are discussed below. Glyceryl trinitrate (GTN) is typically used to prevent spasm, and tolazoline and papaverine to augment flow and reverse spasm. Nifedipine (an antihypertensive) can also be given prophylactically in situations where spasm is anticipated.

### Tolazoline

- **Action**: α-adrenoreceptor blockade.
- **Dose**: 20–50 mg by slow intra-arterial injection.
- **Cautions**: palpitations, angina and nausea are common side effects.
- **Monitor**: pulse, BP and ECG.

### Papaverine

- **Action**: direct smooth muscle relaxant.
- **Dose**: 20–60 mg by slow intra-arterial injection. May be followed by infusion 30–60 mg/h.
- **Cautions**: hypotension.
- **Monitor**: pulse, BP and ECG.

## Glyceryl trinitrate

- **Action**: complex, mixed venous and arterial vasodilator.
- **Dose**: 100–200 µg boluses by selective intra-arterial injection. May be infused at 15–20 µg/min and increased as necessary if the blood pressure allows.
- **Cautions**: hypotension.
- **Monitor**: pulse, BP and ECG.

 **Tip:** GTN typically comes in a solution of 1 mg/mL; to measure small doses accurately, draw up the desired dose of GTN in a 1 mL syringe and dilute to 1 mL with saline.

## Vasoconstrictors

Vasopressin is the only vasoconstrictor in common use.

- **Action**: synthetic, antidiuretic hormone that has direct vasoconstrictor effect.
- **Indication**: used to control variceal and gastrointestinal haemorrhage.
- **Dose**: selective, intra-arterial infusion 0.1–0.4 units/min. May be given IV for variceal bleeding 0.2–0.8 units/min.
- **Cautions**: ischaemic heart disease and peripheral vascular disease.
- **Monitor**: pulse, BP and ECG.
- **Reversal**: the half-life is only 10 minutes.

# Drugs affecting coagulation

## Heparins

The actions of heparins are complex and require a good understanding of the clotting cascades, which are beyond the scope of this book (some excellent references for those wishing to know more are included). What you need to know is as follows.

## Unfractionated heparin

- **Actions**: inactivates multiple clotting enzymes; dominant effect inactivation of thrombin (factor IIa), inhibits platelet function.
- **Indication**: prevention of vascular and peri-catheter thrombosis during endovascular procedures.
- **Dose**: IV, 50–100 units/kg (3000 units for a small woman, 5000 units for a large man). Following IV injection, heparin takes about 3 minutes to take effect. The half-life is about 60 minutes. Give another 1000 units every hour in prolonged procedures.
- **Cautions**: heparin infusions should be stopped 3 hours before the procedure and the activated clotting time (ACT) checked on arrival in the catheter laboratory.
- **Monitor**: ACT, check baseline level, aim for a 2.5× increase for effective anticoagulation. Sheaths can be removed when the ACT has returned to near baseline and is below 200 s.
- **Reversal**: protamine given by slow IV injection to a maximum single dose of 50 mg.

## Low molecular weight heparin

LMWHs are not usually prescribed by interventional radiologists but are relevant as many patients are receiving them.

- **Actions**: major effect is inactivation of factor Xa.
- **Dose**: single daily subcutaneous injection.
- **Monitoring**: not usually clinically necessary due to predictable effect.
- **Reversal**: seek haematology advice if intervention is needed in patients being treated with LMWH.

**Alarm:** Three key facts interventional radiologists should know about LMWH

- LMWH has a long half-life: if a case is not urgent, wait 24 hours.
- APTT does not reflect anticoagulant action.
- Protamine does not reverse LMWH completely. Ask a haematologist to help.

## Platelets

(Ehh. … we know these are not a drug, but they are an essential part of your weaponry.)

- **Indications**: thrombocytopenia. The risk of haematoma following angiography increases when the platelet count is <100 × $10^9$/L. For surgery and invasive procedures, the platelet count should be >50 × $10^9$/L. Below this level, platelet transfusion is advisable.
- **Dose**: each unit of platelets contains the same number of platelets found in 1 unit of fresh blood; 1 unit of platelets raises the platelet count by approximately 5 × $10^9$/L; transfusions of 4–6 units are usually sufficient to cover the procedure.

# Antiplatelet agents

Platelet activation has a central role in thrombus formation and can be inhibited by many agents. Different drugs have different modes of action to inhibit platelets, hence combined therapy may increase effect.

## Aspirin

- **Action**: aspirin irreversibly inhibits platelet cyclo-oxygenase.
- **Indication**: all patients with peripheral vascular disease should take low-dose aspirin.
- **Dose**: 75 mg daily.
- **Caution**: active peptic ulceration, children under 16 years of age, bleeding diathesis.

## Dipyridamole

- **Actions**: reduces platelet aggregation by inhibition of phosphodiesterase.
- **Indications**: patients intolerant to aspirin.
- **Dose**: 75–100 mg qds.
- **Cautions**: other drugs that increase risk of bleeding.

## Clopidogrel

- **Action**: inhibits binding of adenosine diphosphate.
- **Indication**: widely used in coronary and carotid artery stenting.
- **Dose**: 75 mg daily.
  - For full effect, clopidogrel should be started 1 week before the procedure; if the case is more acute give 200 mg 24 hours before the procedure and continue with 75 mg daily, usually continued for at least 1 month.
- **Caution**: active bleeding, planned surgery within 7 days, ischaemic stroke within past 7 days.

## Glycoprotein IIb/IIIa inhibitors (e.g. abciximab)

- **Actions**: inhibition of the GpIIb/IIIa receptor on the surface of the platelets.
- **Indications**: dissolution of platelet aggregates – seriously useful but rarely used in peripheral intervention.
- **Dose**: IV 250 µg/kg, start 10–60 minutes before procedure.
- **Cautions**: use with other drugs affecting coagulation, serious bleeding, surgery.
- **Monitoring**: clotting studies, FBC.

# Thrombolytic agents

Blood clot comprises platelets and blood cells in a mesh of fibrin polymer. Thrombolytic drugs activate plasmin to break down fibrin and factors V and VIII. Fresh clot has less cross-linked fibrin and is more likely to respond to thrombolysis. Several drugs are available for thrombolysis; all cause a systemic lytic state. The most widely used are recombinant tissue plasminogen activator (rt-PA) and urokinase. Streptokinase is cheaper but is associated with more side effects. rt-PA and urokinase are probably safer and more effective than streptokinase. rt-PA has become the favoured drug in the UK and urokinase in the USA.

The indications for thrombolysis and the techniques and dose regimens are discussed in detail in Chapter 19, Thrombolysis and Thrombectomy. All of the drugs cause a systemic lytic state which can result in haemorrhagic complications, which should be treated with FFP.

## Recombinant tissue plasminogen activator

- **Action**: rt-PA is activated by the presence of fibrin and is only weakly active in circulation.
- **Dose**: bolus 5 mg, to a maximum of 20 mg. Infusion 0.5–4 mg/h. Total dose should be kept to 40 mg.

## Urokinase

- **Action**: acts directly on circulating plasminogen to form plasmin.
- **Dose**: bolus 30 000–60 000 units. Infusion 60 000–240 000 units/h.

## Streptokinase

- **Action**: binds to circulating plasminogen; this complex converts free plasminogen to plasmin.
- **Dose**: bolus 50 000 units; infusion 2500–5000 units/h.
- **Cautions**: causes fever (33%) and allergic responses (20%). Circulating antibodies can completely neutralize its action up to 5 years after exposure.

Newer thrombolytic agents are being developed but there is no current evidence that they are any more effective than those currently in use.

# Drugs promoting blood clotting

## Tranexamic acid

- **Actions**: inhibits fibrinolysis.
- **Indications**: haemoptysis, epistaxis, menorrhagia.

- **Dose**: oral 1 g tds up to 7 days, IV slow injection 0.5–1 g tds followed by infusion 25–50 mg/kg/24 h.
- **Cautions**: thromboembolic disease, can cause hypotension.

### Thrombin

- **Indication**: injection of false aneurysm, generation of autologous blood clot.
- **Dose**: variable according to clinical response. Usually given in aliquots of 100 IU in 0.1 mL of saline, repeated until thrombosis achieved.
- **Caution**: thrombin is not licensed for intravascular use in the UK but is widely used to treat false aneurysms. Some haematology departments will generate autologous thrombin from a specimen of the patient's blood. Otherwise there are formulations of human and bovine thrombin available. Bovine thrombin is immunogenic and repeated exposure carries a risk of anaphylactic reaction and coagulopathy due to cross-reactivity with human clotting factors.

## Drugs reducing peristalsis

Antispasmodic drugs are used to abolish bowel peristalsis during DSA and are essential for any serious abdominal and pelvic angiography.

### Hyoscine butylbromide (Buscopan)

- **Action**: antimuscarinic cholinergic blockade.
- **Dose**: 20–40 mg by intra-arterial injection. Maximum total dose 160 mg.
- **Cautions**: heart failure and tachycardia.
- **Monitor**: pulse, BP and ECG.

 **Tip:** There is no point in asking patients whether they have glaucoma. If they do, they will be on treatment and the others will not know!

### Glucagon

- **Action**: polypeptide with direct smooth muscle relaxant mediated by c-AMP.
- **Dose**: 1 mg intra-arterial injection.
- **Cautions**: insulinoma and phaeochromocytoma; may produce hypoglycaemic and hypertensive crises.

## Antibiotics

There is little quality evidence for the use of antibiotics in interventional radiology. However, we use antibiotics when puncturing synthetic vascular grafts, implanting permanent devices and performing biliary manipulation in obstructed biliary or urinary systems.

The use of antibiotics during the insertion of tunnelled lines is not recommended. Local policy will often dictate the individual choice of antibiotics and govern their use. Choose antibiotics targeted at likely causative organisms.

## Antiemetics

Nausea is not an uncommon problem, especially during embolization procedures.

## Metoclopramide

- **Action**: dopamine antagonist with central antiemetic action. It also increases gastrointestinal motility and gastric emptying.
- **Dose**: oral or IV 10 mg tds.

## Prochlorperazine (Stemetil)

- **Action**: phenothiazine with a central antiemetic action.
- **Dose**: oral or IV 10 mg tds.

Both metoclopramide and prochlorperazine can cause dystonic reactions, especially in the young and very old.

- **Reversal**: procyclidine 5–10 mg by IV injection rapidly relieves the dystonic reaction.

## Cyclizine (Valoid)

- **Actions**: antihistaminic.
- **Dose**: 50 mg tds oral, IV or IM.

## Ondansetron (Zofran)

- **Actions**: 5-HT antagonist.
- **Dose**: oral or IV 8 mg and then 12-hourly.

# Drugs to prevent and treat contrast reactions

A crash trolley should be immediately available for the interventional suite. In addition to the standard drugs found in the resuscitation trolley, the following drugs are essential.

## Chlorphenamine (Piriton)

Used in the treatment of generalized urticaria post contrast, and in the emergency treatment of anaphylactic contrast reactions.

- **Action**: blocks the H1 receptor-mediated actions of histamine.
- **Dose**: 10–20 mg by slow IV injection over 1 minute.
- **Cautions**: will cause drowsiness, rapid injection may cause hypotension.

## Hydrocortisone sodium succinate

Used in the treatment and prevention of severe contrast reactions. The mechanism of action is usually too slow to be of immediate benefit in acute reactions, and steroids are used in addition to more immediate treatment such as adrenaline.

- **Action**: multiple effects inhibiting release of a variety of inflammatory mediators.
- **Dose**: 200 mg by slow IV injection repeated at 4-hourly intervals during procedure.

## Prednisolone

Used in prophylaxis against contrast reactions in high-risk patients.

- **Dose**: various regimens have been described including the Greenberger protocol of 50 mg orally 13, 7 and 1 hour(s) before contrast administration.
- **Cautions**: active peptic ulceration.
- **Normal saline**: 1 L rapidly infused if there is hypotension.

## Adrenaline (epinephrine)

A cornerstone to the treatment of severe contrast reactions, adrenaline is used for anaphylactic shock, laryngeal oedema and severe bronchospasm.

- **Action**: multiple actions – cardiac stimulant, vasoconstriction of peripheral vessels and bronchodilation.
- **Dose**: the route of administration is determined by the clinical status of the patient. If the patient remains well perfused, then the subcutaneous route is safest. 0.3–0.5 mL of 1 : 1000 solution is given to a maximum of 2 mL in 5 minutes. In severe shock with peripheral shutdown, IV adrenaline is required: 1 mL of 1 : 10 000 solution (0.1 mg) is given by slow IV injection.
- **Cautions**: ventricular arrhythmias, hypertension and cerebral haemorrhage have all been described. Clearly, the drug carries considerable risks for patients with pre-existing myocardial ischaemia and should only be used in an extreme situation.

## Atropine

Used in the treatment and prevention of bradycardia in the context of vasovagal attack and carotid stenting.

- **Action**: competitive inhibitor for acetylcholine.
- **Dose**: 0.6–1.2 mg by IV injection. Maximum dose is 3 mg.
- **Cautions**: dose-related anticholinergic effects – dry mouth, urinary retention, blurred vision. Contraindicated in closed angle glaucoma.

## Cimetidine

A second-line treatment for severe contrast reactions resistant to adrenaline.

- **Dose**: 300 mg dissolved in 20 mL saline as a slow IV infusion.
- **Cautions**: patients should receive an H1 blocking agent before cimetidine. Rapid infusion may cause cardiac effects.

# Antiarrhythmics

Most of these drugs are best administered by a physician skilled at interpreting the electrocardiogram and managing cardiac arrhythmia – that's not usually a radiologist! Usually best to seek a grown-up but if the patient has supraventricular tachycardia (SVT) consider adenosine, although remember the patient needs to be on ECG monitoring.

## Adenosine

- **Indication**: treatment of choice for SVT. Short duration of action with a half-life of about 10 seconds.
- **Dose**: 3 mg IV over 2 seconds. This may be followed with 6 mg after 1–2 minutes and 12 mg after a further 1–2 minutes.
- **Contraindications**: 2nd or 3rd degree AV block. Patients with heart transplant or taking dipyridamole should receive reduced dose, e.g. 0.5–1 mg.

## Glycopyrronium bromide (glycopyrrolate, Robinul)

- **Actions**: antimuscarinic agent.
- **Indications**: alternative to atropine with fewer cardiac effects, used to prevent bradycardia during carotid stenting.
- **Dose**: intra-arterial or IV 200 µg.
- **Cautions**: as atropine.

# Suggestions for further reading

### Drugs used in the imaging department

Bhatnagar D, Soran H, Durrington PN. Hypercholesterolaemia and its management. BMJ 2008;337:503–508.

McConnell CA. In: Ansell G, et al. eds. Complications in diagnostic imaging and interventional radiology, 3rd edn. Oxford: Blackwell Science, 1996:27–46. A comprehensive overview.

McDermot V, Schuster M, Smith T. Antibiotic prophylaxis in vascular and interventional radiology. AJR Am J Roentgenol 1997;169:31–38.

Schulman S, Beyth RJ, Kearon C, Levine MN. Hemorrhagic complications of anticoagulant and thrombolytic treatment. In: American College of Chest Physicians evidence-based clinical practice guidelines, 8th edn. Chest 2008;133:257S–298S. Available at: www.chestjournal.org/content/133/6_suppl/257S.full.pdf+html. Complications of anticoagulation and lysis.

Scottish Intercollegiate Guidelines Network (SIGN) Guideline 104. Antibiotic prophylaxis in surgery. Available at: www.sign.ac.uk/pdf/sign104.pdf.

# Section Two

# Vascular intervention

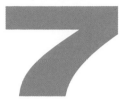

# Non-invasive vascular imaging

Traditionally, vascular imaging has involved some form of assault on the patient with a needle and catheter to obtain a diagnostic angiogram. Diagnostic angiography exposes the patient to the risks of arterial puncture, ionizing radiation and iodinated contrast agents and requires at least a few hours stay in hospital. Non-invasive imaging reduces patient risk, can be performed without a hospital stay and is no more invasive than an intravenous injection of contrast. MRA and ultrasound even avoid the risk of ionizing radiation.

DSA provides a view of the vessel lumen and indirectly the vessel wall. Ultrasound, CT and MRI give a wealth of additional information, including detail of the vessel wall and blood flow, and show adjacent and remote structures. It is therefore no surprise that the focus for vascular diagnosis has moved to non-invasive techniques.

Intra-arterial DSA (IADSA) isn't finished yet – it retains an important role as arbitrator and when imaging of small distal vessels is necessary. This book is no place for a treatise in vascular imaging but we will try to give you a flavour of what can be achieved with contemporary equipment and a guide to prioritizing patients.

This chapter will indicate where we feel each imaging modality should be used in contemporary practice (Table 7.1) and will also give a brief outline of each modality.

## Vascular ultrasound

Ultrasound can show the vessel wall, the flowing lumen and surrounding structures and can image in any plane. Colour Doppler gives physiological information that is not readily available from other modalities and spectral Doppler allows accurate estimation of degree of arterial stenosis.

## Principal uses

*Ultrasound guided intervention* The principles of ultrasound guidance are set out in Chapter 23, Imaging Guidance for Intervention.

*Assessment of abdominal aortic aneurysm (AAA)* There is a tendency for ultrasound to underestimate the diameter of AAA.

*Follow-up of peripheral vascular intervention*

*Assessment of patients with renal arterial disease* Ultrasound is used in the first instance, as it will give information on renal size, parenchyma and upper tract dilatation.

**Table 7.1** Imaging modalities to be used in contemporary practice

| Clinical scenario/aim of investigation | Modality (listed in order of preference) |
|---|---|
| **Intermittent claudication**: assess level and extent of disease to plan treatment; medical ± angioplasty or surgery | MRI: Excellent coverage, stents can cause confusion |
| | US: Good for femoropopliteal segment and follow-up of intervention. Time-consuming for whole leg |
| | CT: Good coverage. High radiation dose. Consider if contraindication to MRA |
| | DSA: If query following other imaging, or postural manoeuvres needed |
| **Critical limb ischaemia**: assess level and extent of disease to plan treatment. Distal disease common | MRI: Good in most patients, May get venous contamination |
| | DSA: May be needed for calf vessels and for intervention |
| | CT: Unproven for calf vessel disease |
| | US: Poor for calf vessels |
| **Assessment of peripheral arterial bypass grafts**: anatomy usually clear look for anastomoses and inflow/outflow | US: Excellent |
| | DSA: Intervention only |
| | MR/CT Minimal role |
| **Assessment of dialysis access**: anatomy usually clear look for anastomoses and inflow/outflow | US: Excellent except for central veins |
| | DSA: Central veins and intervention |
| | MR: Venous contamination problematic |
| **Abdominal aortic aneurysm (AAA)**: Initial screen to establish the diagnosis, follow-up to intervention when AAA big enough. Measurements for EVAR (endovascular aneurysm repair) | CT: Excellent for measurement of AAA, assessment for EVAR, rupture and follow-up post EVAR |
| | US: Screening test, follow-up post EVAR |
| | MR: Follow-up of some stent grafts |
| | DSA: calibrated angiography only if CT with reformats not available |
| **Renovascular disease**: Clear indication for intervention in renal transplantation, flash pulmonary oedema, poorly controlled hypertension and rapidly decreasing renal function | MRI: Technique of choice, poor for small vessel disease and fibromuscular dysplasia |
| | US: Used for renal size, sometimes demonstrates abnormal waveform |
| | DSA: Exclusion of fibromuscular dysplasia (FMD) and intervention |
| | CT: Generally avoided as usually concomitant renal impairment |
| **Mesenteric ischaemia**: mesenteric angina uncommon, usually severe disease of all three vessels. Focal stenosis may cause emboli | MRA Technique of choice for *chronic ischaemia*. Good views of proximal and mid vessels. |
| | CT: Technique of choice for *acute ischaemia*, shows vascular anatomy and intestine |
| | US: Limited role. Can show proximal arteries |
| | DSA: Intervention only |

**Table 7.1** Imaging modalities to be used in contemporary practice—cont'd

| Clinical scenario/aim of Investigation | Modality (listed in order of preference) |
|---|---|
| **Gastrointestinal bleeding**: rapidly evolving interest for interventional radiology. CT becoming investigation of choice | CT: Quicker and more sensitive than DSA for detection of acute bleeding. First choice examination in some centres |
| | DSA: Haemodynamically unstable patients or positive CT. Only radiological modality which will demonstrate angiodysplasia. Chronic blood loss only following negative endoscopy, CT, barium etc. |
| | MR/US: No role |
| **Trauma**: rapidly evolving interest for interventional radiology. CT is the investigation of choice | CT: first choice imaging in major trauma. Demonstrates source of bleeding |
| | DSA: intervention only |
| | MR/US: No role in major trauma. May help in less severe peripheral imaging |
| **Symptomatic carotid artery disease**: Benefit maximum within 2 weeks of event | US: Excellent screen, no information on brain |
| | MR/CT: Excellent for carotid arteries, intracranial circulation and brain |
| | DSA: Discrepancy between US and MR/CT or intervention only |
| **Peripheral veins** | US: Excellent for DVT and varicose veins |
| | DSV: Largely replaced by ultrasound but useful when anatomy confusing and for ovarian vein reflux |
| | CT/MRI: Sledgehammer to crack a walnut. Indirect venography mainly |
| **Portal vein** | US: Good for main portal vein |
| | CT/MRI: Good for portal circulation |
| | Wedged venography: Able to measure pressures and for intervention |
| | DSA: Arterioportography seldom needed |

*Assessment of patients with carotid artery disease* (This is extensively covered in many other publications and will not be considered here.)

This chapter is limited to consideration of peripheral Doppler.

# Basic principles

Ultrasound will only succeed if you choose the correct equipment and settings.

**Probe** Linear array (5–9 MHz) for peripheral and (7–12 MHz) for carotid artery imaging. It is essential to use a linear array as the colour and spectral Doppler can be steered to allow an appropriate angle of insonation of the vessel. Curvilinear array for general renal imaging; the linear array is often still best if the main renal artery is to be interrogated.

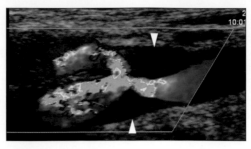

**Fig. 7.1** ■ This figure shows most of the features you need to recognize on colour flow imaging. Type III carotid plaque (white arrowheads) at the carotid artery bifurcation with clear morphological stenosis. The flow changes from uniform velocity (red) in the common carotid artery to turbulent flow with aliasing in the proximal internal and external carotid arteries.

**Settings** Most modern machines have a range of presets; these optimize the greyscale and Doppler parameters for a given type of study. This does not mean that you can rely exclusively on these and a key to success is making adjustments as you scan.

- **Depth and focus**: these are easily forgotten in all the excitement.
- **Colour velocity scale**: this must be appropriate to the flow in the vessel. If the scale is too low then aliasing will be seen with normal flow, too high and sensitivity will be compromised.
- **Colour gain**: should be set to close to the maximum which does not result in colour extending beyond the vessel wall or flow in stationary tissues.
- **Doppler cursor**: should be in the centre of the target vessel and set at an appropriate angle (40–60° is optimal). The cursor width should encompass the centre of the lumen.

**What to look for** With the ultrasound image optimized you are set to find the abnormalities.

- **Greyscale imaging**: plaque morphology and reflectivity may be of some use in the assessment of carotid artery disease but in the main you will be looking for wall thickening, thrombus and mural calcification (Fig. 7.1).
- **Colour flow**: narrowing of the lumen, velocity increases as blood is squeezed through stenoses and the colour becomes lighter. Aliasing is present if the colour changes from red to blue passing through white as it exceeds the range of the velocity scale (Figs 7.1, 7.2).
- **Doppler spectrum**: changes in peak systolic velocity are usually most important with a doubling corresponding to approximately 50% diameter narrowing. The velocities are usually measured on either side of a stenosis as well as at the point of maximal luminal narrowing (Fig. 7.2). In the carotid artery, elevated peak systolic and end diastolic velocities are also used to grade stenosis.

# Peripheral vascular doppler

A complete examination needs the operator to trace the artery from proximal to distal, using colour flow imaging supplemented by spectral Doppler at regular intervals and when areas of higher velocity (lighter colour) are identified.

**Alarm:** A multiphasic common femoral artery waveform will be found in about 10% of patients with significant iliac arterial stenosis.

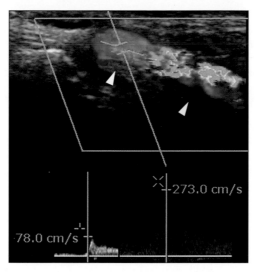

**Fig. 7.2** ■ Significant narrowing in an iliac artery in the absence of morphologically obvious stenosis. Flow changes from uniform (white arrowhead) to turbulent with aliasing (yellow arrowhead). The corresponding velocities increase from 78 cm/s to 273 cm/s, a ratio of 3.5 indicating significant stenosis.

*Iliac vascular ultrasound* This is quite challenging due to the fact that the arteries lie deep in the pelvis, often concealed beneath bowel gas and blubber. Most iliac arteries can be seen with a bit of determination. Start imaging in the transverse plane around the umbilicus and identify the aorta; as you scan caudally the iliac bifurcation will be seen. Unfortunately, this is usually not the best view for a Doppler study. Use this initial position to rotate the probe and follow the common iliac artery inferiorly. There will usually be a favourable angle of insonation with a bit of work.

 **Tip:** In the 'less than lean' patient you will need to press hard. Suddenly pressing very hard always results in tensing of the abdominal muscles. Instead, engage your patient in conversation and gradually press more and more firmly until the vessel comes into range.

*Femoropopliteal segment* The vessel is relatively superficial and imaging is generally straightforward until you reach the adductor canal where the superficial femoral artery (SFA) plunges deeper. Stay calm and adjust the depth, focus and colour flow gain until you find it again. The artery will eventually be too deep to see from this approach. More success can be found by scanning from the popliteal fossa and tracing the vessel superiorly.

*Calf vessels* This is time-consuming and difficult; undoubtedly enthusiasts can succeed but for many centres MR or CT will be required. Ultrasound can be useful to 'problem solve' questionably significant lesions. If you are having trouble following/finding the vessels this is often easiest from the ankle upwards.

## Common pitfalls in peripheral vascular ultrasound

- **Calcification in the vessel wall obscures detail**: try another view but usually not much can be done about this. Fortunately, if there is a significant stenosis there will usually be evidence of turbulence, altered waveform and increased velocity downstream.

- **Unfavourable angle of insonation**: as angles increase the velocities become less reliable. Try adjusting the view and angling the transducer to optimize the angle.
- **Pressing too hard on an artery**: this is surprisingly easy to do and not uncommon in the distal external iliac artery and common femoral artery. The effect is to compress the artery and mimic a stenosis.
- **Incorrect velocity settings**: too high and it will be difficult to demonstrate flow, too low and there will be aliasing everywhere.

# Magnetic resonance angiography

A true understanding of MR physics requires determination, dedication and focus, and while we would like to be sure we lack none of these attributes they just haven't been focused on *k* space equations. Our aim is a level of understanding that permits accurate interpretation of MRA. For all other purposes, read some of the excellent, clever texts listed at the end of the chapter.

The scanning sequences used in contrast enhanced (CE)-MRA:

- **Rely on giving contrast** – gadolinium reduces the t1 of blood
- **Are fast** – enabling data acquisition during breath-holding, and large areas to be scanned in a single study
- **Are flow independent** – enabling scanning to be performed in any plane
- **Suppress the background tissues** – high flip angles and very short pulse repetition times lead to increased signal to noise ratios
- **Are relatively free of artefact** – there is still a tendency to overestimate stenoses but this is nowhere near as marked as in time of flight imaging.

## CE-MRA keys to success

- **Timing data acquisition to correspond to the arterial peak level of gadolinium** (Fig. 7.3) – this is usually achieved by near real-time scanning the aorta at low resolution and starting the angiographic run when there is strong contrast enhancement. Dedicated vascular phased array coils, parallel imaging techniques and variable acquisition

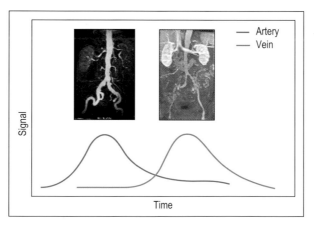

**Fig. 7.3** ■ Variation of arterial and venous signal following intravenous gadolinium. Scanning at the peak of arterial enhancement gives optimal angiographic imaging with peak signal to noise ratio. Scanning too late reduces the signal to noise ratio and results in venous contamination.

parameters permit maximum resolution to be obtained in smaller vessels with reduced risk of venous contamination.

- **Scanning in the coronal and sagittal planes** – this improves resolution, increases the field of view, reduces the number of slices required to cover the area of interest and reduces 'wrap' artefact. Typically, the coronal plane is used for peripheral, renal, arch and carotid MRA, and the sagittal plane for mesenteric MRA.
- **Restricting the volume scanned** – this shortens the time to acquire data and allows thinner slices to increase spatial resolution. The key to volume restriction is to set up the scan carefully by performing localizer sequences that clearly show the position of the target arteries.

 **Alarm:** Don't restrict the volume too much or you will miss part of the artery and the result will be a pseudo-occlusion (Fig. 7.4).

- **Subtraction** – subtracted views can be achieved in the same way as DSA by subtracting preliminary unenhanced images from scans following contrast enhancement.
- **Image review** – don't rely on maximum intensity projection (MIP) images; go to the console and review the unsubtracted source images when there is any doubt!
- **Understand the artefacts and limitations of the technique** – image quality may be degraded by venous contamination, especially in views of the calf in patients with critical limb ischaemia.

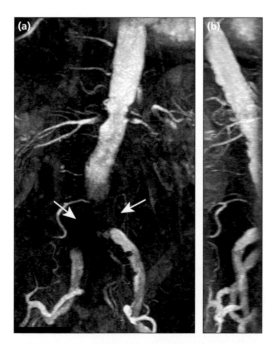

**Fig. 7.4** ■ (A) Pseudo-occlusion due to over-zealous restriction of the scan volume. Apparent occlusion of the distal aorta and both common iliac arteries (arrows); the pattern is atypical in the absence of collateral flow. (B) Pseudo-occlusion due to over-zealous restriction of the scan volume. Lateral view showing that the distal aorta and proximal iliac arteries have not been included in the scan volume.

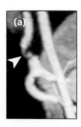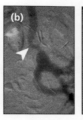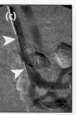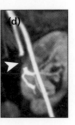

**Fig. 7.5** ■ (A) CE-MR scan and (B) $CO_2$ DSA of a patient with transplant renal artery stenosis (arrowhead). (C) DSA following successful stenting (arrowheads). (D) A follow-up MRA shows apparent occlusion of the artery corresponding to the position of the ferromagnetic stent (arrowhead). Signal dropout due to stents and heavy calcification is a common pitfall during peripheral arterial MRA.

- Interference from metallic objects and vascular calcification. Stainless steel stents and embolization coils will completely obliterate the signal from the vessel (Fig. 7.5).
- The T2 star artefact secondary to concentrated gadolinium in adjacent venous vessels can lead to misdiagnosis of stenosis; classically in the arch vessels secondary to contrast in the subclavian vein post upper limb injection.

## Areas in which CE-MRA is accepted

- Patients with a documented history of severe contrast reaction:
  - With no femoral access, in whom the arm approach would carry a risk of cerebrovascular accident (CVA).
- Carotid artery imaging for carotid arterial stenosis and dissection.
- Renal artery imaging: native renal artery disease, live donor assessment and transplant renal artery.

# Computed tomography angiography (CTA)

CTA has been available since the 1990s but is improving fast with the advent of multislice CT scanners with volumetric image acquisition and fast image reconstruction. CT scanners 16 slice and above are capable of performing rapid angiographic assessment of any vascular territory. The principal advantage of CT is availability and apparent ease of interpretation. CT involves high doses of iodinated contrast and ionizing radiation. Efforts should be made to keep the dose to a minimum by limiting the scan volume, using cardiac gating and reducing the number of phases scanned. At present CTA is the modality of choice for assessment of aneurysm, trauma and gastrointestinal bleeding.

Images are generally produced as MIPs akin to MRA (Fig. 7.6A), 3D shaded surface renderings (Fig. 7.6B); curved and multiplanar (Fig. 7.6C) reformats will also be helpful, especially in dealing with aneurysmal disease (see Chapter 17, Endovascular Aneurysm Repair (EVAR)). Interpretation of source 2D images is vital, particularly because if the scan has encompassed the abdomen and pelvis, significant pathology in the abdominal viscera will be completely overlooked on MIP images alone.

## CTA: keys to success

- **Contrast timing**: scans must be acquired at the peak of arterial enhancement and oral contrast should not be used. A test bolus is usually required to achieve optimal timing. Many scanners feature automatic triggering of contrast injection.

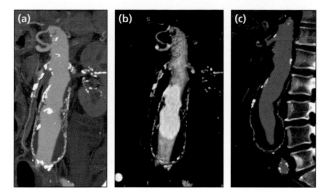

**Fig. 7.6** ■ (A) CT reformats of a patient with AAA and mesenteric ischaemia. MIP – near angiographic image but also shows calcification and areas of high attenuation e.g. kidneys and ureters. (B) CT reformats of a patient with AAA and mesenteric ischaemia. Shaded surface rendering. (C) CT reformats of a patient with AAA and mesenteric ischaemia. Sagittal reformat essentially identical to conventional CT slices.

- **Table timing**: the table can move faster than the contrast bolus, particularly in patients with compromised cardiac function, and therefore tailoring/slowing the speed of acquisition will be required for some patients.
- **Curved plane reformats**: trace a longitudinal centre line through the vessel and give a single view of all but the most tortuous of vessels. If used for interpretation, review of two planes is required to prevent missing eccentric stenoses.
- **Window levels**: calcification and stents cause artefact on CTA and this can lead to misdiagnosis of stenosis if careful window settings are not made. Typically, window level should be 200 and width at least 1000 to minimize these artefacts.
- **Volume rendering** (Fig. 7.6B): these images produce a pseudo-3D appearance and while they look great, they are really only useful to illustrate the most tortuous and complex anatomy. They are poor at quantifying stenotic disease. The workhorses of interpretation are MIPs, and the 2D images with curved plane reformats are the first reserve.

 **Tip:** Remember with CTA reconstruction algorithms are important, and many machines will help by having pre-programmed settings for certain scenarios such as assessing stents.

 **Summary:** Non-invasive vascular imaging is set to replace most of conventional angiography. If you don't want to be left behind, get involved. Think about the most appropriate test and tailor it for each patient.

# Suggestions for further reading

Alkadhi H, Wildermuth S, Despoils L, et al. Vascular emergencies of the thorax after blunt and iatrogenic trauma: multi-row CT and three dimensional imaging. Radiographics 2004;24:1239–1255.

Bruzzi JF, Remy-Jardin M, Delhaye D, et al. Multi-detector row CT of hemoptysis. Radiographics 2006;26:3–22.

Castaner E, Andreu M, Gallardo X, et al. CT in nontraumatic acute thoracic aortic disease: typical and atypical features and complications. Radiographics 2003;23:S93–S110.

Elliot K, Fishman MD, Karen M, et al. Multidetector CT and three-dimensional CT angiography for suspected vascular trauma of the extremities. Radiographics 2008;28:653–667.

Kawashima A, Sandler CM, Corl FM, et al. Trauma: a comprehensive review. Radiographics 2001;21:557–574.

Miller-Thomas MM, West OC, Cohen AM. Diagnosing traumatic arterial injury in the extremities with CT angiography: pearls and pitfalls 1. Radiographics 2005;25:S133–S142.

Neal C, Dalrymple MD, Srinivasa R, et al. Informatics in radiology (infoRAD) introduction to the language of three-dimensional imaging with multidetector CT. Radiographics 2005;25:1409–1428.

Nunex DB Jr, Torres-Leo M, Munear F. Vascular injuries of the neck and inlet: helical CT–angiographic correlation. Radiographics 2004;24:1087–1100.

Poletti PA, Rosset A, Didier D, et al. Subtraction CT angiography of the lower limbs: a new technique for the evaluation of acute arterial occlusion. AJR Am J Roentgenol 2004:183:1445–1448.

Raman SS, Pojchamarnwiputh SS, Muangsomboon K, et al. Utility of 16-MDCT angiography for comprehensive preoperative vascular evaluation of laparoscopic renal donors. AJR Am J Roentgenol 2006;186:1630–1638.

Sammer M, Wang E, Blackmore CC, et al. Indeterminate CT angiography in blunt thoracic trauma: Is CT angiography enough? AJR Am J Roentgenol 2007;189:603–608.

Winston CB, Lee NL, Jarnagin WR, et al. CT angiography for delineation of celiac and superior mesenteric artery variants in patients undergoing hepatobiliary and pancreatic surgery. AJR Am J Roentgenol 2007;188:W13–W19.

# Angiography – getting the picture

This chapter reviews briefly the key areas in image acquisition and manipulation. Angiography is a team sport and a successful angiogram depends on cooperation between the patient and the angiography staff (radiographer, nurse and doctor). A little understanding of the basic principles of angiography can vastly improve the standard of the final study!

## Fluoroscopy

*Fluoroscopy or screening* This is used to provide real-time imaging during catheter and guidewire manipulation. Continuous fluoroscopy is used when optimal image quality is required, e.g. embolization therapy with particles/liquids. Pulsed fluoroscopy is used when less detail is required, e.g. when screening over-sensitive organs, e.g. during uterine fibroid embolization. Radiation dose is reduced as X-ray production is intermittent; the image from each pulse persists on the monitor to give an impression of continuity. At fewer than 7 pulses/s the image is rather jerky (think dancing in a strobe light) and only suitable for crude catheter positioning, e.g. positioning a pigtail catheter. Whenever possible, use fluoroscopy rather than DSA runs, as this keeps the dose to a minimum.

*Last image hold* The fluoroscopic image is automatically stored on the monitor. In systems with two monitors, this image can be transferred to the reference monitor and used for guidance.

**Guide to good fluoroscopy** Aim to keep everyone's radiation exposure to a minimum. You are the person most at risk!

- Keep the image intensifier close to the patient.
- Centre over the area of interest.
- Try to move the table to the position of interest before screening when changing position or using oblique views.
- Use collimation.
- Use pulsed fluoroscopy if available – there is little dose reduction at >7 frames/s (FPS).
- Keep your hands out of the field – you may need your fingers in years to come.
- Use angiographic runs to sort out anatomy and pathology – do not perform repeated fluoroscopic injections.
- Keep your foot off the pedal unless you have a reason to screen and you are actively looking at the fluoroscopic image!

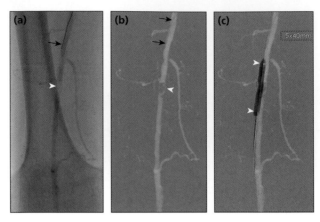

**Fig. 8.1** ■ The principal techniques for guiding catheters and guidewires shown during SFA angioplasty. (A) Fluoroscopy fade: an image of the vessel is superimposed on the standard fluoroscopic image; the guidewire (black arrow), stenosis (white arrowhead) are clearly seen, as is the femur. (B) Roadmap: the background is subtracted, as is the guidewire (black arrows); the tiny channel passing the plaque is clearly shown (white arrowhead), making it easier to traverse the lesion. (C) The lesion has been crossed and a 5 mm balloon (white arrowheads) inflated. Note that the balloon and wire are now seen, as they were not present on the original image. Despite slight movement it is clear that the balloon is in the correct place and appropriately sized.

## Catheter guidance

*Roadmap (non-subtracted fluoroscopy)* An image from a DSA is superimposed on the normal fluoroscopic image (Fig. 8.1A). The density of the superimposed image can be adjusted to suit the application. It is particularly useful in the chest and abdomen as the superimposed image does not move with respiration. Confusingly, this is called by a different name by each of the manufacturers, e.g. on a Siemens' machine it is called fluoroscopy fade.

*Roadmap (subtracted fluoroscopy)* In this mode, a subtracted fluoroscopic image is obtained after a few seconds of fluoroscopy. Contrast is injected to opacify the vessels and fluoroscopy stopped. The next time screening is activated, the catheter and guidewire will be seen on the subtracted image of the blood vessels (Fig. 8.1B). This is used particularly to navigate strictures and avoid branch vessels and also can show that angioplasty balloons are correctly sized (Fig. 8.1C).

 **Tip:** Roadmapping is not effective in the chest and abdomen, as respiration and peristalsis interfere with the subtraction and degrade the image.

# Digital subtraction angiography: basic principles

The vast majority of angiography is now performed using a DSA technique. DSA uses a computer to subtract an image without contrast (mask) from each subsequent image acquired in exactly the same position after contrast injection. The resultant images show only the opacified blood vessels; the underlying bone or soft tissue is not displayed. Movement between the mask image and the contrast image will result in image degradation because of visible bone edges. Most DSA examinations are performed with positive (iodinated) contrast media; however, negative ($CO_2$ gas) contrast can be used.

## Digital subtraction angiography techniques

*Multi-position DSA (MPDSA)* Angiography is performed in discrete sections, each with its own contrast injection. In peripheral angiography, this usually gives the best results at the expense of an increase in radiation dose.

*Stepping table DSA* Only used in peripheral angiography. The table or C-arm moves in a series of overlapping steps. Five positions are usually needed to cover from the abdominal aorta to the feet. Mask images are obtained in each position. A bolus of contrast is injected and the table advanced when the vessels in that position are opacified. The technique only works well with an experienced radiographer and a patient with broadly symmetrical disease. Additional runs are frequently necessary, particularly of the crural vessels.

 **Tip:** Stepping table DSA gives best results when the blood flow is the same in each limb. Use MPDSA if symptoms or pulses are markedly asymmetrical.

*Bolus-chasing DSA* Only used in peripheral angiography. The technique resembles stepping table DSA. Mask images are obtained at multiple levels (approximately every 5 cm); the table is then panned to keep up with the contrast bolus.

*Rotational angiography and angiographic CT* These are variations on MPDSA; the C-arm is rotated in an arc around the patient while masks are acquired. The rotation is repeated during the injection of contrast. The mask is matched with the image acquired at the same obliquity. Modern data reconstruction algorithms allow the angiographic image to be reformatted into a 3D reconstruction akin to a low-resolution CT scan. Rotational angiography is most useful when multiple oblique projections are required, e.g. renal transplant angiography, intracranial aneurysm. Angiographic CT may be useful at completion of EVAR to look for subtle endoleaks.

*Dose reduction* When imaging for guidance rather than diagnosis consider using roadmap imaging and conventional fluoroscopy; this can reduce dose by an order of magnitude.

# Hard copy/archival

The best study in the world can be sabotaged by careless and inadequate hard copy/archival/ post processing. Most images are now stored digitally to PACS.

Angiography is unique in that we discard much of the study almost immediately after acquisition. The hard copy represents only the edited highlights of the angiogram. Vital information may be lost irretrievably if we fail to convey to radiographic staff the essential objectives of the study. In particular, complex or unfamiliar studies should be reviewed at the console with the radiographer and images for hard copy identified.

Suboptimal imaging is most often due to elementary errors. Try to apply the following basic guidelines:

- Image all phases of the run: arterial, capillary and venous.
- Optimal image density is a level of grey that allows overlying vessels to be discriminated from each other. Set window levels accordingly. Too black an image will obscure pathology (Fig. 8.2).

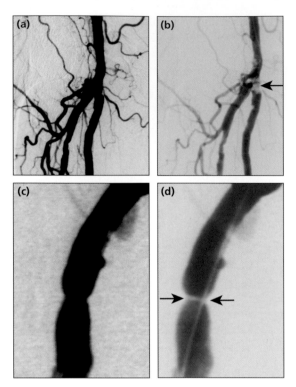

**Fig. 8.2** ■ Effect of incorrect window settings. (A, B) Profunda oblique view: the large posterior plaque (arrow) is obscured by narrow windows. (C, D) Subtle 'web-like' stenosis (arrows) in a vein graft is only appreciated on correct settings.

- Include non-subtracted images to show landmarks.
- Annotate views with relevant information, e.g. tube angulation when it has been difficult to obtain a suitable oblique projection.

 **Tip:** While it's always worth trying to blame the radiographer, no amount of radiographer ingenuity can make up for images that were never there – always review the study on the console before removing the catheter.

*Pixel shifting* If there is no movement between the mask and the run, then a single mask image will suffice. In reality, most patients do not keep completely still, especially if a large volume of contrast has been injected. If there has only been slight movement, then the resultant image can often be markedly improved by pixel shifting (Fig. 8.3). This entails realigning the chosen mask with the image to allow effective subtraction. Pixel shifting is not as helpful when there is considerable movement such as respiration, or when there is rotation.

 **Tip:** If the patient moves during a run, consider continuing imaging after the contrast has passed and use a late image as the mask. If the patient keeps moving then this is futile.

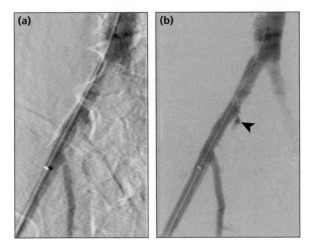

**Fig. 8.3** ■ This patient experienced pain during iliac angioplasty and stenting. (A) Movement has severely degraded the angiographic image. (B) Choosing an appropriate mask and pixel shifting has improved the image and now contrast extravasation (black arrowhead) is clearly seen at the angioplasty site.

*Masking* Some patients cannot stop breathing for the duration of image acquisition, especially if a long sequence is involved. In this case, the solution is multimasking. Multiple masks are made over several respiratory cycles before injecting contrast. Normal respiration is continued throughout the run. Images from the run can then be matched with a mask in the same phase of respiration, allowing subtraction.

 **Tip:** Multimasking is essential in most patients during prolonged runs in the chest and abdomen. No amount of pixel shifting and remasking can compensate for bowel peristalsis. Paralyse the bowel with hyoscine butylbromide (Buscopan) or glucagon.

# Pump injectors

Even the strongest angiographer cannot hand inject rapidly enough for aortic runs. Pump injectors are used to deliver a controlled bolus of contrast while you stand back and reduce your radiation dose. The settings may seem confusing at first but there are only six parameters to consider:

1. **Volume**: this is the total volume of contrast that will be delivered.
2. **Injection rate**: the flow rate in mL/s. Volume/injection rate determines the duration of the bolus.
3. **Maximum pressure (psi)**: the peak pressure the pump will generate during injection.
4. **Pressure rate rise**: the time to peak pressure. In practice, it seems permanently set at 0.4 s.
5. **Inject delay**: delays the injection of contrast to allow mask images to be acquired. This is necessary when contrast will reach the target vessel immediately after injection, e.g. imaging the aorto-iliac segment.
6. **X-ray delay**: delays the X-ray exposure. This avoids unnecessary images prior to the contrast arriving at the area of interest, e.g. injecting in the aorta and imaging the feet.

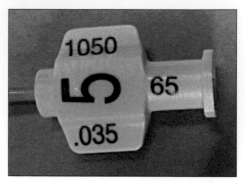

**Fig. 8.4** ■ Closeup of a catheter hub indicating: French size 5, length 65 cm, guidewire 0.035 inches and injection pressure 1050 psi.

**Tip:** Parameters 2–4 are limited by the catheter. Details of the maximum permissible pressure are displayed on the catheter hub (Fig. 8.4) and information about flow rates is on the catheter packaging. The maximum flow rate is only achievable at the maximum pressure (psi).

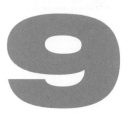

# Equipment for angiography

There is at first a bewildering array of angiographic equipment and terminology. The following section will allow you to make simple rational decisions which will usually be correct.

## Size

As you know, size is everything and in intervention is a question of length and diameter: biggest and longest are not always best. To keep you on your toes, catheters, sheaths and guidewires use different units of measurement including French size, inches and centimetres; to make matters worse, some sizes are outer diameters and some are inner diameters. Read on, all will become clear(er) (Table 9.1).

## Guidewires

Guidewires are a key element to successful intervention. They support and steer catheters to the target and are used to traverse narrowings and blockages. In the majority of cases catheters are advanced over a previously positioned wire.

## Basic properties of guidewires

Guidewires divide into two groups: **non-steerable guidewires** provide a supportive rail that allows the catheter to be advanced into position but are not designed to negotiate stenoses or select branch vessels. **Steerable guidewires** have shaped tips and can be turned easily; some have special slippery 'hydrophilic' coatings that will cross even the tightest stenosis if used properly.

 **Tip:** Membership of the 'whoops Terumo' club is easily obtained by letting the wire slip through your fingers and onto your shoe. Take care when using hydrophilic wires and avoid using them for catheter exchange until you are proficient.

**Hydrophilic guidewires** The key to success with a hydrophilic wire is to keep it wet. The wire is usually flushed while still in its delivery holder (keeping it in this when not in use helps). Wipe the wire with a wet sponge as you remove it and wet it again each time it is used. Dry hydrophilic wires are very sticky, making it hard to advance catheters over them;

**Table 9.1** Sizes made clear

| The following are French sizes (circumference in millimetres) | |
| --- | --- |
| Angiographic catheter size | = outer circumference in mm |
| Guide-catheter size | = outer circumference in mm |
| Sheath size | = inner circumference, i.e. the size of catheter which will pass through it |
| **The following are in inches** | |
| Wire diameter | e.g. 0.014, 0.018, 0.025, 0.035, 0.038 |
| Catheter lumen | e.g. 0.014, 0.018, 0.025, 0.035, 0.038 |
| **The following are in centimetres** | |
| Wire length | |
| Catheter length | |
| Sheath length | |

worse still they will adhere to your gloves and can easily be pulled out from a hard-won position.

 **Tip:** If a catheter sticks on a hydrophilic wire as it is being introduced, try wetting the wire ahead of the tip. If this doesn't do the trick, have an assistant gently inject flush through the catheter hub until the catheter comes free.

**Length** Length is important! The length of the wire becomes critical when trying to exchange catheters, especially if in a hard-fought-for selective position. A standard 180 cm length wire is fine for most uses; however, longer wires, e.g. 260 cm, may be needed when:

- Working in the upper limb from the groin
- Working in the visceral/renal/hepatic circulation and needing to exchange catheters
- Working with 90 cm+ guide-catheters or angioplasty balloons
- Using through and through wires (bodyflossing).

 **Tip:** The minimum length of guidewire necessary to allow catheter exchange = the length of the catheter + the length of the guidewire in the patient.

**Wire tip** Most wires have a soft and atraumatic tip at one end; the other end is rigid and not intended for use. You can tell which end is which by prodding it with a finger, so make sure you use the correct end. The length of the 'floppy tip' is variable, e.g. Amplatz wires come with a 6-cm floppy tip as standard but a wire with a 1-cm floppy tip is also available. The aim is to have the transition between the floppy and stiff portion within the target vessel. The shorter the soft portion of the wire, the more likely it is to cause dissection. As a general rule, choose a wire with a long floppy tip unless there is little wire space in the target vessel to position the wire.

**Stiffness** Stiffness is the biggest factor in the choice of non-steerable wires and there is huge variation between wires. The correct choice is made by matching the stiffness with your task,

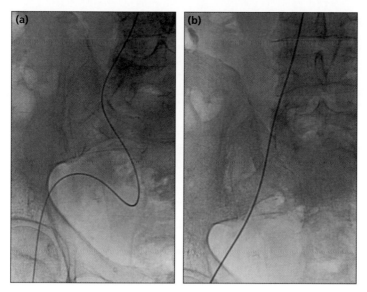

**Fig. 9.1** ■ (A) An extremely tortuous iliac artery with an Amplatz super-stiff guidewire in situ. (B) Following exchange for a Lunderquist guidewire, the artery has straightened markedly.

e.g. a 5Fr catheter can be advanced over a Bentson or standard hydrophilic wire; advancing a 21Fr stent graft needs a wire at the other end of the spectrum, e.g. Lunderquist wire (Fig. 9.1).

*Stiffness ratings of guidewires*
- **Floppy (noodle like)**: Bentson, movable core.
- **Normal**: Hydrophilic guidewire, standard 0.035-inch J or straight guidewire.
- **More supportive**: Heavy duty J or straight guidewire, stiff hydrophilic guidewire.
- **Stiff**: Flexfinder, Amplatz super and extra-stiff wires, 0.018-inch Platinum Plus, V18.
- **Unreasonable force**: Lunderquist wires/Meier back up wire. These are coat hangers with a floppy tip; they are usually reserved for heavy duty work such as aortic stent grafting (Fig. 9.1).

 **Alarm:** Stiff guidewires should always be introduced through a catheter that has been placed over a conventional guidewire. Do not attempt to steer a very stiff wire through even mild curves.

**Diameters** Guidewires come in a range of diameters from 0.014 inches to 0.038 inches. Small calibre wires of 0.014–0.018 inches are used with microcatheters and rapid exchange (monorail) systems; they do not have the same strength as larger wires.

0.035-inch guidewires are used for the majority of cases and will fit through a 4Fr or larger catheter. 0.038-inch wires were used frequently in the past and some 4/5Fr catheters will accommodate this size of wire or a microcatheter.

 **Alarm:** Make sure that your puncture needle will accommodate your intended guidewire. Some central vein catheter sets come with 0.038-inch wires, which will not pass down your standard needle.

# Non-steerable guidewires

*J guidewire* This is one of the most frequently used wires and often the first choice to pass through a puncture needle. The J tip does not dig up plaques and misses small branch vessels. The 3 mm refers to the radius of the curve. Larger (5, 10 and 15-mm) J curves are used to avoid branch vessels, e.g. 15-mm J will avoid the profunda femoris artery during antegrade puncture (Fig. 9.2).

*Bentson wire* This wire has a very floppy, atraumatic 5-cm distal tip. If the end of the wire engages a branch vessel, often gently continuing to advance the wire under fluoroscopy forms an atraumatic loop within the main vessel, which pushes the wire tip out of the branch. It is sometimes used in combination with steerable catheters to negotiate stenoses and occlusions as it does not readily dissect.

*Straight wire* Length of flexible tip varies from 1 cm to 6 cm depending on particular wire type. Take care when passing plaques and branch vessels. Straight wires are not steerable on their own but can be directed using a shaped catheter.

*Other 'heavy-duty' guidewires, e.g. Rosen wire* Come as straight or J and provide extra support for advancing a catheter. This type of wire is useful for inserting a guide-catheter or drainage catheter.

*Amplatz super-stiff wire* A very useful wire for stents, stent-grafts and other devices. Amplatz wires are available with a 1-cm or 6-cm floppy tip; choose the correct length depending on the length of target vessel available as an anchor.

*Meier wire/Lunderquist wire* Serious stuff, essential for large-calibre stiff devices such as stent grafts, but need to be handled with great care.

*Platinum plus* The 0.018-inch equivalent of the Amplatz wire. Excellent and very supportive low-profile wire. The tip can be shaped but there is no torque control.

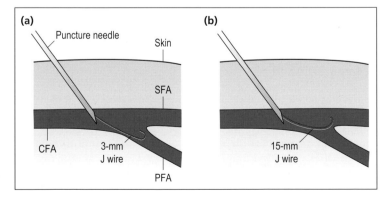

**Fig. 9.2** ■ (A) During antegrade puncture of the common femoral artery (CFA) the 3-mm J wire will often enter the profunda femoris artery (PFA). (B) The increased radius of curve of the 15-mm J wire usually will pass directly down the SFA.

# Steerable guidewires

These wires have a shaped 'angled' tip which is intended to be rotated to face a target vessel. Unless you can defy the laws of physics, this is best achieved using a pin vice attached to the wire shaft a few centimetres behind the catheter hub.

A steerable wire needs some space to work. If only a few millimetres of wire extend beyond the catheter, then the wire will not turn correctly; back the catheter off until you achieve the desired effect.

The tip of some guidewires can be shaped by placing the wire tip over some forceps and pulling it back between the forceps and your thumb.

*Terumo angled hydrophilic wire* The archetypal 0.035-inch steerable wire and benchmark against which others must be judged.

*V18* This has a shapeable floppy tip and can be steered. It is not as supportive as the Platinum plus but isn't as stiff, so will follow more tortuous vessels.

# Catheters

Catheters come in a wide range of shapes, sizes and constructions. Simple rules govern catheter choice. Most angiographers rely on a relatively small selection of catheters to perform almost all cases.

There are three important factors concerning catheter size; fortunately, the catheter packaging should help you find all these values, although you may have to look hard to find it. In addition, size and length are often printed on the catheter hub.

- **Length**: the length of the catheter in centimetres refers to the length from the hub to the tip (obvious really). Beware, some devices, stents in particular, quote both the usable length (X cm) and total length (X + Y cm) of the delivery system. Make a mental note of these and you will be able to select an appropriate-length guidewire.
- **Outer diameter**: the size of the hole or sheath required. This is usually given as the French (Fr) size, which is the outer circumference of the catheter shaft in millimetres.
- **Inner diameter**: relates to the lumen, hence the diameter of catheter or guidewire that will pass through the catheter. To make things confusing, lumen and wire are usually given in inches, e.g. a 0.035 catheter will accommodate a guidewire 0.035 inches or less but will not accept anything larger, such as a 0.038-inch guidewire.

**Tip**

**Translating from French**
For easy reference, the diameter in mm is approximately the French size divided by 3, e.g. 6Fr = 2 mm. The majority of catheters in current use are 5Fr or smaller.

## Essential catheters

Catheters divide into two distinct groups: non-selective (flush) catheters and selective catheters. Non-selective catheters are used to inject contrast in large- to medium-sized vessels and have multiple sideholes to increase the flow rate. Selective catheters are shaped to a wide variety of angles to allow catheterization of branch vessels. Successful catheterization depends on choosing the correct shape for the job.

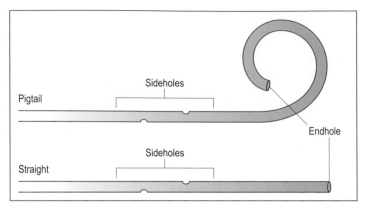

**Fig. 9.3** ■ Pigtail and straight multi-sidehole catheters. Unless the catheter is flushed briskly the flush exits via the proximal sideholes and will not flush the catheter tip, with resultant clot formation.

## Non-selective catheters

*Pigtail catheter* The workhorse of diagnostic angiography. The catheter has an endhole and multiple sideholes extending down onto the distal 1–2 cm of the shaft. The distribution of sideholes produces a homogeneous contrast bolus (Fig. 9.3). In practice, the endhole of the catheter is larger than the sideholes and therefore has greater flow. The pigtail usually forms when the guidewire is withdrawn but if it does not, simply push the catheter forward while twisting. As the pigtail loop measures approximately 15 mm across, this catheter should not be used in vessels smaller than this diameter. The pigtail shape minimizes inadvertent catheterization of small branch vessels.

**Tip:** A test injection of contrast is made to verify the endhole is not in a small branch before the rapid injection of a contrast bolus.

*Straight catheter* Endhole and multiple sideholes on a straight shaft (Fig. 9.3). This catheter is used in vessels too small to form a pigtail but with reasonably rapid flow, e.g. the iliac arteries.

**Tip:** To locate the catheter tip, pull the J wire back until a catch is felt as it begins to straighten on the catheter.

**Flow rates for non-selective catheters** Maximum flow rates vary between catheters, depending on the internal diameter and length and number of sideholes. The maximum flow rate and injection pressure (psi) are usually on the catheter packaging or catheter hub – check them before giving everyone a contrast shower. Typical maximum flow rates for pigtail catheters are:

- 3Fr 6–8 mL/s
- 4Fr 16–18 mL/s
- 5Fr 20–25 mL/s

## Selective catheters

**Endhole vs sideholes** Selective catheters come in two main designs: endhole only and end- and sidehole.

Endhole catheters are used for hand-injected, diagnostic angiograms and embolization procedures. Pump injections are potentially hazardous with endhole only catheters, as the high-flow jet coming out of the single endhole is likely to displace the catheter and may dislodge plaque or cause dissection.

End- and sidehole catheters are used for pump-injected runs (e.g. superior mesenteric artery angiograms), as the multiple sideholes deliver a rapid, safe bolus of contrast; however, sidehole catheters should not be used for embolotherapy: coils may become trapped in the sideholes and particulate matter may escape to non-target territory via the sideholes.

 **Tip:** Endhole catheters will not aspirate if the catheter tip rests against the vessel wall. Gently pull back the catheter and try again.

**Top five selective catheters** These catheters have different shapes in order to point the tip in a specific direction. They only adopt that shape when unconstrained. Passing a wire through a catheter will alter the direction in which the tip points by straightening out any curves. This phenomenon can be used to your advantage to increase the range of directions in which you can aim.

*Cobra* An invaluable catheter for visceral and peripheral selective arteriography (Fig. 9.4). The catheter is pulled down to engage a vessel but is pushed forward over a guidewire to allow deeper catheterization. Cobra catheters come in three flavours, C1–C3, each with a progressively widening curve; in practice, must people simply use a C2. Consider the use of a wider loop if you find the catheter backing out of your selective position when trying to advance a wire; the wider loop can sometimes get support from the contralateral aortic wall. The Cobra is simple to use, does not need to be formed and can be used for selective catheterization.

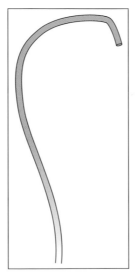

**Fig. 9.4** ■ Cobra catheter.

**Fig. 9.5** ■ Sidewinder catheter.

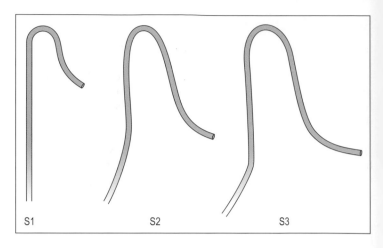

S1 S2 S3

**Fig. 9.6** ■ Berenstein catheter.

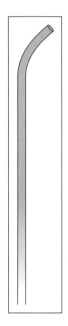

***Sidewinder (a.k.a Simmons)*** This is a very useful tool for visceral angiography. The Sidewinder reverse curve comes in three sizes, S1–S3, with progressively larger curves and longer limbs (Fig. 9.5). There are two other catheters that are very similar in shape and function to the Sidewinder: the Sos Omnicatheter and the Uni Select (USL). Re-forming the reverse curve can be difficult for the uninitiated. The smaller catheters Sidewinder 1, Sos Omni and USL 1 can be formed in the thoracic aorta, within an AAA or sometimes even the abdominal aorta. For the larger catheters there are a variety of techniques and these are outlined below.

***Berenstein*** Endhole only; the tip is angled and therefore at its best when catheterizing forward-facing vessels such as the aortic arch vessels (Fig. 9.6). This is one of the simplest catheters to use – just point and shoot; it is remarkably versatile for super selective catheterization.

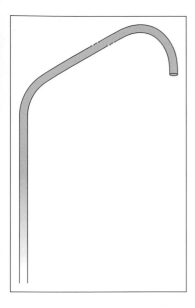

**Fig. 9.7** ▪ Renal double curve catheter.

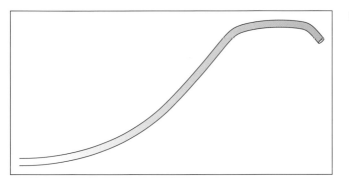

**Fig. 9.8** ▪ Headhunter catheter.

*Renal double curve (RDC)* As the name suggests, this is designed for selective renal work (Fig. 9.7). The tip points downwards and therefore it is very useful for getting across the aortic bifurcation. At least one of the authors thinks this is a useful catheter for inferior mesenteric artery catheterization. The RDC is used much like a Cobra catheter.

*Headhunter* This catheter has a forward-facing primary curve and is available with and without sideholes (Fig. 9.8). It is primarily used to catheterize the head and neck vessels. The catheter is usually advanced beyond the target vessel then slowly withdrawn while applying torque, the catheter tends to spring into vessels, which can be alarming for the unsuspecting.

## Co-axial systems

The term co-axial just refers to the use of one catheter through the lumen of another. The simplest co-axial system is a standard catheter and arterial sheath. Most co-axial systems involve the use of guiding catheters and microcatheters. They are used when they confer specific advantages such as additional support, continuous flushing, etc. A co-axial system may involve multiple catheters, e.g. sheath, guiding catheter, standard catheter and microcatheter.

# Guide-catheters

Guide-catheters are large-calibre catheters that are used to provide a safe and stable conduit for a conventional catheter from the arterial puncture site to the target vessel. The catheters come in a variety of lengths, from ~ 50 cm to 100 cm, and shapes include straight, hockey stick and RDC. Because of its large inner diameter, the guide-catheter does not sit snugly on the wire; this has two important connotations:

1.  They must be introduced through a sheath of the corresponding size
2.  They are intended to be taken to the target vessel ostium rather than rammed through a stenosis; conventional catheters and guidewires should be used for more distal catheterization.

Guide-catheters are most frequently used during stenting procedures when the extra rigidity and increased bail-out options are a reasonable trade off against the increased puncture site size. Occasionally, a guide-catheter can be very useful to take up the torque from tortuous iliac vessels and therefore allow selective visceral catheterization. When selecting a guide-catheter, make sure you choose an appropriate length – too long and your catheter will not pass through it; too short and it will not reach the target vessel.

## Guide-catheters vs introducer guides (long sheaths)

There are many long sheaths on the market, and they broadly serve the same function as guide-catheters. They also have the advantage that they don't need an additional sheath. They do have the disadvantages that they don't come in the same range of shapes. Introducer guides come with a dilator so that they can be advanced directly into an artery.

**Alarm: Guide-catheters** are sized by their outside circumference. Therefore a 6Fr guide-catheter will fit through a 6Fr sheath but will not allow a 6Fr stent through it. Confusingly, their lumen diameter will be given in inches.

**Introducer guides (long sheaths)** are sized according to their lumen. A 6Fr introducer guide will accommodate a 6Fr guide-catheter/stent. This can cause confusion when choosing compatible kit!!

# Microcatheters

Microcatheters are 2–3Fr in size and highly flexible. They allow catheterization of all but the smallest and most tortuous of vessels (Fig. 9.9). Microcatheters are ideal for superselective hepatic, visceral and peripheral catheterization. A conventional catheter is initially used to selectively catheterize a branch of the proximal circulation; it then serves as a guide-catheter through which the co-axial catheter is advanced. A Tuohy–Borst adaptor can be used to maintain haemostasis but in practice may not be needed if the catheter is a snug fit.

**Tip:** It helps to fix the conventional catheter to the drapes using a towel clip. This leaves both hands free to manipulate the microcatheter and wire.

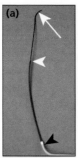
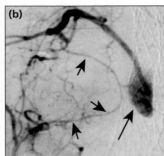
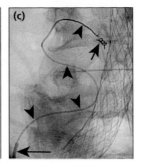

**Fig. 9.9** ■ (A) Microcatheters will negotiate the most tortuous vessels. 4Fr guide-catheter (black arrowhead), microcatheter (white arrowhead) and wire (white arrow). (B) Tiny iliolumbar collaterals (short black arrows) causing type II endoleak (long black arrows) following endovascular aortic aneurysm repair. (C) Microcatheters will negotiate the most tortuous vessels. Microcatheter (arrowheads) delivering embolization coils (short black arrow) into the lumbar artery. 4Fr guide-catheter in the iliolumbar branch of the internal iliac artery (long black arrow).

Microcatheters have improved enormously over the past few years. There are now hydrophilic catheters with integral guidewires (e.g. Progreat, Terumo). There are also additional guidewires which offer greater and lesser degrees of support and steerability.

**Tip:** Avoid being 'so near but yet so far'! Passing a 130-cm long microcatheter through a 100-cm long conventional catheter leaves only about 25 cm free; this may not be sufficient to deeply catheterize the target vessels. Make sure that you choose a catheter combination able to reach the target site.

# Vascular sheaths

Vascular sheaths provide an atraumatic vascular access conduit. Sheaths are invaluable for any case that is likely to use more than one catheter as they greatly simplify catheter exchange, maintain guidewire position and prevent bleeding at the puncture site.

The sheath consists of a hollow plastic tube connected to a haemostatic valve with a side-arm for flushing (Fig. 9.10). The sheath size describes the calibre of catheter it will accept, e.g. a 5Fr sheath takes a 5Fr catheter but actually has an approximately 6Fr outer diameter. Some sheaths have marker bands at the end of the sheath, which can help if you will potentially have to perform an intervention close to the tip of the sheath.

# Other essential equipment

**Vascular access** Puncture needles: most procedures start with a 19G bevelled needle that will accept a 0.035-inch guidewire. A larger bore needle may be needed if 0.038-inch wires are needed. Two-part (Potts) needles have largely been abandoned.

**Mini access set** These sets are used in small vessels or where a less than optimal puncture might cause problems, e.g. anticoagulated patient. The puncture needle is small calibre (21G) and accepts a 0.018-inch wire with a stiff shaft and straight floppy tip. Once the vessel is punctured, a two-part dilator is introduced into the artery. The 3Fr inner component fits

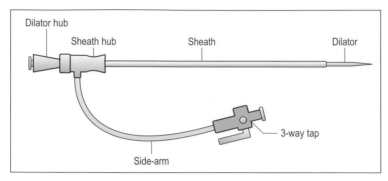

**Fig. 9.10** ■ Vascular sheath with side-arm for flushing.

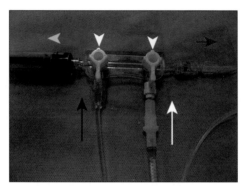

**Fig. 9.11** ■ 'Traffic light' system: two interconnected 3-way taps (yellow arrowheads), with pressurized inflow of contrast (black arrow) and heparinized saline (white arrow). Adjusting the taps allows filling of syringes (turquoise arrowhead) and flushing of catheters/sheaths (red arrow).

snugly on the 0.018-inch wire; the outer component has a 0.035-inch lumen. Once the wire and inner component are removed, a 0.035-inch wire can be passed into the vessel, allowing placement of a vascular sheath.

There are a few miscellaneous pieces of equipment whose existence greatly simplifies yours!

**Haemostatic devices – taps** There are many commercially available taps, and not all have been designed to allow high-pressure injection. Check before you treat everyone to a contrast shower. Only two types of tap are of importance angiographically:

- **2-way taps**. These taps have two positions, on and off, and come in two styles. The standard tap has a rotating valve and is almost ubiquitous. The other variety of tap functions using a 'sliding switch', so that it can be turned on and off very quickly; it is useful for $CO_2$ angiography.
- **3-way taps**. These taps have a sideport. This allows air bubbles to be flushed out when a syringe is connected. It also permits two syringes to be attached together. This allows one to be used as a reservoir, e.g. during embolization. 3-way taps are often used in pressure measurement circuits to allow the system to be calibrated to atmospheric pressure and also within contrast and saline flushing systems (Fig. 9.11).

**Haemostatic valves** Vascular sheaths come with a built-in haemostatic valve. They are also found as standalone devices and are used with guide-catheters when performing thrombus aspiration.

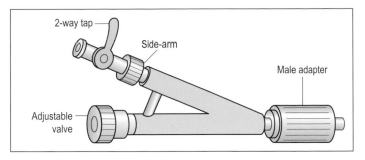

**Fig. 9.12** ▪ Tuohy–Borst adaptor.

Haemostatic valves are also available with a screw-type iris and side-arm for flushing, which can be attached to any catheter and largely take away the need for the more complex Tuohy–Borst adaptors.

**Tuohy–Borst adaptors** This invaluable, but slightly fiddly, Y-shaped device allows a haemostatic seal to be formed around guidewires that are smaller than the catheter lumen (Fig. 9.12). In addition to preventing a puddle of blood on the floor, contrast or drugs can be injected through the side-arm of the Tuohy–Borst around the wire. Tuohy–Borst adaptors are available in sizes that will seal around devices from 0.014 inch to 9Fr (approximately 3 mm). Probably the most frequent use of this device is to permit a 0.018-inch guidewire to be used with a standard catheter without leakage.

Learning to flush the device properly will place you ahead of many of your colleagues:

1. Connect a 2-way tap to the side-arm.
2. Attach the Tuohy–Borst to the catheter.
3. Open the adaptor valve (anticlockwise).
4. Attach a syringe containing heparinized saline to the tap: flushing will expel air through the valve.
5. Now close the valve (clockwise) and flush the catheter.

To use the Tuohy–Borst, the catheter is passed over the guidewire until it stops at the valve. Loosen the valve sufficiently to allow the wire to exit and then tighten it so that it forms a snug haemostatic fit but allows the catheter to slide on the wire.

**Connectors** Connectors should also be used during hand injection to reduce your radiation exposure. Remember the inverse square law, even a small increase in distance results in a significant dose reduction. Get in the habit of taking a step backwards before performing an angiogram.

*High-pressure connectors* These are non-compliant tubes used to connect the catheter to the injection pump. Most incorporate a 2-way tap.

*Low-pressure connectors* Just like their high-pressure cousins but made from compliant tubing, not suitable for use with a power injector.

**Pin-vice** This device is used to grip and steer guidewires and is particularly helpful when using hydrophilic and 0.018-inch wires. Remember to check that the device that you use is the correct size for your wire; a standard pin-vice may not grip a 0.018-inch wire.

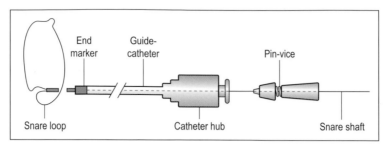

**Fig. 9.13** ◼ Amplatz 'gooseneck' snare.

**Vascular snares** Snares are used to retrieve foreign bodies and to capture guidewires for pull-through procedures; they are dealt with in detail in Chapter 20, Venous Intervention. The best-known and most popular snare is the Amplatz Gooseneck snare (Fig. 9.13). This is made of Nitinol and comes in a range of sizes from 2 mm to 25 mm, which should be matched to the target vessel size. The snare is supplied with its own 6Fr catheter which has a radio-opaque end marker. This catheter can be shaped if necessary to increase manoeuvrability. Gooseneck snares are like lassoes and can be rotated, advanced and withdrawn as well as tightened. The snare is placed around the target object and then the catheter is advanced, shortening the loop and gripping the target. The snare and its prey can now be pulled back to the access site and removed.

Alternative snares are also available with different configurations, e.g. trilobed, which can allegedly simplify capture in some circumstances.

**Puncture site closure devices** These are dealt with separately in Chapter 15, Angioplasty and Stenting.

# 10

# Using catheters and wires

Now you know what everything is, here is what to do with it! Remember that wires go first so the initial step of almost every procedure is to get a guidewire safely to the target zone.

 **Alarm:** Exceptions to the catheter follows the wire are: manoeuvring a pigtail up and down the aorta, moving catheters up and down the aorta to allow them to engage a branch vessel – even then take care in a diseased aorta.

 **Guidewires: a step-by-step guide**

1. Advance the wire smoothly and carefully under fluoroscopic guidance. The wire should slide readily when held between thumb and forefinger.
2. Note the characteristic 'ringing' as wires are passed through a needle and catheters are passed over the wire.
3. STOP if you feel any resistance, withdraw the wire a few cm, then carefully advance again, look for buckling or deviation from the expected path. Inject contrast to show what is wrong.
4. Keep the wire tip in view so that you know it is not causing any harm.
5. If you need to screen away from the tip, e.g. while introducing a catheter, note where the end of the wire reaches on the drapes and make sure it does not migrate.
6. Insert a good length of wire before trying to introduce or exchange a catheter through the skin. You are less likely to lose position and you will have some wire to withdraw if the wire buckles.
7. Never let the wire move forwards when trying to introduce the catheter into the skin. It will buckle at the catheter tip and make the job much harder. Keep the wire out straight under slight tension.
8. Steerable guidewires have good torque control; rotating the shaft will steer the tip in the same direction. Use this in combination with roadmapping to pass branch vessels and enter target vessels. You can use a pin-vice to help torque a steerable guidewire.
9. Do not be fooled by an assistant giving you the wrong end of the straight wire. Always check the flexibility of the end of the wire.

 **Tip:** Always assume that your assistant is determined to pull the guidewire out during catheter exchanges. Get a grip!

In the previous chapter you learnt that wires come in a variety of diameters, lengths and stiffness. There are occasions when even a stiff wire is not enough. In these cases adjunctive methods of providing additional support can be very helpful. Two techniques stand out for this:

**Through and through wire (a.k.a bodyflossing)** This involves two separate vascular access points and is fully described in Chapter 22, Rendezvous and Retrieval Procedures. In essence, a long wire is introduced through one sheath and brought out of a second site. The wire can then be held under tension, affording considerable support like a tight rope! Bodyflossing is used when the wire runs directly across the target site.

**Buddy wire** This is used in situations where bodyflossing is impossible, e.g. when the target vessel is an end artery (for example the renal artery). As the name implies, this requires two separate guidewires.

The 'Buddy wire' is a stiff wire; the first step is to place it deeply in a vessel close to the target. This allows a guide-catheter or sheath to be brought in proximity to the target. The first wire effectively acts as an anchor for the guide-catheter and provides a stable platform to allow the target vessel to be catheterized with the second wire.

 **Alarm:** The observant will have noticed that the sheath must be large enough to accommodate the buddy wire and whatever catheter/delivery system is required for the target vessel. Using an 0.018-inch wire such as the Platinum Plus keeps size to a minimum but this will still require a sheath 1–2 Fr sizes larger than normal.

# Catheter flushing

This is not the most glamorous-sounding task but catheters, like toilets, should be flushed before, during (OK the analogy breaks down here) and after use. The aim of flushing is to fill the catheter lumen with heparinized saline solution rather than alternatives such as air or blood clot. At best these will block the catheter, at worst the next run you perform will fire off a distal clot or air embolus. If you haven't performed a run or flushed the catheter for a few minutes, check for backflow and flush again. Multiple sidehole catheters should be flushed vigorously to ensure adequate flow through both the catheter tip and sideholes. Like many toilets, there are full flush and flush light options.

**Double flush technique** Used in the cerebral circulation where injection of even a small thrombus or air bubble could be disastrous. A syringe with saline is attached to the hub of the catheter and aspiration applied until blood flows freely into the syringe. This syringe is discarded and the catheter is then flushed with a syringe containing clean saline meticulously prepared to exclude air bubbles.

**Single flush technique** This is appropriate outside the cerebral circulation. The objective is to demonstrate that the catheter is free of clot and then to fill it with heparinized saline. Simply slowly aspirate the catheter with a syringe containing saline until a small bead of blood flows into the syringe. If you hold the syringe at 45° to the horizontal, the blood pools near the syringe nozzle at the bottom and any air bubbles rise to lie against the syringe plunger at the top. Now inject saline to flush the catheter; with care, the air bubbles and the blood will stay in the syringe. If the blood mixes with the saline, simply discard the syringe and double flush.

 **Tip:** Remember if you have aspirated flowing blood you know that there is no thrombus in the lumen and can move directly to injection of contrast; heparinized saline is only needed if there will be a delay during which time blood could clot in the catheter.

## Troubleshooting

If you are unable to aspirate blood freely from a catheter then one of the following applies:

- The tip is stuck against the vessel wall (endhole catheters only): try rotating or withdrawing the catheter until free flow resumes, then flush as normal.
- It is blocked: in this case flow will not resume. Presume that you need to remove the catheter and flush its contents outside the patient. UNLESS: you are able to sacrifice the territory the catheter lies in, e.g., during embolization.
- It is wedged in a small vessel: there is usually a giveaway sucking sound when you remove the guidewire. Slowly pull the catheter back until flow resumes.
- It is kinked: use fluoroscopy to check for kinking. Usually a kinked catheter will need to be removed and exchanged, as wires and embolization coils will tend to stick.

# Sheaths

Sheaths have a large dead space and also need to be flushed regularly; it is easy to forget this when concentrating on the catheter. Any clot has a tendency to lodge at the haemostatic valve.

## Troubleshooting

**The sheath will not aspirate** Try to remember to flush the sheath regularly and after every catheter exchange – but it is too late for that now! Adhere to the following guidelines:

- Do not be tempted to clear the sheath with a 'gentle' injection.
- Use fluoroscopy to check if the sheath is kinked.
- Try to aspirate with an empty 50-mL syringe, as this will generate the maximum amount of suction.
- If this fails and there is still a guidewire through the sheath, then the simplest action is to exchange the sheath for a new one.
- If there is no guidewire through the sheath, then apply suction with a 50-mL syringe and insert a straight wire and exchange for a new sheath. This carries a very small risk of distal embolization and should be used cautiously, particularly for patients with diseased run-off.

**Tip:** You can re-use the same sheath: pass a standard guidewire through the sheath. Put the sheath dilator back on the guidewire about 30 cm from the sheath. Aspirate and remove the sheath as above. Compress the puncture site while your assistant flushes the sheath to clear the thrombus. Simply insert the sheath dilator and reinsert the sheath as normal.

**The sheath kinks** Most sheaths are thin-walled and will kink if the sheath enters the vessel at a steep angle, e.g. antegrade puncture in an obese patient. It is almost unavoidable if the abdominal fold was retracted during arterial puncture.

- Try straightening out the sheath by flattening it against the abdomen.
- If this fails, advance a guidewire into the sheath until it stops. Carefully reinsert the dilator to the point of obstruction, then apply traction to straighten the sheath; the guidewire will generally advance.
- If this fails, then remove the sheath and repuncture.

**Tip:** To prevent kinking, try to puncture at a shallow angle; or if a steep puncture is essential, then consider using a reinforced sheath – these have a larger outer diameter. This is one indication for choosing the contralateral CFA for access.

## Selective catheterization: keys to success

### Pre-procedure imaging

- Review the available imaging, e.g. MRA or CTA, to gauge the optimal approach and catheter.
- Make a logical choice of selective catheter.

### Approximate positioning

- Get your catheter into roughly the correct area for the target vessel, e.g. renal artery L1/2.
- Perform a flush angiogram to demonstrate the target.
- Consider oblique views.
- Consider using roadmapping to guide you.

### Catheter manipulation

- Keep the catheter shaft straight. Using the hub, turn the catheter towards the target. If the catheter does not turn readily, then either it is catching on aortic plaque or most of the torque is being taken up in tortuous iliac vessels.
- To improve torque either increase the catheter size, e.g. go from 4Fr to 7Fr, or better still, insert a long sheath or appropriately-shaped guide-catheter.

**Tip:** Check to see if the catheter tip is facing forwards or backwards. If you are working from the leg, rotate the catheter towards you:
- If the tip turns towards you, the catheter faces forwards.
- If the tip turns away from you, the tip faces backwards.

Remember that the opposite applies if you are working from the patient's arm!
- Most shaped catheters are pulled backwards towards the target vessel. If the aorta is relatively free of disease then the catheter can also be pushed forwards. Remember to be gentle as the catheter can be an effective plough and dislodge plaque and thrombus.

# Catheter wire interaction

Catheters and guidewires should work in harmony with each other. Initially, the wire leads the catheter to a large vessel such as the aorta or iliac arteries. The catheter then points the wire in the correct direction such as a branch vessel. The wire is advanced into this and then followed by the catheter. This principle applies whenever a catheter does not simply engage the target.

- Using fluoroscopy, point the catheter at the target, advance the guidewire smoothly and gently; steerable wires can be rotated to aid this process. If the wire starts to buckle or push the catheter back – STOP – do not try to force it. Retract the wire and then try advancing at a different angle.
- Get a reasonable length of guidewire into the target vessel – advancing a catheter across the floppy tip of the guidewire guarantees it will 'spring-out'.
- Keep the guidewire absolutely fixed and under tension when advancing the catheter.
- Advance the catheter smoothly and gently into the target vessel under fluoroscopy. If the catheter/wire start to buckle – STOP – the catheter and wire will spring out of the vessel. Try again, this time with more wire to increase stability or exchange for a different catheter.

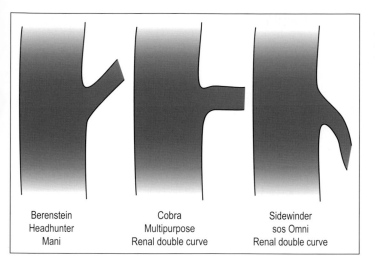

| Berenstein | Cobra | Sidewinder |
|---|---|---|
| Headhunter | Multipurpose | sos Omni |
| Mani | Renal double curve | Renal double curve |

## Choosing your weapon

The most important factor in catheter choice is the angle at which the target vessel arises from the parent vessel. Review the imaging and then choose logically; if the vessel points downwards, then even the most skilled angiographer will struggle with a forward-facing catheter such as the Berenstein. Use Figure 10.1 to aid your catheter choice.

Most catheters adopt their shape as soon as they are in a blood vessel of sufficient size; don't expect a 15-mm pigtail to form in a 6-mm external iliac artery. Similarly, other catheter shapes and effectiveness are affected by the size of vessel you are using them in. Choose the simplest shape most likely to bring the tip close to the target and point it in the correct direction.

## Catheter handling

Small-calibre catheters may be less traumatic in terms of the size of the puncture site but the cost is often reduced turning ability or catheter torque. Catheter torque is also affected by many other factors including catheter material, catheter length and vessel tortuosity. Most non-selective angiograms can be performed with 3Fr catheters but selective catheterization, particularly if tortuous vessels are involved, usually requires 4Fr catheters or larger.

Catheter construction influences handling and manufacturers will tell you of the prowess of their individual devices; experiment with different kits until you find what works for you.

## Construction considerations

**Braiding** Braided catheters have a wire reinforcement which gives increased torque and some kink resistance. The downside is that they tend to be rather rigid and more prone to 'ping in and out of vessels'.

**Coating** Hydrophilic catheters (and wires) have a slippery coating when they are wet; this tends to be most useful at the extremes of scale, e.g. for inserting very large devices such as stent grafts and when using co-axial microcatheter systems.

**Visibility** It can be very difficult to see a small catheter in a large patient. Some catheters have a barium coating or a platinum band to show the tip position.

Many of the common catheters are available with different constructions. These change markedly the handling characteristics, e.g. hydrophilic coatings. Hydrophilic-coated catheters, when used in combination with a hydrophilic wire, can be advanced into small vessels of the distal arterial bed. You may get asked which one you would like; if you are uncertain, a good answer is usually 'which ever one the boss prefers' as this means their favourite is readily available when you call for help.

 **Tip:** A vascular simulator is a good place to learn the concept of selecting an appropriate catheter shape and using it to catheterize branch vessels. Don't be fooled into thinking that success on the simulation will translate into expertise on patients!

# Sidewinder shape catheters

 **Forming a Sidewinder shape catheter**

1. Over the aortic bifurcation: this is very safe. As it does not involve manipulation in the aortic arch, it is recommended in elderly patients and those with aortic arch disease. Unfortunately you cannot do this if there is an iliac occlusion.
   a. Catheterize the contralateral iliac artery using either a Cobra or RDC catheter.
   b. Advance a wire down to the CFA.
   c. Advance the catheter to the CFA and exchange for a J wire.
   d. Exchange the Cobra for a sidewinder catheter.
   e. When the shape forms over the aortic bifurcation, bring the wire back to the 'catheter knee'.
   f. Push the catheter and wire together up into the aorta; the reverse curve shape should be preserved.
2. In the aortic arch: the arch and ascending aorta have the largest diameter, therefore this is used to allow the catheter to form. The '**quick aortic turn**' technique (Fig. 10.2) is perhaps the simplest, but there is a small risk of causing a stroke as the catheter is formed.

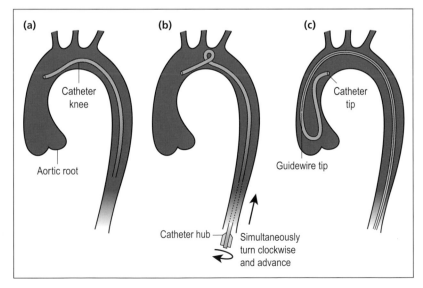

**Fig. 10.2** ■ Using the quick aortic turn to re-form the Sidewinder catheter.

    a. Advance the catheter until the knee of the catheter is across the apex of the aortic arch.

    b. Simultaneously push the catheter forwards and rotate clockwise to re-form the reverse curve.

    c. Under continuous fluoroscopy, pull the catheter down into the aorta. The catheter may occasionally engage vessels on the way down. Remember to push the catheter in to disengage, then withdraw, rotating it slightly.

  The aortic turn manoeuvre can be difficult in the unfolded aortic arch, so insert a guidewire to the level of the 'knee' of the catheter and try again. An alternative is to pass a hydrophilic guidewire around the aortic arch; when it reaches the aortic valve it will tend to double back on itself. Allow a large loop to form and then introduce the Sidewinder catheter until it forms adjacent to the aortic valve (Fig. 10.3).

3. In a branch vessel: this is similar to using the contralateral iliac artery but uses another vessel, such as the subclavian artery or renal artery. Once this has been catheterized and stable wire access obtained, exchange for the Sidewinder catheter. Carefully advance the catheter into the artery as far as the apex of the curve, pull the wire back to the knee then push and rotate clockwise to disengage from the vessel.

  The Sidewinder is a little more complex to use; there are two stages: forming the reverse curve (see box below [Figs 10.2, 10.3]) and using the formed catheter (Fig. 10.4).

**Using the sidewinder** The catheter is positioned above the target vessel and then pulled back down towards the target vessel. It is steered by rotating the shaft (Fig. 10.4). Once at the ostium, pulling it back further will result in the catheter engaging the artery. Once the knee of the catheter has reached the vessel ostium, further traction will start to pull the catheter out! At this stage, deeper catheterization can be achieved by advancing the catheter over a guidewire. This is easiest with an S3, possible for the gifted with an S2 and only for the divine with an S1.

**Tip:** If the catheter loop is too large for the aorta, the tip of the catheter is held away from the aortic wall and will not engage branch vessels. Try introducing a guidewire around the apex of the catheter curve to straighten out the limb; if this fails, choose a smaller curve.

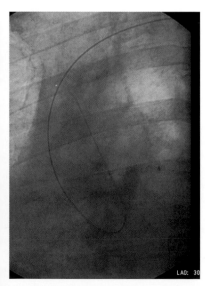

Fig. 10.3 ■ Forming the Sidewinder using the aortic valve. A 260-cm hydrophilic wire is passed around the aortic arch until it doubles back on the aortic valve. The Sidewinder catheter is simply advanced over the wire and will form with its apex at the valve.

LAO: 30

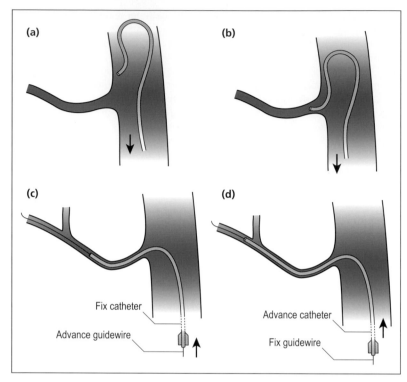

**Fig. 10.4** ■ (A) Using the Sidewinder. Pull back to engage catheter tip in the vessel ostium. (B) The catheter is advanced further by pulling back until the catheter is in as far as the knee. (C) For deeper catheterization, advance a guidewire into the vessel. (D) Push the catheter over the fixed wire.

## Co-axial systems

These include guide-catheters and microcatheter systems. Co-axial systems use all the same basic principles as conventional catheters but are a little more fiddly until you get the hang of them. The key elements to consider are:

- Is everything compatible: no prizes if your working catheter will not fit inside the guiding catheter or is shorter than it!
- Guiding catheters are like sheaths with an even greater dead space for thrombus formation. They need regular flushing or, if working in a high risk environment such as the carotid artery, they can continually be flushed with heparinized saline using a pressure bag.
- Keeping everything tidy: there is an additional catheter to consider. Try to keep the catheters in a straight line. Clipping the guide-catheter to the operative drapes will help hold it in position and free up a hand.
- In critical positions ask your assistant to control either the guide-catheter or the working catheter/guidewire while you manipulate the other.
- The usual rules apply: keep everything out straight, fix the catheter, advance the guidewire, follow with the catheter and so on.

- On occasion, you will want to advance the guide catheter over the smaller inner catheter to give more support. This will only succeed if the guidewire is in place and the inner catheter sufficiently far into the target vessel. Fix the inner catheter/wire combination and use it like the wire for the guiding catheter.

 **Tip:** When using an assistant to fix catheters or wires, explain to them what you are planning to do and how they can recognize what is required of them, e.g. fix the wire so that the tip remains in the same place on the screen.

# 11

# Vascular access

Vascular access is the starting point for all diagnostic and interventional angiography. Several basic principles apply and similar problems are encountered at any access site. Choice of puncture site is dictated by the planned procedure; think what you need to achieve, consider the site of lesion and the size of sheath and catheter required.

The basic technique, first described by Seldinger, has three components:

- Vessel puncture
- Passage of the guidewire
- Introduction of the catheter.

In general, arteries are pressurized and have thick walls, veins are at very low pressure and have thin walls, and this affects the puncture techniques. The following section describes arterial access; venous access is discussed at the end of the chapter.

## Arterial puncture

Puncture sites are points where the artery is relatively fixed and it is compressible over bone to obtain haemostasis. The most commonly used site is the right CFA. However, many factors such as the strength of the pulse and the site of the disease will influence the decision. The shortest, straightest route is nearly always best.

### Arterial puncture: a step-by-step guide

1. Choose the optimal puncture site; take time to find the pulse; clean and drape the area.
2. Palpate the pulse and gently tension the skin. Infiltrate from skin to artery with 1% lidocaine. Leave the needle in situ to mark where to make the skin incision.
3. Make a skin incision appropriate to catheter/sheath size.
4. Place gauze swabs to absorb blood.
5. Insert the needle at 45° to the skin, aiming towards the pulse. Pulsation transmitted to the needle increases as the needle tip approaches the artery wall but falls as the wall is punctured. There is often a change in resistance felt at the arterial wall and on entry to the vessel lumen.
6. Free pulsatile backflow indicates that the needle tip is intraluminal. Poor flow is seen when using a 21G needle or below a high-grade stenosis or occlusion.
7. The needle position is usually quite stable; it does not need to be held with a vice-like grip.

**Tip:** You will occasionally transfix an artery as the needle is introduced. This occurs most often in young thin patients with compressible arteries. Always pull the needle back slowly after a puncture to get a second bite at the cherry.

   If the arterial pulse is not palpable, puncture can be attempted using the normal anatomical landmarks. Fluoroscopy may also demonstrate vascular calcification. If this is unsuccessful, use a form of guidance – either ultrasound or a roadmap image from another catheter. If you cannot get access at your preferred site, use an alternative approach; remember to include the original access site in the subsequent angiogram to clarify the situation.

 **Consent issue:** The main complications of arterial puncture can be readily remembered as the three Bs: **bruising, bleeding** and **blockage** of the vessel. <1% of patients should need either a blood transfusion or an operation to put things right.

# Passage of the guidewire

The 3-mm J wire is the most frequently used initial guidewire. Arterial sheaths often come with guidewires with straight and J tips; the straight end is useful in small vessels, e.g. the radial and brachial arteries. Use the introducer to advance the wire into the needle. If the introducer is not immediately available, which usually means it has migrated to the floor, it is possible to straighten the J wire by applying tension to the inner mandrel (Fig. 11.1). The wire should advance smoothly and without resistance when held loosely between finger and thumb. There is a very characteristic feeling when a guidewire is passed through a needle or has a catheter passed over it – you will learn to recognize it but it is still best to use fluoroscopic guidance to ensure that the wire follows the expected path without buckling or deforming (Fig. 11.2). It is better to put plenty of wire in the vessel rather than too little!

 **Alarm:** Never use force on a guidewire; something is wrong; STOP and CHECK. Use fluoroscopy to check wire passage. Force is never necessary and always harmful.

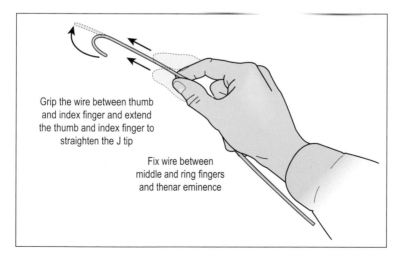

Grip the wire between thumb and index finger and extend the thumb and index finger to straighten the J tip

Fix wire between middle and ring fingers and thenar eminence

**Fig. 11.1** ■ Straightening the J wire. Fix the wire between the middle and ring fingers and the thenar eminence. Grip the wire between thumb and index finger and extend the thumb and index finger to straighten the J tip.

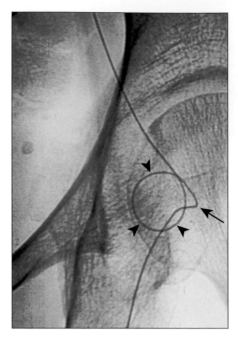

**Fig. 11.2** ■ A 0.018-inch guidewire has kinked at the end of the catheter (arrow). Further pressure has caused a subcutaneous loop to form (arrowheads). The wire was pulled back and straightened to allow the catheter to be advanced.

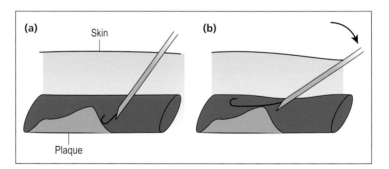

**Fig. 11.3** ■ Flattening the needle against the skin will often allow the wire to negotiate plaque adjacent to the puncture site.

## Troubleshooting

### The wire will not advance beyond the needle tip

- It is not intraluminal; usually the needle has been advanced too far and is in the far wall of the vessel. Remove the wire and verify pulsatile backflow; reposition as necessary.
- The needle tip is abutting plaque; alter the angle of the needle: flattening towards the skin is often helpful (Fig. 11.3). Try straightening the wire tip and redirecting.

Use a test injection of contrast via the puncture needle to confirm intraluminal position. A roadmap may help guide the wire. Use tight collimation; keep your fingers out of the main beam (you may need them in years to come).

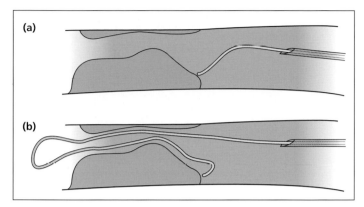

**Fig. 11.4** ▪ The very floppy tip of the Bentson wire will negotiate plaque with minimal risk of dissection.

- Try another wire: many sheath wires have both a 'J' and a straight tip. The straight end will often pass when the 'J' tip will not advance. The Bentson wire often finds its way past plaque (Fig. 11.4) that the J wire will not negotiate. Never use a Terumo wire because the hydrophilic coating may shear off in the cutting bevel of the needle.

  If no success, obtain haemostasis and try again or consider another approach.

## The wire stops after a short distance

- Confirm that the wire is taking the expected route and is not in a branch vessel. Redirect as necessary.
- Insert a 4Fr dilator to secure vascular access.
- Make sure blood can be aspirated from the dilator.
- Using fluoroscopy, gently inject contrast to confirm intraluminal position.
- Perform a hand-injected angiogram to identify the problem.
- Use a roadmap and steerable hydrophilic wire to negotiate diseased and tortuous vessels.
- Make sure that you have plenty of wire in the artery before exchanging the dilator for a catheter. If necessary, replace the hydrophilic wire with a standard wire for stability.
- If all fails, try again using a shaped catheter (e.g. Cobra II).

## Introduction of the catheter

The choice of catheter depends on the procedure. If the guidewire is held straight under slight tension, the catheter should slide smoothly along it. In a scarred groin, it often pays to use a dilator and consider changing for a stiff guidewire. Use the following basic rules:

- Always insert plenty of guidewire.
- The guidewire should be held out straight and under slight tension.
- Hold the catheter close to its tip within 1–2 cm of skin.
- Push and twist the catheter to advance it.
- Feel the catheter slide freely along the wire.

 **Alarm:** If the catheter seems to stick and pulls on the wire as it is advanced then the wire has kinked. Stop. Use fluoroscopy to show the problem (Fig. 11.5).
   **Solution**: This was why you put in lots of wire! Pull back the catheter and wire until the kink is outside the skin (Fig. 11.5). Try again, using a 4Fr dilator and then change the wire that has been damaged.

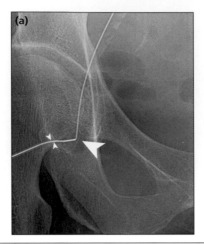

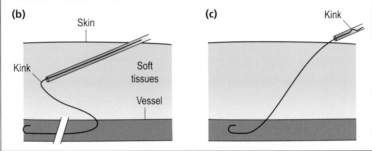

**Fig. 11.5** ■ (A) If the catheter (small arrows) is difficult to advance through the skin, the wire may have kinked (large arrow). (B) Schematic view. (C) The wire is pulled back until the kink lies outside the skin.

The catheter tip is often difficult to see, especially when using 3Fr catheters in obese patients. Pull back the guidewire until it takes the shape of the catheter tip; J wires can be felt to engage the catheter tip. The position is now readily seen on fluoroscopy. Use a test injection of contrast to confirm intraluminal position before flushing the catheter or performing a run. If the catheter is extraluminal, an extensive dissection will be avoided!

## Commonly used arterial puncture sites

*Common femoral artery* The CFA runs over the medial half of the femoral head. When the pulse is weak (Fig. 11.6) it is worth checking your position on fluoroscopy. Always aim to puncture the artery at the level of the midpoint of the femoral head whether for retrograde or antegrade puncture. This is usually the point where the pulse is most readily palpated.

**Alarm:**
- Puncturing too high, above the inguinal ligament, increases the risk of bleeding.
- Puncturing too low, i.e. superficial or profunda femoral artery puncture, increases the risk of false aneurysm and arteriovenous fistula (Fig. 11.7).

The wire generally does not need any steering to enter the external iliac artery; however, occasionally a plaque may deflect the wire into the deep circumflex iliac artery, which comes off the CFA at approximately 10 o'clock. This is usually easily appreciated on fluoroscopy;

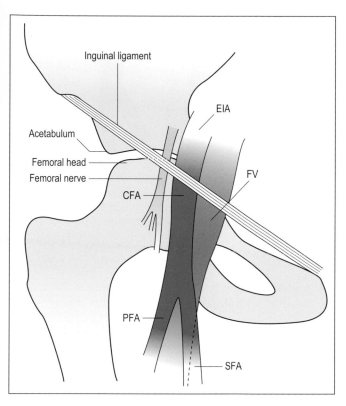

**Fig. 11.6** ■ The femoral anatomy. Note the femoral vein (blue) lies medial to the artery (red) in the groin but then passes deep to the superficial femoral artery (SFA). CFA, common femoral artery; EIA, external iliac artery; FV, femoral vein; PFA, profunda femoris artery.

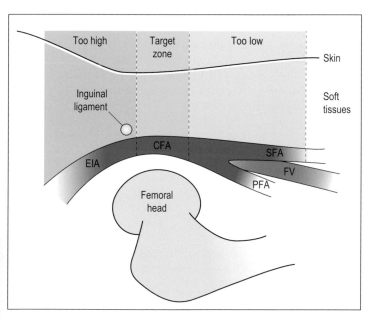

**Fig. 11.7** ■ Target puncture zone in the common femoral artery (CFA). Puncture at sites too low or high cannot be effectively compressed. Puncture above the inguinal ligament is especially dangerous. EIA, external iliac artery; FV, femoral vein; PFA, profunda femoris artery; SFA, superficial femoral artery.

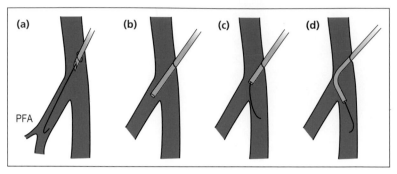

**Fig. 11.8** ■ Antegrade common femoral artery (CFA). (A) Wire repeatedly enters profunda femoris artery. Insert a 4Fr dilator. (B) Perform an angiogram in the profunda oblique to confirm puncture is proximal to superficial femoral artery. (C) Carefully pull back the dilator to CFA and try to direct an angled hydrophilic wire down the superficial femoral artery. (D) If still unsuccessful, exchange for a Cobra catheter and use this to direct the wire into the superficial femoral artery.

take care in this vessel as it is prone to severe spasm, which will retain the wire in a vice-like grip. The spasm usually responds to vasodilation with nitrates and the passage of time.

*Antegrade puncture (*Fig. 11.8*)* Antegrade puncture is more difficult and carries increased risk as dissection flaps tend to be elevated by the flow and may occlude the vessel lumen. The point of skin puncture is always higher than you expect. Aim to hit the artery at the level of the midpoint of the femoral head. In obese patients, it may help if an assistant holds back the abdominal folds. The profunda femoris artery (PFA) arises posterolaterally. This is in line with the needle; hence, the guidewire tends to pass preferentially into it. To catheterize the SFA under these circumstances:

- Flatten the needle and point it towards the SFA. If the wire still passes into the PFA, try steering by straightening the wire tip.
- Put a 4Fr dilator into the PFA. Withdraw it slowly into the proximal PFA, injecting contrast to show catheter position.
- Obtain a roadmap image in the profunda oblique projection (ipsilateral anterior oblique 25°). Inject hard enough so that contrast refluxes into the CFA and then opacifies the SFA. Ensure that the puncture site is proximal to the SFA origin. If it is not, start again.
- Try using an angled hydrophilic wire or a 15-mm J wire to select the SFA. Do not exchange over a hydrophilic wire; put the dilator into the SFA and change to a safer wire.
- No luck? Put a J-guidewire deep into the PFA and exchange for either a 4Fr Cobra or RDC. The catheter is pulled back into the CFA and the wire is directed into the SFA.

## Arm approaches

 **Consent issue:** An additional risk of the arm approach is causing a stroke as the catheter passes across the great vessels of the arch. Patients should be reassured that the risk is low (1%) but even that will be too high for some. Consider using non-invasive arterial imaging if the femoral approach is contraindicated

*Brachial artery (*Fig. 11.9*)* This is used when the femoral approach is precluded; it is often the best route for upper limb angioplasty, stenting and fistulography. For diagnostic angiography, the left brachial artery is the preferred approach as it is usually the

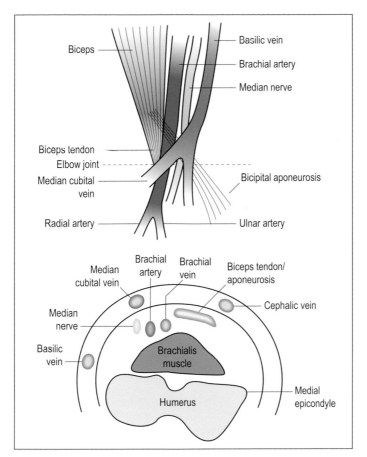

**Fig. 11.9** ■ Anatomy of the antecubital fossa. The brachial artery is punctured in the antecubital fossa above the elbow joint; it lies medial to the biceps tendon.

non-dominant arm and this route crosses the fewest cerebral vessels. The brachial artery is a small muscular artery and is prone to spasm. To prevent spasm, use a micropuncture set and straight guidewire, and administer prophylactic intra-arterial glyceryl trinitrate (GTN). Consider a surgical cutdown for sheaths larger than 7Fr.

 **Tip:** From the arm, the guidewire tends to pass into the ascending aorta. Use the left anterior oblique (LAO) 30° projection and a Berenstein catheter to direct the wire into the descending aorta.

*Radial artery* This is an alternative route for diagnostic angiography. It is fiddlier than other approaches but has advantages for haemostasis. Bedrest is not necessary, so it is well suited to outpatient procedures. Use a micropuncture set, a 4 Fr sheath and prophylactic GTN. A 120-cm long catheter is needed, which restricts flow rates to 6 mL/s. Long-term rates of thrombosis are not known.

 **Tip:** Perform Allen's test to confirm the ulnar arterial supply to hand. Alternatively, place a pulse oximeter on the middle finger. Compress the radial and ulnar arteries:

desaturation will occur. Release the ulnar artery; resaturation confirms dual blood supply to the hand. The reverse Allen's test involves release of the radial artery to confirm its contribution to supply.

## Esoteric arterial access sites

These are well recognized but seldom needed. In the past 15 years the authors have needed to use the translumbar, popliteal and pedal arteries on a few occasions but have never required the axillary artery. Our advice is to keep an open mind and be prepared to try novel approaches if they will solve a particular problem.

*Popliteal artery* (Fig. 11.10) Occasionally used to access the SFA and CFA when angioplasty via the CFA has failed. SFA occlusions may be easier to traverse from below, especially in the presence of collaterals. Balloons up to 8 mm can be used through a 4Fr sheath. With the patient prone, use ultrasound guidance to puncture the artery at the level of the patella.

*Pedal arteries* Occasionally it is simpler to traverse a calf artery occlusion from a retrograde puncture of the dorsalis pedis or posterior tibial artery. Use a mini access set and consider making a separate antegrade puncture with a through and through wire to perform angioplasty.

*Translumbar aortic puncture* The translumbar aortogram has long been superseded by non-invasive approaches. With the advent of endovascular aneurysm repair, it is occasionally helpful to puncture the aneurysm sac to treat a type II endoleak. In this case, CT is usually used to target the actual leak rather than a blind puncture into the aorta.

*Axillary artery* Puncturing the mobile axillary artery can be difficult and haemostasis no easier. There is a significant risk of brachial plexus injury secondary to haematoma. This approach is less safe than brachial puncture and is rarely needed and seldom used nowadays.

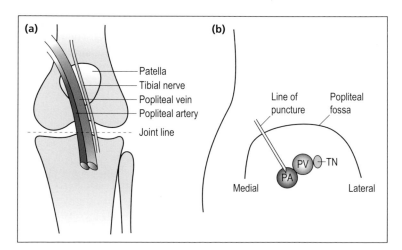

**Fig. 11.10** ▪ The popliteal fossa. (A) The popliteal vein (PV) lies superficial and lateral to the popliteal artery (PA). (B) Puncture at the level of the patella, medial to the popliteal vein and tibial nerve (TN).

# Venous puncture

The principles of venous access are similar to arterial access, but remember that veins are thin walled, highly compressible and prone to spasm. Venous spasm is readily provoked by injudicious catheter and wire manipulation. This can be a real catheter-gripping affair. Do not be tempted to start a tug-of-war – completely avulsing part of the venous system is seldom a satisfactory outcome. STOP and let the vein settle down for at least 5 minutes. If this does not work, try either GTN via the catheter or oral nifedipine. Blood pressure monitoring is advisable. Veins are more fragile and prone to dissection than a correspondingly sized artery, but fortunately bleeding is less severe.

**Venous puncture: a step-by-step guide**
1. Choose the optimal site depending on the planned procedure.
2. Consider using a tourniquet, Valsalva or Trendelenburg manoeuvres to distend the vein.
3. Clean and drape the area. Infiltrate the skin with 1% lidocaine. Leave the needle in situ to mark where to make the skin incision.
4. Make a skin incision appropriate to the catheter/sheath size.
5. Attach a 5-mL syringe to the puncture needle. Advance the needle at 45° to skin, aspirating as you go – a change in resistance may be felt on entry to vessel lumen.
6. Confirm intraluminal position by aspirating blood. If the tip is not in the vein, aspirate as the needle is slowly withdrawn. Flush the needle between attempts.
7. Guidewire passage and catheterization are the same as for arterial puncture.

*Ultrasound guided vein puncture* Ultrasound guidance is invaluable in some circumstances. Use ultrasound guidance if:

- The vein is not visible or palpable. Ultrasound should be used for all elective central venous access and also other superficial veins and visceral veins, such as the portal vein
- There is any difficulty or when there is a contraindication to arterial puncture, e.g. coagulopathy
- Access options are limited; even just one failed entry to the venous system is usually enough to cause a haematoma that will compress the vein and make subsequent puncture difficult.

**Tip:** Watch the needle advance to abut the vein wall and then advance quickly to puncture.

There are several signs on ultrasound that suggest a downstream stenosis or occlusion, especially with jugular vein puncture:

- Thrombus in vein
- Spontaneous contrast, swirling echo pattern from slow-moving blood
- Presence of collateral veins
- Abnormal distension
- Loss of pulsatility or respiratory variation.

Only absence of the vein precludes puncture; the rest should make you anticipate trouble and consider an alternative approach.

## Commonly used venous access sites

The approach chosen depends on the objective of the procedure.

*Common femoral vein (CFV)* The CFV lies medial to the CFA (Fig. 11.6). Palpate the CFA and infiltrate local anaesthetic 1–2 cm medial to it. Aim to puncture the vein at the level of the midpoint of the femoral head. The right femoral vein is preferred to the left as it has a straighter course to the inferior vena cava (IVC).

 **Tip:** Remember veins are easily compressed. Do not palpate over the vein during puncture because this just flattens the vein. Always aspirate as the needle is withdrawn since sometimes a compressed vein has been transfixed during puncture and opens as the needle is pulled back.

*Internal jugular vein (IJV)* The IJV is one of the most important venous access points; it is used for central venous catheterization, hepatic venous intervention and IVC filter insertion. The right IJV provides a straight path to the right atrium and IVC. The left IJV detours via the (left) brachiocephalic vein; this angled course limits its utility for interventional procedures. The vein is punctured 1–5 cm above the clavicle using either traditional anatomical landmarks or guided by ultrasound. Guidance makes the procedure simpler, safer and quicker.

*Subclavian vein and axillary vein* These are usually punctured under ultrasound guidance. The subclavian vein is usually punctured approximately two-thirds of the way along the clavicle and 1 cm inferior to its inferior margin. The axillary vein is punctured at a point just lateral to the first rib.

*'Blind' central vein puncture* In the UK, the National Institute for Clinical Excellence (NICE) has recommended that all central venous punctures should be made with ultrasound guidance. You are expert at this and have access to ultrasound so there is little justification for blind puncture.

*Ultrasound-guided jugular vein puncture* A 5–7.5-MHz ultrasound probe offers the best combination of resolution and depth for guidance. Turn the patient's head away from the side to be punctured and scan the neck to identify the vein lateral to the carotid artery and infiltrate local anaesthetic. It is usually easiest to position the probe transversely unless your probe has a very small footprint. Position the transducer 1–2 cm below the skin puncture site and line up the vein with the midpoint of the probe head. Slowly advance the needle into the scan plane and onto the anterior vein wall. The vein is easily compressed and should be punctured with a quick stab. Free aspiration of blood confirms intraluminal position.

*Median cubital vein* This is the medial superficial vein in the antecubital fossa (Fig. 11.9); it drains into the basilic vein and is the best arm vein for obtaining central venous access for IVDSA. The cephalic vein can also be used but it may be difficult to negotiate from it into the subclavian vein. A hydrophilic guidewire and catheter are indispensable in this situation.

## Esoteric venous access sites

These sites are not used in daily practice but may be useful for some forms of intervention and also in cases where there are no options left.

*Inferior vena cava* The IVC can be used for long-term central venous access. It is punctured using fluoroscopic guidance from a posterior approach to the right of the spine. If possible, place a pigtail catheter in the IVC below the renal vein; this provides a target to aim at and also helps to hold the vein open during puncture.

*Hepatic vein* The hepatic veins are another approach for long-term venous access and may also be used for intervention in Budd–Chiari syndrome. The target vein is punctured peripherally under ultrasound guidance. It is helpful to have colour Doppler to clarify that the vein is patent and that it is not a portal vein radicle. The mini-access set is very useful in these circumstances. The initial puncture uses a 21G needle, which is relatively atraumatic.

*Portal vein* Portal venous access is required for pre-operative portal vein embolization and also to treat post-transplant stenosis. The transhepatic and trans-splenic approaches can both be used. It is also possible to access mesenteric radicles via a mini-laparotomy.

*Renal vein* Rarely used for placement of a dialysis catheter in a defunct native kidney.

*Collateral veins* These are a last resort for central venous access. They are usually identified and punctured with ultrasound guidance. Preliminary venography will help plan the path through to the central veins. Even using hydrophilic catheters and wires, it can be very difficult to navigate through these small tortuous vessels.

# Suggestions for further reading

Kaufman JA, Kazanjian SA, Rivitz SM, et al. Long-term central venous catheterization in patients with limited access: A pictorial essay. AJR Am J Roentgenol 1996;167:1327–1333.

Spies JB, Berlin L. Complications of femoral artery puncture. AJR Am J Roentgenol 1998;170:9–11.

Trerotola SO. Management of hemorrhagic complications. J Vasc Intervent Radiol 1996;7:92–94.

What to do when the wheels come off, or how to keep your head while all around are losing theirs.

# 12

# Haemostasis

Even if you enjoy talking to your patients, obtaining haemostasis after a diagnostic or therapeutic angiogram is tedious. Hence the art of staunching the flow is often neglected or delegated to the most junior member of staff in the vicinity. This approach risks haematoma or haemorrhage; make sure you give as much importance to haemostasis as you do to arterial access (Fig. 12.1). In reality, haematoma is a much more common complication of arterial procedures than any other.

Stopping the bleeding is usually straightforward unless:

- The patient is severely hypertensive
- The patient is obese
- The patient is excessively anticoagulated or has a bleeding diathesis
- You didn't puncture the artery in the correct place
- You made a bigger hole than normal, i.e. >7Fr
- Or, as is often the case, a full house of the above.

 **Tip:** If you are anticipating problems call for help before you remove the sheath. Consider using an arterial closure device. If necessary leave the sheath in situ, keep the patient heparinized and have it removed surgically. Less than 1% of patients should require transfusion or emergency surgery.

## How to prevent haemorrhage and haematoma

If you have only recently given 5000 units of heparin, stop and have a cup of tea before taking out the sheath. When both you and the patient are ready, and have emptied your bladders, you can start.

Remember that the skin entry point is not directly above the arterial puncture site! In antegrade punctures the skin entry point is above (in well-padded patients it may be considerably higher, in retrograde punctures it will be lower.

1. Place a finger to either side of the catheter proximal and distal to the hole in the artery. You should be able to feel the pulse – this confirms that it is the correct place to press.
2. Press firmly down until the pulse reduces; if increasing the pressure abolishes the pulse, you are in control.
3. Look at a clock and check the time.
4. Remove the sheath and continue pressing, feeling the pulse. Don't forget to watch the puncture site or the patient will develop a haematoma.
5. After 5 minutes, slowly reduce the pressure and check the puncture site.

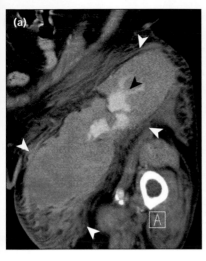
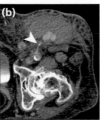
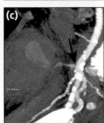

**Fig. 12.1** ■ Fatal haematoma following SFA angioplasty through a 4Fr sheath. The patient was resuscitated following cardiorespiratory arrest and had the artery repaired but succumbed to a CVA. (A) Coronal reformat showing massive haematoma in the left thigh (white arrowheads) with active bleeding (black arrowhead). (B) The point of extravasation is seen anterior to the femoral head. (C) Coronal oblique reformat clearly demonstrating active bleeding from the CFA.

6.  Still pulsatile bleeding? – press for at least another 10 minutes before you check again.
7.  Gentle ooze? – then press for another 5 minutes before checking.
8.  If the bleeding has stopped, get someone else who understands the principles of haemostasis to press for a further 5 minutes just to be on the safe side.
9.  When the bleeding has completely stopped, the puncture site will remain dry. Place a swab over it, place the patient's hand on the pulse, check that they can feel it. Instruct them to keep pressing until they get back to the ward and to remember to press if they cough, sneeze, etc.

*Bedrest post angiography* There is no scientific formula and precious little evidence to tell us what the optimum period of rest is before mobilizing. For uncomplicated 3/4Fr punctures it is probably reasonable to sit up after 30 minutes and get out of bed after about 1 hour. For larger punctures a period of 4 hours bedrest is probably prudent. Make sure that you advise patients to rest as much as possible for the remainder of the day. Day case and outpatients should be given clear instructions to rest up and only to exercise the remote control. They and their carer should be shown how to press on the puncture site and told how to contact help if bleeding starts again after discharge.

# Troubleshooting

## The bleeding doesn't stop – there's a range of escalation here

### Every time I release the pressure bleeding starts

- Stay calm and look calm – it reassures the patient.
- If your fingers are numb ask someone to help you.
- Check pulse, BP and venous access is working.
- Think about the clotting time and consider checking it.
- Make sure you know the vascular surgery phone number.
- If it's still like this after 30–40 minutes, it's time to make that call.

**The groin is okay but the BP is dropping**
- Keep pressure on the groin.
- Get help now.
- If the pulse is slow – is this vasovagal? Having someone push on your groin is not pleasant.
- If the pulse if high – then consider retroperitoneal bleeding.
- Check the venous access and get some IV fluids open.
- Check BP and pulse and adjust fluid support accordingly.
- Ultrasound can be useful for a quick assessment, CT is definitive.
- It's time to get vascular surgery on speed dial again.

**A large haematoma develops**
- Stay calm and reassure the patient.
- Make frequent observations of the pulse and blood pressure.
- Try to find the pulse and continue compression.
- If you can't do this, ultrasound and colour Doppler are useful to check for continuing bleeding or false aneurysm. Use the ultrasound probe to direct compression.
- A large haematoma will be painful, so give strong analgesics as necessary.
- Inform the vascular surgeon and assess the patient.
- If you achieve control, mark the haematoma margin – it's easier for the ward to assess then.

**I can't stop the bleeding no matter how hard I press**
- Stay calm and look calm – but it's time to move quickly.
- Get help now – you need at least two other people.
- Try to get the groin pressure on the pulse – often a minor adjustment will get control.
- Check the venous access and get some IV fluids open.
- Check BP and pulse and adjust fluid support accordingly.
- If it comes under control, great – but don't let your helpers disappear for at least 10 minutes.
- If it doesn't come under control within a few minutes – it's time to summon the vascular cavalry.

**Tip:** Remember, if bleeding will not stop you can always tamponade the puncture site by placing an angioplasty balloon from another access point. This will stop the bleeding and allow the patient to be stabilized and everyone else to compose themselves and work out the best solution.

**Alarm:** If there is any doubt, perform a contrast-enhanced CT scan. This will show the extent of any haematoma, whether there is ongoing bleeding and where it is from (Fig. 12.1).

## Arterial closure devices

These will not help you once the above problems have set in but they can help prevent them occurring. Closure devices are relatively expensive and are not without their own problems; they are not a panacea. Obviously we cannot give details or recommendations on every device and hence we recommend that you should become familiar with the use and indications for one or two of the devices. As a general rule, larger holes need more complex

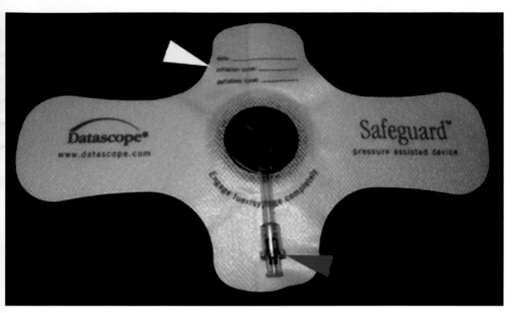

**Fig. 12.2** ■ Safeguard external compression device can be used in two ways. (1) Once haemostasis is achieved in the conventional fashion the device is applied over the puncture site (exactly where you would normally press) and the bladder is inflated with air (red arrow). The time and inflation pressure are recorded (yellow arrow). (2) The device is positioned and the bulb inflated prior to removal of the arterial sheath. Pressure is applied to the bulb until bleeding stops and the device left in position. In either case the puncture site can be observed through the transparent window. The device is left in position as long as necessary and can be periodically deflated to check for bleeding and the skin condition.

devices. Most interventionalists should know a simple device for small punctures (5–8Fr) and some will need a second device for bigger holes.

Devices for helping obtain haemostasis can be divided into passive and active.

**Passive devices** These are not directly applied to the arterial puncture.

There are a variety of devices which apply external pressure over the puncture site, some of which should be outlawed by the Human Rights Act. Essentially, they are no better than manual compression, but they do have the advantage that they do not tire. It's essential to realize the patient still needs the same level of observation and the device needs to be removed promptly. One device that can be helpful for superficial punctures that continue to gently ooze is the Safeguard (Fig. 12.2). The device is stuck to the patient over the puncture site and the balloon inflated. As the balloon is transparent, the puncture site can be observed while the device is in place. The balloon is deflated periodically to check whether the bleeding has stopped; when it has ceased, the device is simply removed.

Alternatives include materials that promote blood coagulation; these are quite effective when placed directly on a site of bleeding, e.g. a vascular anastomosis. But remember it's just possible that application on the skin does not directly affect the bleeding artery.

**Active devices** These devices are directly applied to the hole in the artery. There are three basic types: suture-mediated, vascular plugs and external clips.

The devices and the techniques for deploying are evolving and improving, making them more reliable; the following descriptions are a general overview and are not a substitute for hands-on training. Each system has its own idiosyncrasies and limitations, and these require familiarity and understanding, which should be obtained through specific training.

**Alarm:** None of the active devices is infallible and problems most commonly occur when the common femoral artery is diseased.

*Suture-mediated closure devices* These devices are typified by the Perclose, Proglide, Prostar (Abbott Laboratories) and the SuperStitch (Sutura). With a suture device there is immediate haemostasis and the artery may be punctured again immediately afterwards. These devices are capable of closing the largest punctures as the sutures appose the edges of the hole in the vessel just as they would in surgical repair. There are two clear impediments to this when the vessel is several centimetres deep and accessible only through a small hole in the skin:

- **How do you pass a suture through the correct part of the vessel wall?** The answer is to think of crochet. Figure 12.3 illustrates the process. A suture is introduced into the vessel through the 'arteriotomy' made by the sheath. Subsequently, a system of needles fires through the vessel wall adjacent to the arteriotomy and 'catches' the suture. The ends of the suture are pulled back through the needle holes and exteriorized ready for fastening.
- **How do you secure a knot at the vessel surface?** The answer is to think of slip knots. Each device has a system for apposing the sutures that starts with the suture ends outside the patient and then slides this down to the vessel surface and locks it in place.

Perclose and SuperStitch devices have to be correctly sized to be effective. If the 'arteriotomy' is too big, the needles will just pass through it rather than puncturing through the adjacent vessel wall. Clearly if this happened the suture would simply pull straight out again. As there is a chance of the device not working, this would be an unattractive proposition when dealing with very large holes such as those associated with stent grafting and percutaneous cardiac valve placement. To get around this problem, the concept of 'preclosure' has been developed. This simply involves deploying the suture after placing a small sheath. The ends of the suture are not tied at this stage and the puncture is up-sized to the larger sheath. When the procedure is finished, the knot is deployed. For really large sheaths, such as those used to deliver stent grafts, two sutures can be predeployed at an angle to each other to give an extra measure of security. Even then it is prudent not to attempt this unless you are able to control a 20Fr puncture site. In other words, if the suture fails you will need to be able to control the bleeding and then perform an open repair of the artery.

The design of the Perclose is quite complex. In essence it passes two needles through the vessel wall adjacent to the puncture site; these retrieve a suture loop. Pulling the button out

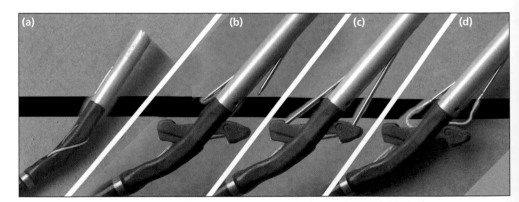

**Fig. 12.3** ■ How the Perclose works. (A) The device is inserted into the artery and held at an angle of 45°. (B) The footplate is opened and the needles advanced. (C) The needles pass through the wall and 'dock' in the footplate. (D) The needles are retracted, bringing the sutures back through the artery wall with them.

of the handle pulls the suture through and out of the skin. A slipknot is formed and as it is tightened it closes the hole in the artery. The current device has the knot already tied within the device. Sounds easy? Using the Perclose is not actually difficult but there are quite a few elements to remember and carry out in the correct order.

The device needs a minimum of a 5-mm vessel to allow the footplate to open properly. The manufacturer recommends an angiogram of the puncture site in the oblique plane to be certain that the vessel is a suitable size and the puncture is through the CFA.

### Basic steps in using the Perclose

### Phase 1: introducing the catheter

1. Introduce the monorail suture device over a standard 0.035-inch guidewire up to the wire exit channel. Do not use a hydrophilic wire as the catheter also has a hydrophilic coating and is quite slippery. The metal handle is not.
2. Remove the guidewire.
3. Continue introducing the device. When the transition point between flexible plastic and rigid metal is reached, it usually helps to change the angle of approach from about 45° to a shallower angle. When pulsatile blood flow is seen from the clear plastic sidearm, the device is far enough into the artery.

### Phase 2: catching the suture (Fig. 12.2)

1. Lift up the lever on the front of the device to open the footplate.
2. Hold the device at an angle of approximately 45° to the skin and gently pull the device back until resistance is felt; this opposes the footplate to the inner wall of the artery.
3. Firmly depress the button on the end of the device until it stops.
4. Pull the button right back out of the handle; the two needles will appear and hopefully one will have a green suture attached.
5. Cut the suture close to the needle.
6. Push down the lever on the front of the device to retract the footplate.
7. Pull the device back until the guidewire channel is visible and replace the guidewire – this is useful if the device fails.

### Phase 3: tying the knot

1. The knot and sutures will now be visible.
2. Harvest the sutures from the device window. Don't pull hard on either of them until you know which is which.
3. Irrigate the sutures with a syringe full of saline; this makes it easier for the knot to slide and to see the colours.
4. The green suture (the longer one) is the rail suture, i.e. the knot slides down this suture.
5. The white suture is the locking suture; place it carefully to one side.
6. **DO NOT PULL THE WHITE SUTURE.**

### Phase 4: advancing the knot

1. Attach the knot pusher to the rail suture above the knot.
2. Keep tension on the **rail** suture while pulling the delivery catheter out. The suture should slide progressively further into the puncture site as you do this. If the bleeding stops, maintain tension on the rail suture and remove the guidewire.
3. Advance the knot pusher along the rail suture to deliver the knot against the arterial wall. It is usually possible to feel the knot against the wall.
4. Relax the pressure and inspect.
5. No bleeding? Ask the patient to cough, if still no bleeding then proceed to cut the suture.
6. If there is still some bleeding, try steps 3, 4 again.
7. Now is the moment to pull on the **WHITE** suture; this locks the knot tight.

**Phase 5: the final cut**

1. Advance the knot pusher down onto the knot and by pressing the red lever a tiny blade will cut the suture – above the knot not through it – honest!
2. If there is no bleeding after 10 minutes, allow the patient to sit up.

# Troubleshooting

*Only one suture end is captured* Well, we warned that it was not perfect. Replace the guidewire and consider using an Angioseal or compressing as normal. Sometimes rotating the angle of fire of the needles will be successful with a second Perclose.

 **Alarm:** Remember with the latest version of Perclose only the longer 'rail' suture emerges with the needle – look to see if the knot is tied; if it is, both sutures were captured.

*The suture won't slip* Wet it and try again. Unfortunately, this is usually a prelude to the suture snapping and failure. Did you leave the wire in place?

*The suture snaps* See above.

*Bleeding continues despite your best efforts* If the wire is still in, try an Angioseal if the puncture site is 8Fr or smaller; if not, press on (literally).

# External plug

These devices deploy material on the surface of the artery to promote thrombosis. There are different variations on the theme, depending on whether there is a temporary intra-arterial balloon that is withdrawn at the time or an absorbable intra-arterial anchor that dissolves over time.

Temporary balloons, e.g. Mynx (AccessClosure), Duett Pro(Vascular Solutions), are devices that use a low-profile semicompliant balloon, which is inserted just into the artery lumen, inflated and then pulled back until it abuts the vessel wall. This 'presses on the inside of the artery' and stops bleeding. With the balloon in place, the procoagulant haemostatic material is deployed outside the vessel. This forms a plug which solidifies. The balloon is deflated and pulled out, leaving the plug in place to seal the hole.

The Boomerang ClosureWire Vascular Closure System (VCS) system is a variation on this theme. Instead of a balloon, a Nitinol 'button' on a guidewire is opened and pulled back against the puncture to stop bleeding. There is no haemostatic agent. Instead, you are intended to go away for a few minutes to write the notes and have a beverage while the puncture hole contracts. The button is closed and the device withdrawn, leaving you to press on a 3Fr puncture for a few minutes. This mechanism is probably only effective in vessels that are not heavily calcified.

 **Collagen plug and anchor:** Typified by the Angioseal (St Jude Medical). The Angioseal comes in 6Fr and 8Fr sizes. This system resembles the plastic tag used to attach price tags to clothing. A collagen footplate is deployed in the artery lumen using a version of a pusher system. The anchor is attached to a thread with collagen 'wadding' on it. The wadding is tamped down the thread with a pusher to form a plug at the puncture site (Fig. 12.4). Haemostasis is rapid. The collagen footplate dissolves over about 10 weeks and the artery should not be punctured again within three months, as there is a risk of dislodging the anchor plate. This subsequently forms an effective embolus.

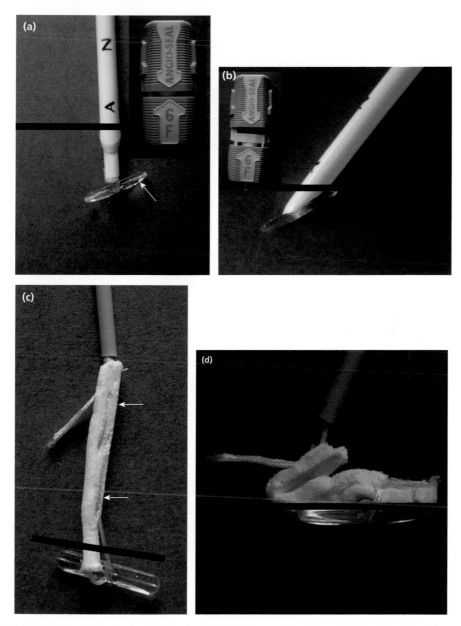

**Fig. 12.4** ■ Angioseal: the basics. (A) The footplate (white arrow) is released in the artery. Black line (arrowhead) represents the artery wall. Insert shows the delivery mechanism. (B) The footplate is retracted to the end of the delivery catheter (insert shows the delivery mechanism). (C) The catheter is withdrawn to leave the footplate in the artery and the collagen 'wadding' (white arrows) outside the artery. (D) The wadding is tamped down to affect a seal.

**Tip:** If you do need to access the artery again, the plug can be identified with ultrasound and a puncture made as far away from it as possible.

Using the Angioseal is not actually difficult. There are just a few elements to remember and carry out in the correct order.

**Basic steps in using the Angioseal**

**Phase 1: assembling the delivery catheter**
1. Open the packaging and you will find: a green dilator, a delivery catheter which has Angioseal written on it with the letters conveniently spaced 1 cm apart, a guidewire and a sealed foil packet. This contains the seal itself; open it as well.
2. The catheter is basically like a sheath. Pass the green dilator into the catheter until it engages. Note that there is a hole in the side of the catheter just beyond the distal end of the sheath and another proximal to the sheath.

**Phase 2: inserting the delivery catheter**
1. Keep the side with the writing facing up. The catheter is introduced just like a conventional sheath over a guidewire.
2. Continue to introduce until pulsatile flow is seen from the proximal sidehole.
3. Pull the catheter back until pulsatile flow stops – this indicates that the distal end lies just outside the artery. Note which letter of 'ANGIOSEAL' is at the skin surface (usually G unless the patient is large).
4. Advance the catheter in 1 cm (to the next letter). Pulsatile flow should start again.
5. Fix the delivery catheter firmly in place and remove the wire and dilator.

**Phase 3: deploying the 'footplate' (Fig. 12.4)**
1. Take the component containing the seal and introduce it into the sheath until the two components positively engage with a click. Do this quickly for the first few centimetres or the collagen plug will get wet and won't advance. The footplate is now dangling freely in the artery lumen.
2. Keeping the delivery catheter still, disengage the two components you just clicked together. Pull back the second catheter about 5 mm; it usually makes two clicks as you do this. The footplate is held taut sitting across the end of the delivery catheter.

**Phase 4: deployment of the device**
1. Press gently over the puncture site as if to obtain haemostasis.
2. Pull back the delivery catheter and second catheter together until they stop. A firm steady pull is usually required. A thread will be seen coming out of the puncture site. The collagen sponge can be seen on this and behind it a green plastic pusher.
3. Keeping the thread taut use the pusher to tamp down the collagen sponge until bleeding stops or a black transition is seen on the thread, which indicates that the plug is packed firmly enough.
4. Check the femoral pulse.

**Phase 5: the final cut**
1. Place a clip on the thread just behind the green plastic. This will keep the plug in place; it is probably unnecessary but will remind everyone to be careful of the puncture site.
2. Transfer the patient to the recovery area.
3. If there is no bleeding, tension the suture and cut it close to the skin.
4. Wait a few more minutes and make the patient sit up.
5. Tell them that the artery should not be punctured for 3 months and give them the patient information sheet. It does no harm to place the same information in their case notes!

# Troubleshooting

*Bleeding continues after deployment* A minor degree of bleeding isn't that unusual and usually resolves with a bit of groin pushing after 5 minutes.

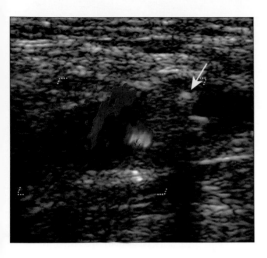

**Fig. 12.5** ■ Occlusion of the CFA by Angioseal. Colour flow is seen proximal to the footplate (yellow arrow). At surgery the footplate caught on plaque in the artery and did not pull back to the deployment catheter tip during phase 3; the collagen plug was partly inside the artery.

*There is no pulse after deployment* Perform an immediate Doppler ultrasound of the groin. The footplate can usually be easily seen; if there is no flow then contact vascular surgery immediately (Fig. 12.5).

# Suggestions for further reading

Dauerman HL, Applegate RJ, Cohen DJ. Vascular closure devices the second decade. An overview of the use of arterial closure devices. J Am Coll Cardiol 2007;50:1617–1626. Available at: www.medcompare.com/matrix/988/Active-Closure-Devices.html
The site lists a variety of closure devices with links to the appropriate websites; www.vascularsolutions.com/ information on the Duett; www.accessclosure.com/ information on the Mynx.

Korney M, Riedmüller E, Nikfardjam M, et al. Arterial puncture closing devices compared with standard manual compression after cardiac catheterization: systematic review and meta-analysis. JAMA 2004;291:350–357.
Paul T, Vaitkus MD. A meta-analysis of percutaneous vascular closure devices after diagnostic catheterization and percutaneous coronary intervention. J Invasive Cardiol 2004;16:243–246.

# 13

# Complications of angiography and vascular intervention

Puncturing arteries and blowing up balloons in them can and does occasionally cause problems. They never seem so bad if you know what to expect and what to do. Basically, most mishaps can be categorized into immediate and delayed and, with retrospect, predictable and unpredictable. Immediate and unpredictable complications are often more spectacular and the delayed are more sinister.

 **Alarm:** Try to avoid repeating others' mistakes! What seems unpredictable to you may be well recognized, so consult others before trying something new. Whenever you experience a complication, review the case and make sure that you and your colleagues learn from your mistakes.

Teamwork is essential in a crisis and an actual disaster is not the time to rehearse roles. Does everyone know what they will be expected to do? Has someone got the keys to the drug cupboard? Who will perform basic life support? Is it safe to perform cardiopulmonary resuscitation (CPR) on your angiography table? It is a good idea to consider what would happen in some common scenarios such as severe contrast reaction, severe hypotension, chest pain, difficulty breathing, fire, etc.

Remember the central tenets of crisis management:

- Stay calm
- Reassure your patient
- Stop and think what is likely to be the problem
- Plan your action
- Get help
- Action your plan.

## Immediate complications

Whenever a complication occurs, stay calm and try to think logically. A downward spiral of disaster can easily set in; ask for help sooner rather than later. Carefully document the episode in the patient's notes and explain what has happened to the patient or the patient's relatives. Many misunderstandings occur because of poor communication, and patients frequently complain about not being told what was happening.

Immediate complications can be grouped according to the site affected:

- Puncture site
- Intervention site
- Remote.

# Puncture site complications

These are the commonest and most predictable.

## Haematoma

Some bruising is inevitable but significant haematoma requiring either transfusion or surgery is rare (<1%). The risks increase with increasing catheter size, increasing patient size, hypertension, anticoagulation and low platelets. Think carefully before you deputize removal of an 8Fr sheath in an obese, hypertensive patient who has just been heparinized.

## Bleeding

Haemorrhage at the puncture site almost always occurs during haemostasis. A large haematoma (Fig. 13.1) can accumulate very quickly and will alert you to the problem. More sinister is occult bleeding into the pelvis. This happens when the arterial puncture is above the inguinal ligament. Be alert for signs of blood loss, yawning, confusion, agitation, faintness, tachycardia and hypotension; these can be a prelude to cardiac arrest. **Act quickly as soon as you suspect a problem**.
  Basic survival strategy:

- Do not struggle alone – call for assistance. By the time the surgeon arrives, the situation is usually under control and you can have a nice chat. If not, don't hesitate – the patient should have an urgent arterial repair, usually requiring just one or two sutures.

### First aid

- Lie the patient down and elevate their legs if necessary.
- Attempt to control the bleeding, try to find the pulse and apply local pressure.
- If local pressure does not work, place a balloon from the contralateral side into either the iliac artery or aorta.
- Resuscitate the patient, put in a large drip and take blood for cross-match and clotting studies. Start a rapid infusion of a plasma substitute or saline and give oxygen by mask.
- Closely monitor the patient's pulse, BP, oxygen saturation and ECG.

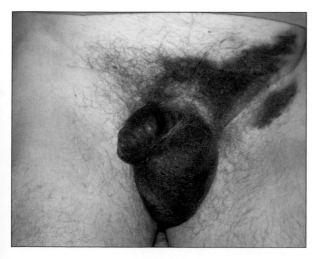

**Fig. 13.1** ■ Large haematoma in left groin, penis and scrotum following bilateral iliac stenting. Note right groin puncture site is free of bruising. No transfusion was required but moderate discomfort persisted for several weeks.

- Correct any clotting abnormality, e.g. protamine to reverse heparin (Chapter 6, Drugs Used in Interventional Radiology).
- Use ultrasound to document the site of the bleeding and the extent of any haematoma.
- Ultrasound-guided compression can be very effective when there is a large haematoma and the pulse is difficult to feel. If the bleeding has been occult, look in the pelvis for haematoma displacing the bladder.
- Don't hesitate to get a CT; extensive retroperitoneal haematoma can be very difficult to see on ultrasound.

 **Tip: The radiological tourniquet**: an angioplasty balloon inflated across the site of bleeding or in the inflow vessel can be lifesaving!

## False aneurysm

False aneurysm most often occurs when there has been inadequate haemostasis. Fortunately, this complication is usually caused by someone else (frequently a cardiologist). There are reasons for this, principally vigorous use of anticoagulation and antiplatelet drugs, large sheaths, early mobilization of patients and low puncture where the artery cannot be compressed against the femoral head. Whatever the aetiology, it frequently falls to us to remedy the situation.

**Management of puncture site false aneurysms** The first step is to reverse anticoagulation whenever clinically possible. Ultrasound is an excellent guide for the treatment of acute false aneurysms. Typically, false aneurysms will have an echo-poor area of unclotted blood and have 'in and out' blood flow on colour Doppler. The following features should be noted:

- Size of the chamber: >2 cm should be treated.
- Length of the neck: longer are more likely to respond to interventional therapy.
- Diameter of the defect in the artery wall: <2 mm most likely to respond.
- Complexity: false aneurysms can have more than one lobe, and the jet of flow arising from the hole in the artery identifies the primary chamber.

*Ultrasound-guided compression* This works best for acute false aneurysms, so is the first thing to do if you have just caused one. It is much less likely to succeed if the false aneurysm is a few days old. Compression is first choice where there is a documented reaction to thrombin or there is no thrombin available.

Compression is a simple technique that works because you press in the correct place! Scan the puncture site until you find the artery and use colour flow to look for the jet of flow in and out of the false aneurysm. Keep the colour on and use the probe to compress over this point. The aim is to press hard enough to occlude the flow in the false aneurysm whilst preserving flow in the main artery. In simple cases, this is just like obtaining haemostasis, and the aneurysm will thrombose after a few minutes. If you do succeed, bring the patient back for a follow-up scan after 24 hours to ensure that the false aneurysm has not recurred.

Commonly, the patient will have a large and tender haematoma and find the whole procedure very uncomfortable. Some patients will either not tolerate this or only manage a few minutes despite analgesia/sedation. Both you and the patient will be very uncomfortable if you need to press hard for more than about 15 minutes. If this is the case then consider the other options.

*Thrombin injection* This technique has been widely adopted as it is quick and easy. It is not cheap, and complications have been reported, including anaphylactic reactions to the thrombin (especially the bovine preparation) and thrombosis of the donor artery. Direct a 21

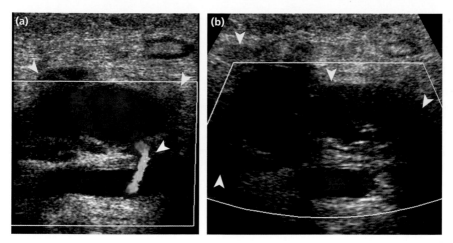

**Fig. 13.2** ■ CFA false aneurysm following coronary artery stenting. (A) The turbulent jet (white arrowhead) in the neck of the false aneurysm is seen arising from the front of the CFA, as is typical 'yin-yang' flow in the false aneurysm (yellow arrowheads). (B) Following injection of 100 units of thrombin, the false aneurysm (yellow arrowheads) and the neck are thrombosed, and flow is preserved in the CFA.

or 23G needle into the false aneurysm under ultrasound guidance; you may need a long needle if there is a lot of bruising in a large patient. Attach a 1-mL tuberculin syringe containing 1000 IU of thrombin. Aim towards the inflow defect and inject in 0.1-mL aliquots, keeping the colour flow on throughout (Fig. 13.2). Multilocular false aneurysms may need to be injected at more than one site. Thrombosis usually occurs very suddenly and further injection will risk thrombus or, worse, thrombin being injected into the artery with potentially calamitous results.

 **Alarm:** There are three rules for thrombin injection:
- **You must be able to see the needle tip in the false aneurysm during injection of thrombin.**
- **Do not aspirate blood into the thrombin syringe or you will need to start again.**
- **Do not stop if there is still visible flow.**

## Troubleshooting

*If thrombosis does not occur* Confirm that the needle tip is in the false aneurysm by injecting saline and looking for turbulence. Reposition as necessary and try again.

- Check that it is thrombin, not just saline in the syringe.
- Consider placing an angioplasty balloon across the defect from an alternative access point. Inflate the balloon to cover the hole and inject a small volume of thrombin. Slowly deflate the balloon and check for thrombosis. **Do not** overinject the false aneurysm sac or you will simply inject a bolus of thrombin into the artery when the balloon is deflated.
- Check the clotting and reverse coagulopathy if necessary.
- If it still won't thrombose, it's back to surgery.

*The false aneurysm thromboses but a tongue of thrombus is seen in the artery* If this is a small amount and there is no problem with limb ischaemia, accept this and stop. Consider heparinizing the patient. Rescan the patient after 24 hours.

*The artery thromboses* This is usually time to call the vascular surgeon and explain what has happened.

## Other puncture site complications

*Thrombosis* This usually occurs if the artery is severely diseased at the puncture site or if there has been arterial dissection during antegrade puncture. Check the condition of the limb; if there is acute ischaemia, then urgent surgical revascularization is required. If you have vascular access, get an angiogram to demonstrate the extent of the problem. If the situation is less urgent, thrombolysis may be appropriate; fresh thrombus is particularly likely to lyse. If the patient is asymptomatic, consider terminating the procedure and reviewing the patient's clinical progress.

*Arteriovenous fistula* This is very uncommon with a CFA puncture and is much more likely if the SFA is punctured, as the femoral vein lies deep to it. This is not the time to inject thrombin.

*Nerve damage* This is very uncommon and may result from direct injury, ischaemia, local anaesthetic and compression by haematoma. Occasionally, patients will develop femoral neuralgia.

# Intervention site complications

It is hardly surprising that occasional arterial injuries occur when you consider what we are doing inside these structures with catheters, guidewires and balloons.

*Arterial dissection* As angioplasty works by stretching and tearing the vessel lining, some dissection is expected. It is important if it is flow-limiting, and most commonly happens with antegrade approaches; retrograde dissections are usually self-limiting. If a dissection flap is causing significant obstruction, make sure that the patient is heparinized. In these circumstances there are four treatment options:

- Do nothing: only a consideration if the problem is unlikely to lead to a clinical deterioration.
- Perform a prolonged (5–10 minutes) low-pressure balloon inflation: try to stick the dissection flap back to the wall (Fig. 13.3).
- Stent the dissection: this provides an immediate and durable solution but is not advisable if the dissection involves a point of arterial flexion.
- Call your friend the vascular surgeon again: most of the time you should be able to leave the surgeon untroubled by using one of the three above options.

*Arterial occlusion* This is not uncommon when treating severely diseased vessels and may be of little clinical significance, e.g. when a severely narrowed artery becomes occluded. Occlusion is important if it:

- **Results in an acute decrease in perfusion** such as when important collaterals are blocked. In this case, a bail-out procedure such as stenting, thrombolysis or surgery is indicated
- **Modifies the treatment options** for the patient, e.g. when the length of an occlusion is increased, affecting the type of surgery required.

Heparinize the patient and consider the treatment options, stenting and surgery.

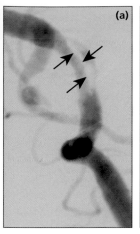 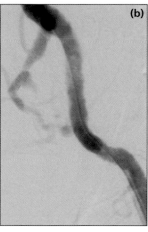

**Fig. 13.3** ■ (A) External iliac artery showing extensive post-angioplasty dissection (arrows) with residual 30 mmHg pressure gradient. (B) Abolition of pressure gradient and improved angiographic appearance post-prolonged low pressure inflation.

*Arterial rupture* Minimize the chances of this occurring by using a correctly sized balloon and asking the patient to let you know if discomfort is experienced during balloon inflation. Mild discomfort is normal but marked pain is not; do not be surprised if the vessel splits if you stretch the adventitia much more. Arterial rupture is an emergency and can lead to rapid destabilization of the patient's clinical condition (Fig. 13.4). **Apply the basic survival strategy as above.** Whatever you do, keep control of the bleeding by gently inflating an angioplasty balloon across or proximal to the injury. If you have a correctly sized stent-graft, now is the time to use it.

*Venous filling* A little filling of the venae comitantes is nothing to worry about, but stop and think if there is a brisk arteriovenous shunt. This is unlikely to happen, as rupture is much more common.

# Remote problems

This means that the problems are not at the sites above and not that they are remote from you.

*Distal macroembolization* Thrombus or atheroma may break off from the wall of a diseased vessel and will migrate distally until it occludes a vessel of a suitable diameter, usually at a bifurcation. Once again, the treatment should be based on the clinical scenario. If a small and unimportant vessel is affected, do nothing. If the limb has become ischaemic or a vital vessel has been blocked, then some action is necessary:

- Heparinize the patient.
- Attempt to aspirate the embolus (Fig. 13.5) (thrombo-aspiration, Chapter 19, Thrombolysis and Thrombectomy).
- Stent over the embolus.
- Call 0800 Fogarty.

*Distal microembolization* Microembolization can affect any organ system, and cholesterol, thrombus and atheroma can all cause severe problems. Catheter manipulation in the diseased aorta is the most common cause, with the resultant microemboli causing occlusion of the distal vascular bed. If the patient experiences sudden severe back or abdominal pain during the procedure, this indicates massive embolization and has a poor prognosis. More

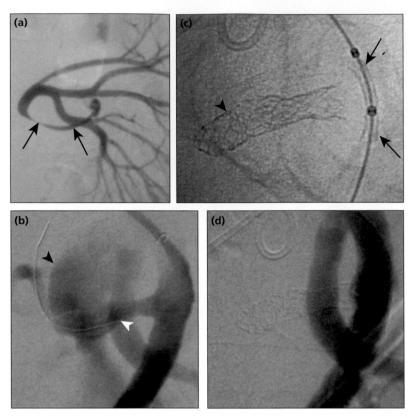

**Fig. 13.4** ■ Rupture of a renal transplant artery. (A) An unusual 5-cm long high-grade stricture (black arrows) in an acutely non-functioning transplant. (B) Arterial rupture (white arrowhead) following placement of three stents; extensive extravasation (black arrowhead). (C) Site of the rupture (black arrowhead). Unfortunately it was impossible to place a stent graft in the ruptured artery. A covered stent is being deployed over the origin of the transplant artery (black arrows). (D) Completion angiogram shows complete occlusion of the artery.

**Fig. 13.5** ■ (A) Distal embolization of atheroma into the crural vessels post angioplasty. (B) Flow is restored after thrombosuction with a 5Fr catheter.

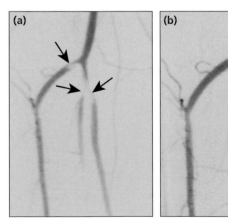

commonly, there will be cutaneous manifestations (livido reticularis) which come on after a few hours. Renal dysfunction is common; this may be abrupt in onset or manifest by a progressive, often irreversible, loss in renal function starting days after the procedure. 'Trash foot' is a serious outcome, frequently requiring amputation and it presents classically as distal tissue necrosis in the presence of palpable pulses.

*Cardiorespiratory failure* This can result from fluid overload, bronchospasm, drugs, sedation and contrast reaction. A vicious cycle is set up with hypoxia and myocardial ischaemia. The patient should be given oxygen and vigorously resuscitated.

# 14

# Angiographic diagnosis

Having a high-quality route map of the target vascular bed and, if necessary, the access to it are the keys to successful vascular intervention. They determine the choice of approach, the best equipment to use and the suitability for intervention. A preliminary diagnostic angiogram was the traditional way to obtain this information and 'test the water' regarding access. This is seldom now the case and preliminary imaging is typically performed non-invasively (see Chapter 7, Non-Invasive Vascular Imaging) using ultrasound, magnetic resonance angiography and CT angiography. Therapeutic decisions and approach are planned on this basis.

The skills necessary to perform high-quality angiography are still mandatory as DSA is required in the following contexts:

- Intervention
- When small vessel detail is required
- In many acute cases
- Where non-invasive imaging has failed or cannot be tolerated
- To arbitrate when non-invasive imaging is not conclusive and a definitive answer is needed.

This chapter has been divided into elective and acute presentations and will describe which test is usually required in the most important clinical scenarios that you are likely to encounter.

## Diagnostic digital subtraction angiography

Obtaining good quality diagnostic angiograms is the first step to any successful intervention. The principles of getting a good picture can be checked in Chapter 8, Angiography – Getting the Picture. This chapter details the indications, equipment, procedural details and views for all the common sites.

If the pump injector is recommended, then we have assumed 300 mg/mL-strength iodine will be used. When hand injections are recommended, 300 mg/mL is too viscous for rapid injection and we would suggest dilution with saline to approximately 200 mg/mL.

## Lower limb arterial diagnosis

The imaging modality of choice will depend on local availability, expertise, clinical urgency, level of detail required and the need for immediate intervention (see Table 14.1).

# Indications

Imaging the lower limb arteries is most frequently requested to investigate chronic ischaemia (intermittent claudication, rest pain and ulceration) or acute ischaemia (Fig. 14.1). Less common reasons are trauma, vascular malformation and tumour. The study should be dedicated to obtain the information necessary for the clinical scenario, with additional images, e.g. of the vessels in the feet, if necessary.

**Table 14.1** Lower limb arterial imaging depends on the clinical scenario

| Scenario | Modality |
|---|---|
| **Elective** | |
| Intermittent claudication | MRA > CTA > Ultrasound* > DSA |
| Chronic critical limb ischaemia | MRA > CTA > DSA |
| Assessment of bypass graft | Ultrasound then DSA for intervention |
| Popliteal aneurysm | Ultrasound for diagnosis and size, MRA for inflow/outflow |
| Popliteal entrapment | Ultrasound initial diagnosis, MR/MRA for delineation of type |
| Tumour/vascular malformation | Ultrasound for flow (high or low), MRA for extent, DSA for intervention |
| **Acute** | |
| Acute limb ischaemia | MRA, DSA depending on availability and expertise |
| Trauma | CTA for vascular and non-vascular injury, DSA for intervention |

*Ultrasound can be used to perform a basic screen of the femoropopliteal segment but this does not answer issues regarding inflow and outflow, hence MRA is the preferred tool due to speed and increased coverage.*

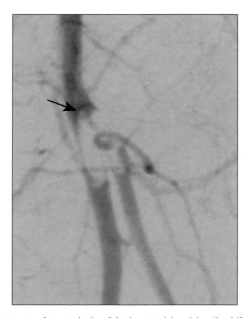

**Fig. 14.1** ■ Typical appearance of an embolus (black arrow) involving the bifurcation of the common femoral artery. The filling defect has a convex meniscus and is sited at a bifurcation. The underlying artery is normal and there are no collaterals.

## Equipment

- Basic angiography set.
- Catheter: pigtail or straight, 3Fr 30-cm length, 4Fr 60-cm, 90-cm or 120-cm (femoral, brachial and radial approach, respectively). Always use the femoral route unless contraindicated.

## Procedure

*Access* Tailor to the specific indication.

Diagnostic angiography for peripheral vascular disease is traditionally performed from the symptomatic leg unless the femoral pulse is absent or very weak. This ensures optimal images of the affected side. Straight catheters can be pulled back into the external iliac artery for single leg views. There is no risk to the asymptomatic limb.

 **Tip:** If the patient has had a duplex scan indicating a treatable femoropopliteal lesion, then approaching from the contralateral side allows both diagnostic views of the iliac inflow and treatment of the lesion from a single puncture and leaves options open for an ipsilateral antegrade puncture if necessary.

*Catheterization* Position the catheter below the renal arteries unless there is a reason to image them, i.e. renal impairment or hypertension.

*Runs* Our standard angiogram covers from the infrarenal abdominal aorta to the ankle (see Table 14.2). Tailor the examination to the individual patient. It is not routinely necessary to image the renal arteries. Lateral foot views are mandatory if distal reconstructive surgery is being considered.

To obtain high quality views of the aorto-iliac segments, always paralyse the bowel using hyoscine butylbromide (Buscopan) and use breath-hold or multimasking to eliminate misregistration.

## Additional views

Oblique views are not really additional and should be routinely used in the iliac arteries. In other circumstances, use your skill and judgement to decide whether they are required. A problem commonly occurs due to prosthetic joints obscuring a vessel; try an oblique view to see around the metalwork. In the presence of a TKR flexing the contralateral leg will give an unimpeded lateral view (Fig. 14.2).

**Table 14.2** Typical parameters for a lower limb angiogram

| View | Contrast volume (mL) | Injection rate (mL/s) | Frame rate (FPS) | Field size (cm) | Inject delay (s) | X-ray delay (s) |
|---|---|---|---|---|---|---|
| AP aorto-iliac | 15 | 8 | 2 | 40 | 1.5 | 0 |
| Oblique aorto-iliac | 15 | 8 | 2 | 28 | 1.5 | 0 |
| AP proximal thigh | 10 | 5 | 2 | 40 | 0 | 0 |
| AP distal thigh | 10–15 | 5 | 1 | 40 | 0 | Increase as necessary |
| AP calf vessels | 10–20 | 5 | 1 | 40 | 0 | Increase as necessary |
| Lateral foot | 10–20 | 5 | 1 | 28 | 0 | Increase as necessary |

*AP, anteroposterior; FPS, frames per second.*

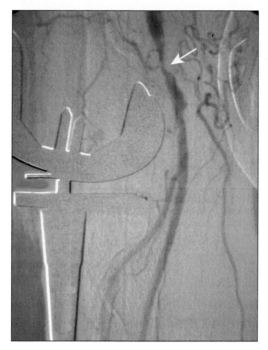

**Fig. 14.2** ■ High-grade stenosis behind a knee prosthesis (white arrow) seen on the lateral knee view. This was not seen on AP or shallower obliques.

 **Tip:** Remember the diagnostic maxim: one view is one view too few. We are trying to visualize 3D structures. If in doubt, try another run at 90° to the original.

*Iliac obliques* The iliac vessels are tortuous and oblique views are essential to allow full assessment and to see the origins of the internal iliac arteries in profile, i.e. LAO 25° for the right iliac system.

*Profunda oblique* To see the origins of the PFA, SFA and femoropopliteal/distal grafts, i.e. right anterior oblique (RAO) 30–50° for the right PFA.

*Focal stenoses* Any stenosis can be more accurately assessed if an additional oblique view is taken. Experiment with 30° obliques in either direction to try to profile the lesion.

*Lateral foot views* 'Charlie Chaplin' – place both heels together, turn toes out, 40-cm field.
Single foot – externally rotate the foot and rotate C-arm to obtain lateral projection, 28-cm field.

## Troubleshooting

- Poor views of the distal run-off: increase the volume and strength of contrast delivered.
- Collimate to a single limb.
- In the ipsilateral limb, pull back a straight, multisidehole catheter into the EIA to direct all of the contrast to the area of interest.

- In the contralateral limb, use a shaped catheter (e.g. Cobra II or RDC) to catheterize the contralateral EIA.
- Use a vasodilator such as tolazoline or GTN.
- Consider performing an antegrade puncture so that contrast will be directed solely to the run-off vessels.

**Tip:** Use iso-osmolar contrast in patients with critical ischaemia. This reduces the pain/heat associated with contrast injection. Everyone is happy, the patient stays still, you save time and improve your images!

# Arterial bypass graft diagnosis

Most graft assessment is performed with ultrasound as routine screening or for recurrent symptoms. Graft angiography is almost exclusively combined with intervention. Due to scarring and limited access, graft angiography can be difficult. Success is much more likely if you spend time ascertaining the graft anatomy, material and the results of the Duplex ultrasound before you start.

## Aims of graft angiography

Angiography is a prelude to treatment and aims to demonstrate mechanical problems:

- Confirm findings of non-invasive imaging.
- Anastomotic stenoses caused by neointimal hyperplasia. Usually within the first year.
- Intragraft stenosis, particularly at valve cusps and in composite vein grafts.
- Progression of disease in the arterial inflow or outflow. Usually after the first year.
- Graft kinking during knee flexion. This should always be excluded following thrombolysis if no other abnormality is found (Fig. 14.3). The graft usually kinks a few centimetres above the knee joint; this is best appreciated in the lateral projection.
- Give prophylactic antibiotics when puncturing synthetic grafts, e.g. cefuroxime 750 mg IV.

## Equipment

- Basic angiography set.

**Fig. 14.3** ■ Following thrombolysis, lateral views with the knee straight (A) and flexed (B) reveal kinking as the underlying problem.

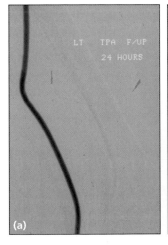
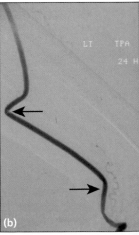

# Procedure

*Access* Use Table 14.3 as a guideline.

*Catheterization* The majority of at-risk grafts will be infra-inguinal, and antegrade puncture is usually required. Most grafts come off the CFA anteriorly. Steep ipsilateral anterior oblique views are useful to profile their origins and to guide selective catheterization (Fig. 14.4).

**Table 14.3** Access sites for graft angiography

| Graft configuration | Angiography approach | Intervention approach | Tips |
|---|---|---|---|
| Axillofemoral | Radial or brachial* | Brachial for proximal lesions<br>Graft or CFA for distal problems | |
| Aortofemoral | CFA or brachial* | CFA or brachial | |
| Iliofemoral crossover | Donor side CFA | Either CFA or graft | Angulation at origin, use Amplatz wire, long sheath or guide-catheter |
| Femorofemoral crossover | Donor CFA | Either CFA or graft | Use ultrasound to avoid direct graft puncture at groin |
| Femoropopliteal/ distal | Antegrade CFA | Antegrade CFA for distal problem, retrograde for inflow | Cobra or RDC useful to access graft origin |

*Consider MRA whenever there are no femoral pulses and it would be necessary to use the arm approach.*

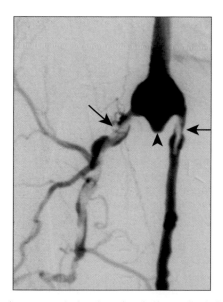

**Fig. 14.4** ■ Oblique view showing non-occlusive thrombus in the profunda femoris artery (black arrows) and origin of the femoropopliteal vein graft. The stump of the native SFA (arrowhead) lies in between.

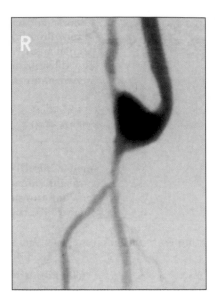

**Fig. 14.5** ■ Profile view of the distal cuff of a below-knee femoropopliteal vein graft. The popliteal artery is diffusely narrowed below the graft.

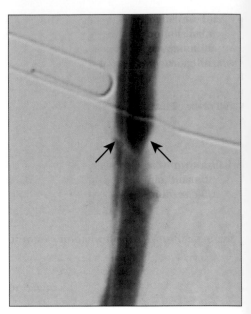

**Fig. 14.6** ■ A valve cusp (arrows) that was causing significant stenosis in a vein graft.

*Runs* A satisfactory angiogram must show the graft inflow and run-off and include views of the proximal and distal anastomoses in profile (Fig. 14.5). Magnified oblique views should be used to demonstrate stenoses. When imaging vein grafts, demonstration of contrast jetting as a result of valve cusps requires runs at 6 FPS. These should be viewed with a wide contrast window (Fig. 14.6).

**Tip:** The Doppler is right! If the lesion cannot be identified at angiography, it should be marked under ultrasound guidance.

## Troubleshooting

**Difficulty inserting the sheath** Heavy scarring at the puncture site is a predictable problem. Remember the basics of vascular access and insert plenty of wire. Keep the guidewire taut and push and twist the catheter from close to the skin. Try a 4Fr dilator. A judiciously inserted Amplatz wire is often helpful.

**Difficulty catheterizing the graft origin** Remember to use a steep oblique projection; roadmap or fluoroscopy fade are invaluable for guidance. A shaped catheter, usually a Cobra or RDC, can be directed towards the graft origin.

**Difficulty visualizing the graft origin** Contrast in the CFA patch, the stump of the SFA or in the PFA may obscure the graft origin. Position the catheter with its tip in the proximal graft; contrast can then be refluxed to show the graft origin. A frame rate of ≥2 FPS is necessary. Laterally running grafts are best shown with the ipsilateral posterior oblique view.

# Upper limb arterial diagnosis

Upper limb ischaemia represents only 4% of peripheral vascular disease and is not as frequently associated with generalized atherosclerosis as lower limb ischaemia. Disease is usually focal affecting the origins of the great vessels. In thoracic outlet syndrome (TOS), vascular compression by bone or ligament is associated with distal embolization, Raynaud's syndrome and subclavian aneurysm. Imaging depends on the clinical scenario (Table 14.4).

 **Alarm:** Arch aortography and selective catheterization of the great vessels carry a risk of stroke, so particular care must be taken during catheter and wire manipulation and catheter flushing. **Never flush a blocked catheter in the aortic arch**.

## Equipment

- Basic angiography set.
- Catheters: 90-cm 4Fr pigtail, Berenstein, Headhunter, Sidewinder.
- Guidewires: angled hydrophilic guidewire.
- GTN or other vasodilator.

## Procedure

*Access* Diagnostic angiography is usually performed from the femoral approach. Therapeutic intervention is often easier from the brachial artery or with combined femoral and brachial access.

*Catheterization* Use a pigtail catheter for arch aortography. A Berenstein catheter will engage the vast majority of arch vessels if used properly. Use a guidewire to advance the catheter tip beyond the target vessel. Withdraw the guidewire and rotate the catheter until the tip points cranially; the catheter tip will flick into the vessel origin as it is withdrawn. More distal catheterization requires the catheter to be advanced over a guidewire.

**Table 14.4** Upper limb arterial imaging depends on the clinical scenario

| Scenario | Modality |
| --- | --- |
| Elective | |
| Chronic upper limb ischaemia | Measure blood pressure in both arms; MRA* > CTA > ultrasound**; DSA for intervention and for detail of small vessels |
| Thoracic outlet syndrome | Ultrasound with postural manoeuvres as initial screen. MRA using blood pool agent and postural manoeuvres subsequently |
| Acute | |
| Acute limb ischaemia | MRA, DSA depending on availability and expertise |
| Trauma/dissection | CTA for vascular and non-vascular injury, DSA for intervention |

*Dedicated MRA is needed for the hand vessels.
**Ultrasound does not demonstrate origins of the great vessels.

*Runs* Begin with an arch aortogram to show the origins of the great vessels. Additional views may be needed to show the proximal subclavian arteries, particularly when they are tortuous. In suspected thoracic outlet syndrome (TOS), perform runs with the arms raised and also in the Roos position (elbow flexed 90°, shoulder abducted 90° and dorsiflexed). It is possible to see as far as the elbow from an arch injection; a selective catheter should be advanced peripherally to image the distal arm vessels. Use iso-osmolar contrast when imaging the digital arteries. The radial and ulnar arteries may arise from the axillary or brachial arteries; failure to recognize this will lead to misinterpretation.

 **Tip:** To obtain high-quality images of the digital arteries, invert the C-arm and place the hand on the image intensifier, immobilizing it with a sandbag. Use a vasodilator to increase flow (Fig. 14.7).

## Interpretation

Vascular compression during postural manoeuvres occurs in about 30% of normal subjects; subclavian artery irregularity or aneurysm is a more valuable sign of TOS (Fig. 14.8). Diffuse atheroma affecting the subclavian and axillary arteries is most commonly caused by radiotherapy. A proximal high-grade stenosis or occlusion may cause a subclavian steal; this is usually asymptomatic. You should expect reversed flow in the vertebral artery from the duplex; if not, it will only be seen on late images from the arch aortogram.

## Troubleshooting

### Unable to catheterize an arch vessel

- Remember the basic rules; identify the target vessel on an overview.
- If the arch is unfolded, the Berenstein catheter may be difficult to control; try using a Headhunter 1 catheter which has a wider primary curve.
- If the target vessel is angulated backwards, then a reverse curve catheter such as a Sidewinder may be helpful.

**Fig. 14.7** ■ 'Blue digit syndrome', hand arteriogram following intra-arterial GTN. There are multiple digital artery occlusions (arrows) secondary to microemboli from a subclavian stenosis. The middle finger is particularly ischaemic.

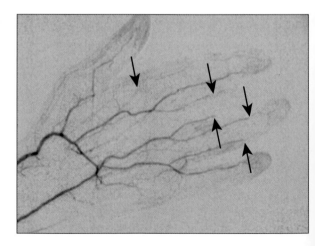

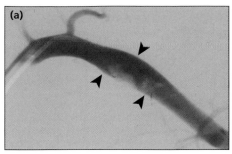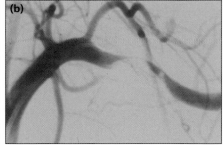

**Fig. 14.8** ■ Thoracic outlet stenosis presenting with distal embolization. (A) There is a subclavian aneurysm containing thrombus (arrowheads). (B) Arm abduction results in marked compression of the subclavian artery.

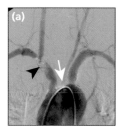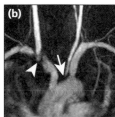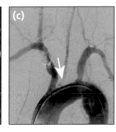

**Fig. 14.9** ■ (A, B) AP projections from arch aortogram and MRA showing calcified plaque causing innominate (arrowhead) and left CCA (arrows) stenosis. (C) LAO 30° projection gives a better view of the final line arch morphology and the left CFA (arrow) but obscures the innominate.

## Poor visualization of the distal vessels

- Use a vasodilator to increase flow and also to discriminate spasm from irreversible fibrosis.
- Use iso-osmolar contrast and try increased contrast strength.

# Aortic arch arterial diagnosis

Arch aortography is seldom performed for diagnosis and has been almost completely replaced by CTA and MRA when looking for patients with aortic syndromes, penetrating ulcer, dissection, intramural haematoma and traumatic injury. Paradoxically, arch angiography has become more frequent in the context of thoracic aortic stent grafting and carotid artery intervention (Fig. 14.9). Don't be tempted to perform arch aortography unless you have a C-arm which will allow sufficient angulation.

Consider MRA or CTA for studies of the aortic arch and proximal great vessels. Cardiac-gated acquisitions can improve image quality further.

## Equipment

- Basic angiography set.
- Catheter: 90-cm 4Fr or 5Fr pigtail.

## Procedure

*Catheterization* Position the pigtail catheter in the ascending aorta just above the aortic valve.

*Runs* A 30° LAO to show aortic arch and origin of the great vessels (centre on the aortic arch); a 60° LAO may be helpful in trauma cases. See Table 14.5.

## Interpretation

Look for irregularity in the lumen in the region of the ligamentum arteriosum as this is the usual site of injury (Fig. 14.10). If there is evidence of dissection, demonstrate the origin of the dissection flap and the site of re-entry into the aortic lumen, and document visceral artery involvement.

## Troubleshooting

The ductus bump can mimic aortic rupture. It appears as a smooth bulge at the site of the ligamentum arteriosum.

**Table 14.5** Suggested runs for arch aortography

| View | Contrast volume (mL) | Injection rate (mL/s) | Frame rate (FPS) | Field size (cm) |
|------|----------------------|------------------------|-------------------|-----------------|
| LAO 30°, LAO 60° AP | 40 | 18–25 | 2–4 | 28–40 |

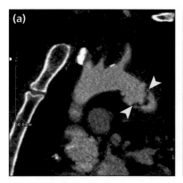
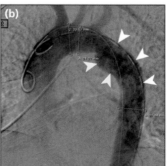
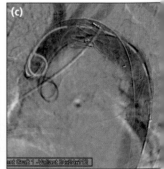

**Fig. 14.10** ■ Aortic trauma: the chest X-ray showed mediastinal widening. (A) CT reformat showing intimal/medial tear (yellow arrow) and adjacent haematoma. (B) Arch angiography with calibrated catheter (white arrows) shows false aneurysm (yellow arrows) distal to the left subclavian artery. (C) Following stent-graft repair.

# Renal arterial diagnosis

Renal arterial imaging is needed in three groups of patients:

- Those with renal vascular pathology
- Those with renal transplants
- Potential live renal donors.

Diagnostic renal angiography is being replaced by magnetic resonance and CT angiography. DSA remains the 'gold standard' and is still required in case of doubt or to demonstrate distal disease such as fibromuscular dysplasia (FMD) (Fig. 14.11).

Renal arterial imaging is most frequently requested to investigate renal artery stenosis (RAS) even though the benefits of renal revascularization are uncertain. The remainder of referrals are for trauma, tumour, pretransplantation assessment or, rarely, arteritis (Table 14.6).

 **Tip:** Remember 15% of people will have accessory renal arteries; they are often multiple and may arise almost anywhere in the abdominal aorta or iliac arteries.

**Table 14.6** Renal arterial imaging depends on the clinical scenario

| Scenario | Modality |
| --- | --- |
| **Elective** | |
| Renal artery stenosis | MRA*, DSA for intervention and for detail of small vessels |
| Live renal donor assessment | MRA, including venous and ureteric phases. DSA if *any* doubt |
| Renal tumour embolization | Check the contralateral kidney and plan approach on CT/MRA |
| Renal artery aneurysm | CTA or MRA for roadmap and assessment |
| **Acute** | |
| Trauma/bleeding | CTA for vascular and non-vascular injury, DSA for intervention |

*MRA is unable to exclude subtle lesions of FMD.*

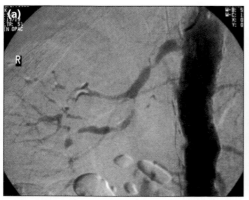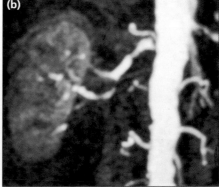

**Fig. 14.11** ■ Multifocal renal artery stenosis: (A) DSA; (B) MRA. Note that the MRA does not demonstrate the calcification in the aorta and renal arteries.

# Equipment

- Basic angiography set.
- Flush aortogram: 4Fr pigtail catheter.
- Selective angiography: Cobra II, RDC, Sidewinder II.

# Procedure

*Access* The right CFA is usual for diagnostic angiography; the contralateral CFA often provides better access for selective angiography and intervention as the catheters tend to deflect towards the contralateral side of the aorta.

*Catheterization* Start with a flush arteriogram! This is good, safe practice; an aortic injection will answer most questions. Position the catheter at L1.

 **Tip:** Use the cross-sectional imaging to predict the optimal approach and also the angiographic projection.

*Runs* See Table 14.7.

Selective catheterization should be avoided when there is RAS as it increases the risk of thrombosis and embolization. Use selective renal angiography to resolve detailed intrarenal anatomy or in rare instances when the renal artery origin cannot be seen in profile.

*Flush aortogram* Aim to show the origins of the renal arteries in profile (Fig. 14.12). The renal arteries arise at L1/2. On a clock face, the right renal artery typically arises from the aorta at 10 o'clock and the left renal artery at 3 o'clock. In theory, an LAO 15° projection

**Table 14.7** Typical parameters for renal angiography

| Run | Field size (cm) | Catheter position | Contrast volume (mL) | Injection rate (mL/s) | Frame rate (FPS) |
|-----|-----------------|-------------------|----------------------|------------------------|-------------------|
| AP aortogram | 40 | L1 adjust | 15–20 | 15–20 | 2 |
| 20° oblique | 28 | As needed | 15–20 | 15–20 | 2 |
| Selective | 28–20 | Proximal renal | 10 | 5 | 2 |

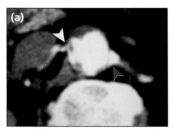 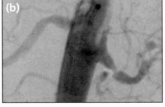 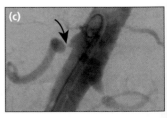

**Fig. 14.12** ■ (A) Axial CT in a patient with bilateral renal artery stenosis showing typical position of the origins of the renal arteries, right (yellow arrowhead), left (red arrowhead). (B) The right renal artery appears normal on first run (RAO) but the origin is not seen. (C) The LAO view reveals a high-grade stenosis of the right renal artery (arrow). It is essential to obtain views of both renal artery ostia in profile. The same applies to MRA images.

should suffice. Unfortunately, this does not hold true in the diseased or aneurysmal aorta. In practice, other projections are frequently necessary. In these cases, rotational angiography is helpful if it is available.

*Selective angiography* A Cobra II or RDC catheter will usually select the renal artery, and should be the first-choice catheters. Occasionally, a Sidewinder or arm approach will be necessary to deal with an acutely angled artery. Hand injection of 10 mL of contrast is usually satisfactory.

## Troubleshooting

**Only one kidney seen, time to check how many were on the non-invasive imaging?**
Only 1 – relax; however, if there were 2:

- Ensure the catheter is high enough.
- Fluoroscope to check for an ectopic kidney.
- Check late-phase angiogram for renal perfusion via collaterals.

**Contrast in the superior mesenteric artery (SMA) obscures the right renal artery** If the catheter is too high, contrast fills the SMA. For subsequent runs, pull back the catheter and try alternative oblique tube positions.

**Unable to profile the renal artery ostia** If all else fails, catheterize selectively.

**Angiography for potential live renal donors** This is the same as for native kidneys but the objective is to select the appropriate kidney for donation. The left kidney is usually chosen as it has the longer renal vein. The transplant surgeon needs to know:

- The number and position of renal arteries
- The presence of any disease in the renal vessels
- The number and position of the renal veins
- The ureteric anatomy.

# Renal transplant angiography

In **established transplants**, chronic deterioration in function or hypertension may indicate RAS. In a **recent transplant**, angiography usually follows an abnormal MRA or duplex. Acute graft failure occurs secondary to rejection, thrombosis of the artery or vein, or less commonly, a poorly fashioned anastomosis.

## Equipment

- Basic angiography set.
- Catheters: 4Fr straight, RDC for selective angiography.
- Wires: 3-mm J, Terumo.

## Procedure

*Access* Ipsilateral CFA for diagnosis; the contralateral CFA is often better for intervention.

*Catheterization* Contrast in the internal iliac artery or the contralateral iliac artery often obscures the transplant renal artery. To minimize this, use a hand injection run to establish the position of the catheter just proximal to the transplant artery.

*Runs* A hand injection is mandatory for selective catheterization. See Table 14.8.

## Interpretation

In **adults**, cadaveric transplants are often taken with an aortic patch (Carel patch, Fig. 14.13) and anastomosed to the side of the EIA. Live related donor transplants may be anastomosed to the internal iliac artery. In **children**, because of the small calibre of the iliac vessels, the graft is often anastomosed to the lower aorta. RAS occurs at the anastomosis, and focal smooth stenoses distal to this are often clamp injuries. In transplant rejection, there is pruning of the intrarenal vessels. If there is early venous filling, look hard for a post biopsy arteriovenous fistula.

 **Tip:** Look at the operative note to see the site of anastomosis and the number of renal arteries.

## Troubleshooting

- The transplant artery is tortuous or overlapped by other vessels.
- Craniocaudal tilt and rotational angiography may be necessary.
- If satisfactory views cannot be obtained, try selective catheterization. Contrast can be refluxed to show the anastomosis.
- Try a higher frame rate.

**Table 14.8** Suggested runs for renal transplant angiography

| Position | View | Contrast volume (mL) | Inject rate (mL/s) | Field size (cm) | Centring |
|---|---|---|---|---|---|
| Above renal artery | AP, multiple obliques | 10–15 | 5 | 28–20 | Over renal artery and kidney |

**Fig. 14.13** ■ (A) MRA and (B) $CO_2$ angiogram of a cadaveric renal transplant showing typical appearance of the Carel patch (long arrows) and stenosis (arrowheads) distal to this.

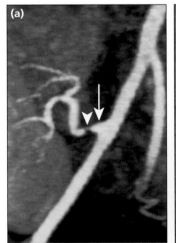
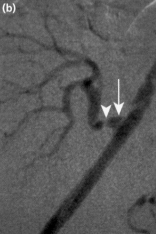

# Hepatic arterial diagnosis

Diagnostic hepatic angiography has been superseded by CT, MRI and ultrasound. Angiography is requested only when intervention is an option (Table 14.9).

## Equipment

- Basic angiography set.
- Catheters: Cobra II, Sidewinder II (hydrophilic Cobra catheter, microcatheter).
- Guidewires: 3-mm J, angled Terumo.

## Procedure

*Access* Usually the right CFA, but sometimes the arm approach will be necessary due to the angulation of the coeliac axis.

*Catheterization* The coeliac axis arises anteriorly from the aorta at T12/L1. A Cobra catheter will be successful in most cases; if it will not engage the ostium or remain stable, a Sidewinder is the next choice. Perform a diagnostic angiogram to ensure the arterial anatomy is conventional. Anatomical variants of the hepatic arterial supply are common (Fig. 14.14). Transplant vascular anatomy may be surprising; the transplant hepatic artery may be anastomosed to the recipient hepatic artery or via a conduit to the aorta or iliac artery. Check the operative note before starting! Selective catheterization of the common hepatic artery and its branches may be required, particularly when assessing tumours or embolizing.

 **Tip:** Catheters often pass preferentially into the splenic artery, which comes more anteriorly off the coeliac axis. A Terumo wire can usually be negotiated into the hepatic artery and the catheter will follow it. If this fails, the Sidewinder tip can be shaped with a bend to the right.

*Runs* Runs should be centred to include all of the liver, including the right hemidiaphragm and chest wall. Less contrast is required for distal selective angiograms. Magnified oblique views of the liver hilum are often required. See Table 14.10.

Most secondary liver tumours are hypovascular and angiographic signs are subtle. Mass effect displaces vessels; constant vessel irregularity or occlusion suggests arterial invasion. Vascular tumours (e.g. hepatoma and carcinoid) show neovascularity and an abnormal

**Table 14.9** Hepatic arterial imaging depends on the clinical scenario

| Scenario | Modality |
| --- | --- |
| **Elective** | |
| Liver tumour embolization | MR/MRA; Check the portal vein is patent, DSA for intervention |
| Liver transplant artery stenosis | Ultrasound diagnosis, DSA for intervention |
| **Acute** | |
| Trauma | CTA for vascular and non-vascular injury, DSA for intervention |
| Haemobilia | CTA unless secondary to percutaneous transhepatic procedure |

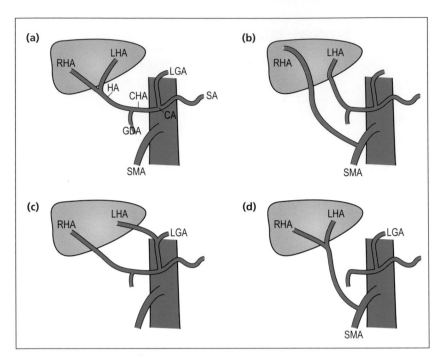

**Fig. 14.14** ■ Common variants of hepatic arterial supply. (A) Conventional anatomy – 55%. (B) Replaced right hepatic artery (RHA) arises from the superior mesenteric artery (SMA) – 16%. (C) Replaced left hepatic artery (LHA) arises from the left gastric artery (LGA) – ~20%. (D) Replaced common hepatic artery (CHA) arising from the SMA – ~2%. CA, coeliac artery; GDA, gastroduodenal artery; HA, hepatic artery; SA, splenic artery.

**Table 14.10** Typical parameters for hepatic angiography

| Catheter position | Contrast volume (mL) | Injection rate (mL/s) | Frame rate (FPS) | Field size (cm) | Projection | Run length (s) |
|---|---|---|---|---|---|---|
| Coeliac axis | 32 | 8 | 2–1 | 40 | AP | To portal vein ≈20 |
| Selective Hepatic artery | 5–15 | Hand | 2 | 20–28 | AP and RAO 20° | ≈5 |
| Splenic artery | 20 | 5 | 2–1 | 40 | AP | To portal vein |

parenchymal stain (Fig. 14.15). Arterial injury following percutaneous transhepatic cholangiography (PTC) usually manifests as a small pseudoaneurysm, which can almost always be selectively embolized.

**Tip:** The hepatic artery is prone to spasm when catheterized. Have a low threshold for prophylactic antispasmodic agents. Take care not to misdiagnose spasm as encasement.

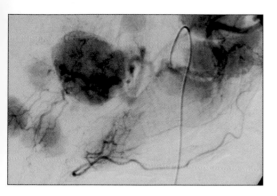

**Fig. 14.15** ■ Carcinoid syndrome. Late arterial phase image from a coeliac axis injection showing multiple hypervascular liver metastases.

# Troubleshooting

## Unable to pass a guidewire into the hepatic artery

- Check that the catheter tip is not in the splenic artery by gently injecting contrast and avoiding reflux.
- If the Cobra catheter is pushed out by the wire, try a reverse curve catheter.

## Unable to selectively catheterize the hepatic artery

- Put plenty of guidewire into a peripheral hepatic branch or the gastroduodenal artery.
- Keep the wire under tension while gently rocking the catheter from side to side; only apply gentle forward pressure, and let the catheter find its own way in.
- Try a softer catheter, e.g. a hydrophilic Cobra.
- Try from the radial or brachial artery; the caudal angulation of the mesenteric vessels lends itself to this approach.
- If all else fails, dust off a 7Fr Sidewinder III – the superior torque control often helps.

**Spasm in the hepatic artery**
- This is very common and minimized by administering prophylactic GTN and using microcatheters.

# Mesenteric arterial diagnosis

Three categories of condition will require your input:

- Mesenteric ischaemia
- Mesenteric aneurysm
- Gastrointestinal bleeding.

There is a move to non-invasive imaging, not least because the production of satisfactory mesenteric angiograms is challenging, particularly in patients with acute gastrointestinal bleeding (Table 14.1).

## Mesenteric ischaemia

Once again, MRA and CTA are the first choice investigations and will demonstrate the site and extent of disease and allow planning of surgical and radiological intervention. At least two of the visceral arteries will be diseased, and the SMA and coeliac axis are both almost always involved. Visceral angiography is virtually confined to treatment and pressure measurements in cases of uncertainty.

## Equipment

- Basic angiography set.
- 4Fr pigtail catheter.

## Procedure

*Catheterization* Begin with a pigtail catheter above the coeliac axis (T11/12).

*Runs* Start with a lateral flush aortogram. The visceral arteries arise anteriorly from the aorta. Contrast layers posteriorly in the aorta, so it is sometimes necessary to use a larger, faster contrast bolus (20–30 mL at 15–20 mL/s). Centre on L2/3 just anterior to the spine and use filters to eliminate flare caused by bowel gas. An additional AP flush aortogram is often all that is required to demonstrate the integrity of the distal SMA.

 **Tip:** Mesenteric vascular stenosis should be suspected when a large marginal artery of Drummond is seen during peripheral angiography (Fig. 14.16). Similarly, large pancreaticoduodenal arteries suggest stenosis of the coeliac axis or SMA (Fig. 14.17).

## Troubleshooting

**A vessel is seen on the AP arteriogram but cannot be identified on the lateral aortogram**
- This is usually due to proximal occlusion with reconstitution via collaterals. The coeliac axis and SMA often communicate via a hypertrophied pancreaticoduodenal arcade.

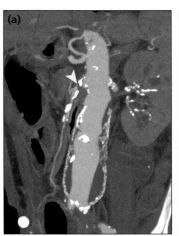
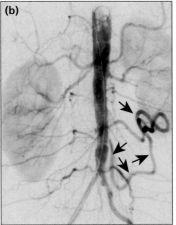
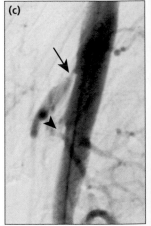

**Fig. 14.16** ■ Images from patients with 'intestinal angina'. (A) Reformat from CTA showing high grade stenosis (yellow arrowhead) of the superior mesenteric artery (SMA), which is heavily calcified. (B) AP DSA in a different patient shows hypertrophy of the inferior mesenteric artery (IMA) (arrows). Branches of the SMA are filling via the IMA. Lateral flush aortogram (C) showing high-grade stenosis of the coeliac axis (arrow) and occlusion of the SMA (arrowhead).

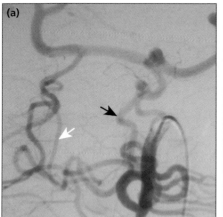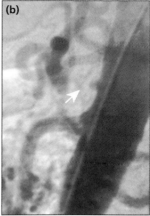

**Fig. 14.17** ■ (A) SMA injection showing filling of the coeliac axis via hypertrophied pancreaticoduodenal (white arrow) and pancreatic collaterals (black arrow). (B) Lateral flush aortogram showing occlusion of the coeliac axis (white arrow).

**A smooth impression is seen on the superior aspect of the coeliac axis**
- This is the result of extrinsic compression by the median arcuate ligament of the diaphragm. The diagnosis is confirmed by showing a normal appearance on a lateral flush aortogram with the patient in the right lateral decubitus position. This finding is seen in 20% of asymptomatic patients. A few patients have severe compression of both coeliac axis and SMA and are candidates for surgery.

 **Tip:** Selective catheterization is only required when distal disease is suspected on the flush angiogram.

## Mesenteric aneurysm

These are uncommon and often diagnosed incidentally on CT performed for other indications. Less is known about them than renal artery aneurysm. As described above, high-flow aneurysms can be associated with stenosis of the coeliac axis or SMA. When identified, it is usual to perform a CTA to delineate the anatomy. DSA is usually only necessary during intervention (embolization or stent grafting).

## Chronic gastrointestinal bleeding

Improvements in diagnostic and therapeutic colonoscopy and new developments such as capsule endoscopy have reduced the need for mesenteric angiography in recent years. Just as well, as angiography in patients who were not actively bleeding was frequently negative.

  If persuaded to undertake angiography in this group, the patient's history may give important clues to the source of the bleeding. There are two forms of long-term blood loss:
- **Repeated episodes of brisk bleeding** are often associated with a structural lesion such as angiodysplasia. Herald symptoms, typically abdominal pain, are usually associated with heavy bleeding, e.g. from a pseudoaneurysm. These cases should be treated as repeated episodes of acute bleeding and angiography performed during active bleeding.

- **Chronic insidious blood loss** In these patients, a cause is unlikely to be found by angiography. The patient will already have had multiple negative investigations, so do not expect to solve the problem in 5 minutes. Do not perform angiography unless you know the results of all the previous investigations.

Angiography should be performed as an elective procedure by the most experienced gastrointestinal angiographer available. Catheterization of all three main visceral arteries and multiple selective views will be necessary. Even with excellent technique, the study is likely to be negative!

# Acute lower gastrointestinal bleeding (LGIB)

It is essential to recognize that the role of angiography has moved from one of diagnosis to one of treatment; this is not recognized by all clinicians. One of the most important facts to know is that LGIB is almost always intermittent and the clinical picture of active bleeding is one of **hypotension and tachycardia**. This allows calculation of the shock index.

 **Tip:**

$$\text{Shock index} = \frac{\text{Heart rate (beats per minute)}}{\text{Systolic BP mmHg}}$$

Investigating patients with a shock index <1 has a very low positive yield. If the shock index has normalized by the time the patient reaches you, then don't do the angiogram; it will be negative and you will probably be called again when there is re-bleeding.

 **Alarm:** The shock index will sometimes normalize during vigorous resuscitation. In this 'metastable' condition, fluid replacement is keeping up with the bleeding and the patient still requires urgent investigation.

Patients with a shock index >1 are typically elderly, agitated and by definition haemodynamically unstable. Don't be fobbed off with delaying tactics such as: the patient 'is too sick to move', 'needs a central line', etc. Delays lead to missing the bleeding. Start resuscitation and go directly to DSA or CT (Table 14.11). If the patient is too unwell for investigation, they require immediate laparotomy and bowel resection with the associated morbidity and mortality.

The passage of fresh or altered blood often continues in between bleeds. This has important connotations for imaging and intervention, which are geared towards detecting, localizing and stopping bleeding. The sign of bleeding is contrast extravasation into the bowel lumen. Imaging the patient between bleeds is usually a fruitless task as there are no signs of the underlying cause. The exception to this is post-operative bleeding, which is often associated with structural abnormalities such as false aneurysm. It is important to work to an agreed algorithm (Box 14.1).

 **Alarm:** In patients with diffuse bleeding, embolization can be positively harmful, especially in the colon. Sometimes embolization can allow the patient to be stabilized before bowel resection but embolization of a significant amount of intestine will lead to infarction, perforation and death if untreated.

Most centres will choose CT as the primary investigation (providing they have at least a four-slice machine); it's more contrast sensitive and at least as sensitive as an angiography for

**Box 14.1 Algorithm for managing lower gastrointestinal bleeding**

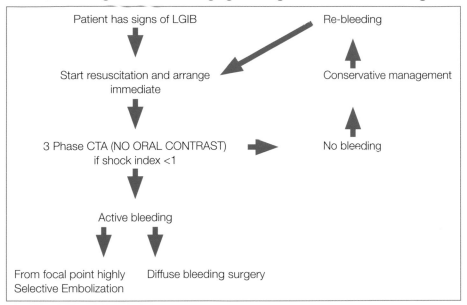

**Table 14.11** Mesenteric arterial imaging depends on the clinical scenario

| Scenario | Modality |
| --- | --- |
| **Elective** | |
| Chronic mesenteric ischaemia | US as rapid screen for proximal disease; MRA, CTA |
| Mesenteric aneurysm | Usually incidental finding on CT, further assessment with dedicated CTA, DSA for intervention |
| Chronic gastrointestinal bleeding | Angiography almost completely replaced by non-invasive studies, conventional and capsule endoscopy |
| **Acute** | |
| Upper gastrointestinal bleeding | Endoscopy is first choice for diagnosis and therapy. CT if negative endoscopy or if post-operative. DSA if endoscopy positive and embolization needed |
| Lower gastrointestinal bleeding* | Bleeding rectal varices should be excluded first. Apart from this, endoscopy is rarely helpful due to lumen full of blood. Three-phase CTA will demonstrate active bleeding and site and allows targeted angiography |
| Acute mesenteric ischaemia | CTA – don't forget to look at the intestine as well as the vessels as there is no point in revascularizing a 'black pudding' |

*More philosophical musings on lower gastrointestinal bleeding later!*

active bleeding. The biggest advantage, however, is that almost everywhere it's also quicker to get a CT, so we catch the site of intermittent bleeding more readily. In addition, if it is negative, there is now sufficient evidence to support conservative management only, for this patient group. We can't go into the detail of the best CT technique here but there are some good links in the bibliography.

**Table 14.12** Likely sources of gastrointestinal bleeding

| Blood loss | Likely source | Target vessel |
| --- | --- | --- |
| Red blood PR* | Left colon | IMA (Fig. 14.18) |
| | Right colon | SMA (Fig. 14.19) |
| Altered blood PR | Small intestine | SMA/Coeliac axis |
| Haematemesis/malaena** | Oesophagus, stomach or duodenum | Coeliac axis (Fig. 14.20) |
| | | SMA (pancreaticoduodenal arcade) |

*PR per rectum.*
**The patient should have oesophagogastroduodenoscopy first.*

Regardless of the exquisite anatomical detail of multi-slice CT, you will have to be able to catheterize mesenteric arteries and demonstrate the point of extravasation to target embolization.

Like any emergency investigation, studies for LGIB may be performed out of hours with relatively inexperienced staff. Using a systematic approach to acquire and interpret the images will greatly increase the chances of success.

## Before starting

* Ensure that the patient is being adequately resuscitated, has large-calibre IV access and appropriate blood product and electrolyte replacement available. Someone from the clinical team should be available to manage the patient's haemodynamic status as you will be concentrating too hard on the angiogram to do this.
* If you don't have the luxury of endoscopic or CT localization, target the angiogram to the suspected source of bleeding (see Table 14.12).
* Check the plan of action for the patient. What will happen if the angiogram is positive or negative? Will embolization or laparotomy be appropriate? Has the patient given appropriate consent?

## Equipment

Personal preference is important here:

* 5Fr sheath.
* Catheters:
  * 4Fr pigtail catheter for flush aortography
  * Cobra II, RDC, Sidewinder, Sos Omni for selective catheterization.
* Hydrophilic guidewire.

A hydrophilic catheter or microcatheter may be useful for distal catheterization.

## Procedure

*Access* Right CFA is easiest.

*Catheterization* If the patient has had a CT showing bleeding, head straight to the vessel of interest. If not, perform an overview of each target arterial territory before proceeding to more selective angiography. It used to be advised to start with the IMA to avoid bladder contrast obscuring detail of the sigmoid arteries. In practice, DSA will usually subtract the bladder out

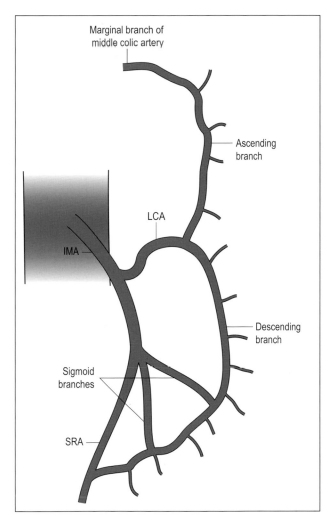

**Fig. 14.18** ■ The inferior mesenteric artery (IMA). LCA, left colic artery; SRA, superior rectal artery.

and a sufficiently unwell patient should have a bladder catheter in situ already. Starting with the SMA will be a winner in many more cases.

Selective catheterization of the mesenteric vessels can be frustrating for even the most experienced angiographer. Start with the right tool:

- The **IMA** arises acutely from the anterolateral aspect of the distal aorta (Fig. 14.18). Perform a steep RAO angiogram of the distal aorta to show its origin; there is often a 'sentinel plaque' adjacent to the origin. Catheterization is easiest with a short reverse curve catheter such as the Sos Omni or Sidewinder I.
- The **SMA** can usually be catheterized with a Cobra II. It can be advanced distally over a hydrophilic wire for superselective views of the ileocolic and right colic arteries, which are the most common sites of bleeding (Fig. 14.19).
- A Cobra II will often engage the **coeliac axis** (Fig. 14.20 ). If this fails, try a Sidewinder II catheter.

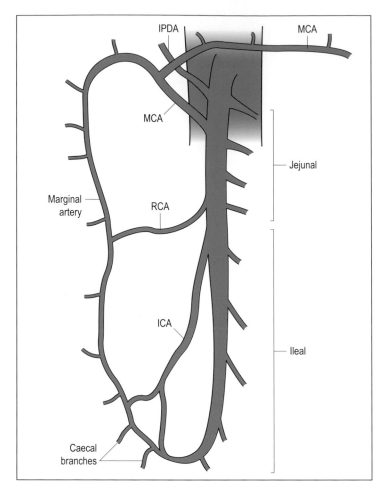

**Fig. 14.19** ■ The principal branches of the superior mesenteric artery: ICA, ileocolic artery; IPDA, inferior pancreaticoduodenal artery; MCA, middle colic artery; RCA, right colic artery. The origin of the ICA marks the transition between jejunal and ileal branches.

- The **gastroduodenal artery** is most easily catheterized with a forward-facing catheter such as the Cobra II or RDC.
- For a virtuoso finish, the **left gastric artery** (LGA) can be catheterized using a Sidewinder II. The catheter is initially advanced into the splenic artery and then slowly pulled back until the tip flicks up and engages the LGA. In reality, this vessel is seldom catheterized unless there is a very strong clinical suspicion of gastric bleeding (Fig. 14.21).

*Runs*  See Table 14.13.

- Paralyse the intestine. If you cannot abolish peristalsis with Buscopan or glucagon, there is little hope of success!
- Use breath-hold if the patient's condition permits. If not, wake the radiographer and try multimasking.

*What to look for*  Gastrointestinal bleeding – A few conditions are responsible for the majority of cases and it is essential to know what to look for.

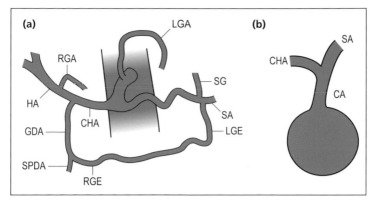

**Fig. 14.20** ▇ The coeliac artery (CA). (A) Principal arterial branches. (B) Cross-section showing why catheters and wires preferentially enter the splenic artery (SA). CHA, common hepatic artery; GDA, gastroduodenal artery; HA, hepatic artery; LGA, left gastric artery; LGE, left gastroepiploic artery; RGA, right gastric artery; RGE, right gastroepiploic artery; SG, short gastric artery; SPDA, superior pancreaticoduodenal artery.

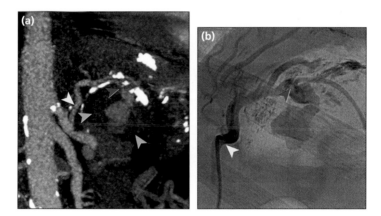

**Fig. 14.21** ▇ (A) CT reformat and (B) DSA showing haemorrhage into the stomach (red arrow head) from a pseudoaneurysm (turquoise arrowheads) of the left gastric artery (yellow arrowheads).

**Table 14.13** Suggested runs for mesenteric angiography

| Run | Field size (cm) | Centring | Contrast volume (mL) | Injection rate (mL/s) | Frame rate (FPS) |
|---|---|---|---|---|---|
| SMA AP | 40 | Mid-abdomen | 30 | 6 | 2–1 |
| IMA AP | 28 | Rectosigmoid | 10 | Hand | 2–1 |
| IMA RAO 25° | 28 | Rectosigmoid | 10 | Hand | 2–1 |
| IMA LAO 30° | 28 | Ascending colon and splenic flexure | 10 | Hand | 2–1 |
| Coeliac axis | 40 | Epigastrium | 30 | 6 | 2–1 |
| Gastro-duodenal artery | 28 | Epigastrium | 15 | Hand | 2 |
| LGA | 28 | Epigastrium | 8–10 | Hand | 2 |

- **Active bleeding**: contrast extravasating into the bowel lumen.
- **Spasm**: vessels which appear truncated.
- **Early venous filling**: a sign of angiodysplasia.
- **Abnormal vessels**: false aneurysm, chaotic tumour circulation, collaterals, encasement etc.

 **Tip:** $CO_2$ may demonstrate the site of extravasation from a flush aortogram and will sometimes display bleeding that is not readily shown with conventional contrast (Fig. 14.22).

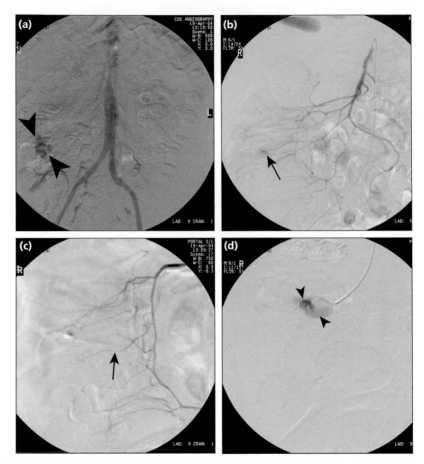

**Fig. 14.22** ■ Intermittent gastrointestinal bleeding. (A) Initial aortic run $CO_2$ angiogram showing extravasation in the caecum (arrowheads). (B) Selective SMA contrast angiogram: the extravasation is just visible (arrow). (C) Highly selective run from the right colic artery. The bleeding has stopped (arrow = target artery). (D) Extravasation (arrowheads) is seen again immediately prior to embolization.

## The usual suspects

*Angiodysplasia* Almost universally suspected in the elderly, but less frequently convincingly demonstrated. Angiodysplasia most often occurs in the caecum and ascending colon, though it can occur elsewhere, and is seen as a focal area of increased vascularity with dilated tiny arterioles with a prominent early draining vein (Fig. 14.23).

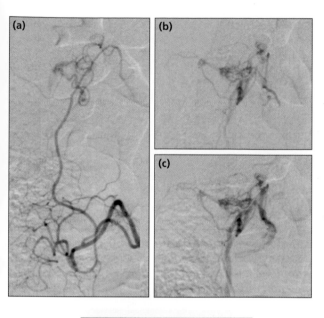

**Fig. 14.23** ■ Angiodysplasia in the ascending colon. (A) Early arterial phase shows a subtle blush. (B) Mid arterial phase. Note the dilated arterioles and venous staining. (C) Late arterial phase shows prominent draining veins.

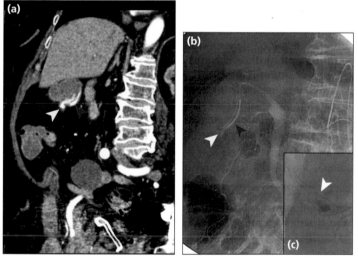

**Fig. 14.24** ■ Diverticular bleeding. (A) CT reformat (B) non-subtracted angiogram showing typical appearance of blood filling the diverticulum (yellow arrowhead) before 'spilling' into the colon (red arrowhead). (C) Highly selective angiogram immediately prior to embolization, showing the supplying vessel (white arrowhead).

*Diverticular disease* Bleeding is often venous and therefore difficult to demonstrate. Arterial bleeding characteristically fills the diverticulum before spilling into the colon (Fig. 14.24). Inflamed diverticula will give a patchy hyperaemic blush.

*Meckel's diverticulum* Bleeding rarely occurs in the absence of ectopic gastric mucosa, hence the diagnosis is usually made on technetium isotope scanning. The feeding vitelline artery characteristically extends beyond the mesenteric border, has no side branches and ends in a corkscrew appearance (Fig. 14.25).

**Fig. 14.25** ■ Meckel's diverticulum. (A) The superior mesenteric artery run shows a vessel (arrows) extending beyond the mesentery; not all of the vessel is seen. (B) The subsequent run shows the typical blush (arrows) of a large Meckel's diverticulum; the vessel is the vitelline artery.

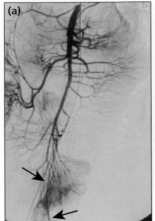
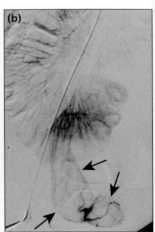

**Fig. 14.26** ■ Carcinoid tumour. There is a blush in the right iliac fossa (arrows). Invasion of the mesentery is demonstrated by occlusion of the ileocolic artery and distortion of the adjacent vessels (arrowheads).

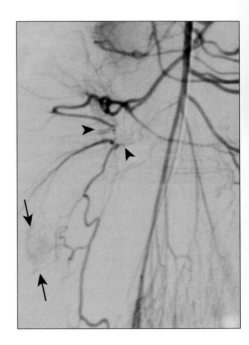

***Tumour*** A rare cause of acute gastrointestinal bleeding. Angiographic signs of bowel tumours are often subtle. Examine the venous phase carefully – veins are larger and thinner walled than arteries and therefore involved earlier. Look for vascular displacement, encasement (constant narrowing – be careful not to misdiagnose spasm) and truncation (Fig. 14.26).

## Interpretation

Examine the run frame by frame, looking carefully at the whole field. Take the time to remask each image. Review each phase of the angiogram, looking for the following abnormalities:

1. Arterial phase
   a. Active bleeding: extravasation appears as an irregularly shaped contrast stain that persists beyond the arterial phase of the angiogram (Fig. 14.27). Is the bleeding from a named vessel? This will localize the site of bleeding and aid the surgeon.
   b. Structural vascular abnormalities: look for false aneurysm, arterial encasement, displacement or occlusion.
   c. Early venous return: the appearance of a vein in the arterial phase is abnormal and may indicate angiodysplasia. The ileocolic vein often opacifies before other mesenteric veins in normal subjects.
2. Capillary phase
   a. An area of increased capillary stain may indicate angiodysplasia or inflammatory or neoplastic involvement; look for supporting evidence. Beware, in the normal intestine, the capillary phase may appear patchy, particularly in the large bowel.
   b. Remember, areas of overlapping bowel can simulate increased vascularity – be particularly careful in the sigmoid colon. If there is a genuine lesion, the abnormality will be seen on every view.
3. Venous phase
   a. Look carefully for evidence of venous invasion, occlusion or hypertrophied collateral veins, as these may be the first angiographic evidence of a tumour.
   b. Normal veins have a similar branching pattern to the arterial tree; tumour venous circulation is often chaotic and tortuous.

*If a bleeding site is identified*
- Inform the surgeon (ideally the surgeon is watching from the control room).
- Embolize the bleeding vessel if it can be catheterized highly selectively. Non-selective embolization is likely to result in bowel infarction in the colon and may not be effective in the small intestine due to collateral flow. Remember, the surgical alternative is likely to be quite extensive bowel resection, e.g. hemicolectomy.

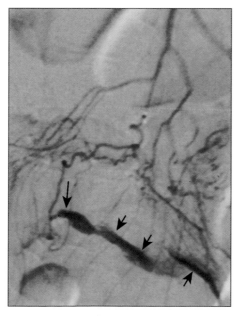

**Fig. 14.27** ▪ Bleeding from the inferior mesenteric artery; contrast is extravasating (arrows) into the sigmoid colon.

- If the site will be difficult for the surgeon to identify in theatre, consider marking the abnormal area with a guidewire or coils, or by leaving a microcatheter in situ for injection of methylene blue or saline.

## Troubleshooting

The commonest causes for failing to spot an identifiable lesion are due to poor imaging:

- Failure to get good subtracted images owing to peristalsis and respiratory artefact
- Missing out part of the intestine
- Failing to image through to the venous phase
- Lack of understanding of the relevant pathologies.

# Bronchial and pulmonary angiographic diagnosis

Pulmonary angiography is another victim of the success of non-invasive imaging and is very rarely required as a diagnostic modality. Once again, the therapeutic importance of pulmonary and bronchial embolization has come to the fore (Table 14.14).

## Bronchial artery angiography

Before setting forth, it is crucial to appreciate that the bronchial circulation is complex tiger country. A little knowledge will help you and the patient survive.

### Bronchial artery anatomy

Most bronchial arteries arise at the T5/6 level but variations are common, including multiple and conjointed bronchial arteries and common bronchointercostal arteries. Like the gut arteries, the bronchial arteries arise anteriorly. Combined bronchointercostal arteries arise posteriorly. Bronchial arteries also supply oesophagus, mediastinum and pulmonary arteries and have anastomoses with the anterior spinal artery. The latter is essential to recognize if

**Table 14.14** Bronchial and pulmonary imaging depends on the clinical scenario

| Scenario | Modality |
|---|---|
| **Elective** | |
| Recurrent haemoptysis | CT and bronchoscopy to evaluate lungs. Bronchial artery embolization (BAE) if underlying pathology. Pulmonary angiography if suspected tuberculosis Rasmussen aneurysm |
| Pulmonary arteriovenous malformation (PAVM) | CT for diagnosis. Pulmonary embolization for treatment |
| **Acute** | |
| Suspected pulmonary embolism | CTPA, DSA only for insertion of IVC filter and mechanical thrombectomy |
| Active haemoptysis | Bronchoscopy CTA for vascular and non-vascular injury, DSA for bronchial artery embolization |

embolizing! The bronchial arteries also anastomose with arteries that supply anything in contact with the pleura, including the subclavian arteries and their branches, internal mammary arteries, intercostal arteries, phrenic arteries and even coronary arteries. These variant anatomies are particularly relevant if embolization has been performed.

 **Tip:** The majority of bronchial arteries are found within the air lucency of the L main bronchus, i.e. where you can see the L main bronchus when screening.

## Equipment

- 5Fr sheath.
- 3-mm J guidewire.
- 5Fr 90–100 cm-long pigtail catheter.
- Terumo wire.
- A variety of selective catheters – multipurpose and reverse curve shapes can be effective but the variable anatomy of the bronchial arteries makes prediction of the correct tools something of a lottery!

## Procedure

*Access* The right femoral is normal but consider any approach that simplifies selective catheterization.

*Catheterization* No holds barred here, be prepared to try a variety of catheters until you find one that fits. Microcatheters are often necessary for embolization.

*Runs* Start with a flush aortogram (40 mL at 20 mL/s) with the catheter just beyond the left subclavian artery centred on T6. Then play it by ear.

*What to look for* Conventional bronchial arteries branch away from hilum and are not normally seen beyond the medial half of the lung. Abnormal bronchial arteries are hypertrophied and may reach further into the parenchyma (Fig. 14.28). Anterior spinal branches arise close to the midline and have a characteristic course, initially running cranially and medially, then bending suddenly downwards to pursue a midline vertical course.

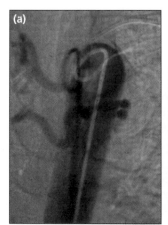
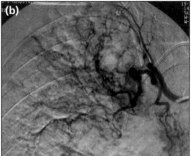

**Fig. 14.28** ■ Bronchial angiography. (A) Flush aortogram showing origins of a right bronchial artery and a combined trunk. (B) Selective catheterization of the right upper bronchial artery prior to embolization.

## Troubleshooting

**Unable to see bronchial arteries**
- Check you have included the aorta from the left subclavian onwards.
- Try another run in a magnified oblique projection.
- If this fails, then try 'systematically trawling' the aorta around T5/6, injecting contrast as you do. Start at 12 o'clock and work your way round the clockface, paying particular attention to the area of the air shadow of the left main bronchus. Feel for the catheter engaging and look for filling of the bronchial arteries.
- If still no success, then time to search for aberrant arterial supply from one of the vessels above.

**Unable to catheterize the bronchial arteries**
- Go back to basic principles and ensure that you have a catheter pointing in the correct direction.
- It might be that they are tiny – check the previous CT to try to identify them.
- Try a reverse curve catheter such a Sos Omni.

 **Alarm:** Be careful not to wedge the catheter; with your luck, it will be a vessel feeding the anterior spinal artery. If you think the catheter might be tight in the vessel then place the hub of the catheter in a bowl of saline before removing the guidewire. If the catheter is wedged in the vessel, saline rather than air is sucked in, preventing an air embolus.

# Pulmonary angiography

Seldom required for diagnosis in contemporary practice but lifesaving when combined with pulmonary thrombectomy in massive pulmonary embolism or occluding symptomatic PAVM.

## Equipment

- 5Fr sheath.
- 3-mm J guidewire.
- 5Fr 90–100 cm-long pigtail catheter.
- Terumo wire.
- ECG monitoring and pressure kit required.

## Procedure

Access can either be from the femoral vein or from the basilic or jugular vein. Most practitioners use femoral venous access.

 **Alarm:** It should go without saying: **do not puncture a grossly swollen leg**. Embolization of the underlying ileofemoral thrombus may cause embarrassment to both the patient and you. Stop and consider alternative access points such as other groin, jugular vein or basilic vein.

1. Obtain an IV cavogram. Use a hand injection of 20 mL non-ionic contrast via the side-arm of the sheath. Use Buscopan or glucagon to paralyse the gut. If there are filling defects within the IVC, consider an alternative access point from above.
2. Advance the 5Fr pigtail catheter over the J wire until the loop of the pigtail lies at the level of the suprarenal IVC.
3. Insert the Terumo wire into the pigtail catheter and advance (Fig. 14.29). The wire will progressively unfurl the pigtail until the wire points to about 1 o'clock, almost invariably

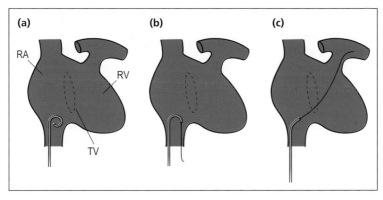

**Fig. 14.29** ■ Technique for pulmonary artery catheterization. (A) Pigtail and hydrophilic wire at the upper inferior vena cava. (B) Advance the guidewire which opens the pigtail loop. (C) The wire usually goes through the tricuspid valve into the pulmonary artery. RA, right atrium; RV, right ventricle; TV, tricuspid valve.

straight at the pulmonary trunk. Carefully advance the wire across the tricuspid valve – get your assistant to watch the ECG – and the wire almost always goes into the left main pulmonary artery. Advance the catheter until it is in the left main pulmonary artery.

4.  Measure the pulmonary artery pressures:
    a.  Systolic pulmonary artery pressure <50 mmHg, then angiography is safe.
    b.  Systolic pulmonary artery pressure >50 mmHg, then pull the catheter back into the right ventricle.
    c.  Measure the right ventricular pressures – if the right ventricular end diastolic pressure (RVEDP) is greater than 20 mmHg, non-selective pulmonary angiography is dangerous.
5.  If this is your first pulmonary angiogram, now is a good time to shout very loudly for help. If you remain determined, selective pulmonary angiography with hand injections of contrast into areas identified by the V/Q scan may be very useful.
6.  Give a test injection with 10 mL of contrast, and make sure the end of the pigtail catheter is not in a small pulmonary artery branch. Connect the catheter to a pump injector. Set the pump for 40 mL at 20 mL/s.
7   Assuming you are using DSA, ask for 6 FPS – the faster frame rate will help overcome misregistration secondary to cardiac motion. Start with an AP view.
8.  Look carefully through the first run. If you have definitely identified an embolus, then you have finished the examination and may proceed to item 12.
9.  Proceed to perform further runs in RAO 30° and LAO 30°.
10. Pulling the pigtail catheter back into the pulmonary trunk, then gently advancing, the Terumo guidewire enters the right pulmonary artery. The guidewire often loops into the right pulmonary artery; by gently manipulating the wire, a right lower lobe pulmonary artery can be entered with the wire. Make sure you advance the catheter well into the right main pulmonary artery at least as far as the hilum, as the catheter always tends to come back slightly when the wire is withdrawn.
11. Repeat the AP, LAO and RAO projections for the right lung.
12. Look through the standard projections. If there are any questionable areas, consider a repeat run, possibly magnified or in a different projection.
13. Before withdrawing the catheter, **straighten out the pigtail** with the Terumo wire. This prevents an unnecessary thoracotomy to retrieve a catheter firmly entangled in the chordae tendinae of the tricuspid valve.

## Troubleshooting

### Failure to catheterize the pulmonary artery

- Bad luck! Did you really use the rules in Chapter 9, Equipment for Angiography? Enlarged right ventricles can cause difficulty with the wire repeatedly entering the apex of the right ventricle.
- *Carefully use* a Headhunter or Berenstein catheter with a Terumo wire to manipulate into the pulmonary artery.

### Pulsatile injection with poor peripheral pulmonary artery filling despite 40 mL at 20 mL/s

- Check the psi rate on the pump – fast injections require higher psi. The catheter packaging will tell you the maximum rate for that catheter. Rarely, 50 mL at 25 mL/s is required.

### Breathless patient and poor DSA images

- Ask the radiographer to get more mask images at the beginning of the run. It may be better to do a run at 2 FPS with the patient breathing or consider selective angiography of relevant areas from the V/Q scan.

## Complications

- Pulmonary angiography is a relatively safe procedure. Overall mortality rate is 0.2%.
- Cardiopulmonary collapse is the main cause of death. It usually occurs in patients with severe pulmonary hypertension and right ventricular end diastolic pressure >20 mmHg or right ventricular strain diagnosed echocardiographically.
- Right ventricle perforation 1% – usually no sequelae.
- Symptomatic persistent arrhythmia.

# Carotid arterial diagnosis

Until recently, carotid and cerebral angiography were frequently performed diagnostic tests in the investigation of cerebrovascular disease. Advances in CT, MRI and ultrasound have now greatly reduced the indications for angiography. In most centres, carotid angiography is now the domain of neuroradiologists as part of cerebral angiography for the investigation and treatment of aneurysmal disease and vascular malformations (Table 14.15).

**Table 14.15** Carotid arterial imaging depends on the clinical scenario

| Scenario | Modality |
| --- | --- |
| **Elective** | |
| Recent TIA | Ultrasound, CT and MRA to look for carotid artery stenosis and also cerebral lesions. Carotid angiography when US/MRA are discordant or to assess origins of great vessels and arch |
| Post dissection aneurysm | MRA/CTA. DSA for carotid stent grafting |
| **Acute** | |
| Suspected CVA | CT/MR perfusion scans and assessment of carotid arteries DSA for thrombolysis (some centres only) or stenting |
| Suspected carotid dissection | US, MRA, CTA. DSA for stenting |

# Equipment

- Basic angiography set.
- 5Fr sheath.
- Catheters: **non-selective** – 90-cm 4Fr pigtail; **selective** – personal preference is important, options include Berenstein, Headhunter, Sidewinder and Mani.
- Guidewires: 3-mm J and angled Terumo.

# Procedure

*Access*   Usually via the right CFA.

*Catheterization*   In presence of carotid disease, there is an approximately 2% stroke risk associated with selective carotid angiography. The risk of cerebrovascular accident (CVA) is probably less for aortic arch injection but image quality is reduced. It is best practice to avoid catheterizing the carotid and vertebral arteries unless absolutely necessary for the test. To minimize the risk of CVA, scrupulous angiographic technique and attention to catheter flushing are mandatory. This is the time to use the double flush technique – **aspirate flowing blood and discard, flush with a fresh syringe with no air bubbles.**

*Arch aortogram*   Position a pigtail catheter in the ascending aorta just above the aortic root.

*Carotid and vertebral artery catheterization*   The difficulty of this procedure depends on the curvature of the aortic arch and the presence of any disease within it. In general, it is easiest to start with an LAO 30° projection to 'open up the arch'. An arch aortogram may help to localize the vessel ostia. Choose the most suitable catheter for the configuration of the arch; remember the basic rules of catheter selection. The Berenstein catheter is forward facing and can be used for most arch vessels unless they are angled acutely retrogradely. In unfolded arches or when the vessel is awkwardly angulated, use the Headhunter, Sidewinder or Mani catheter.

When selective catheterization is necessary to investigate carotid stenosis, position the catheter in the common carotid artery (CCA). For a vertebrobasilar problem, start with the catheter in the proximal subclavian artery to show vertebral origin. Then perform selective vertebral catheterization. Cerebral angiography requires selective internal carotid artery (ICA) catheterization.

*Runs*   **The runs performed depend on the clinical indication. Perform the minimum number of runs to achieve a diagnostic examination.** See Table 11.16. Additional runs may be required to demonstrate specific intracerebral vessels. These are beyond the scope of this book and may be found in textbooks of neuroradiology.

# Interpretation

Stenoses should be measured accurately using calipers and analysed according to the NASCET study criteria, which form the basis for treatment (Fig. 14.30). Dissection of the carotid artery causes string-like narrowing (Fig. 14.31).

Flush catheters in the descending aorta whenever possible; that way, any emboli will not affect the cerebral circulation. Make sure that there are no air bubbles in the flush solution. Never flush a blocked catheter in the aortic arch!

**Table 14.16** Typical parameters for carotid angiography

| Position | Runs | Contrast volume (mL) | Injection rate (mL/s) | Frame rate (FPS) | Centring | Field size (cm) |
|---|---|---|---|---|---|---|
| Aortic arch | LAO 30° | 30–40 | 15–20 | 2 | Aortic root upwards | 40–28 |
| Carotid | AP and lateral | 10 | Hand | 2 | Over carotid bifurcation (ant to C4) | 28 |
| Internal carotid extracranial | AP and lateral | 10 | Hand | 2 | Over ipsilateral carotid | 28–40 |
| Internal carotid intracranial | AP and lateral | 10 | Hand | 2–1 for venous phase | Lateral skull and Townes view | 28–40 |
| Vertebral | AP and lateral | 10 | Hand | 2–1 for venous phase | Intracranial– lateral skull and Townes view | 28–40 |

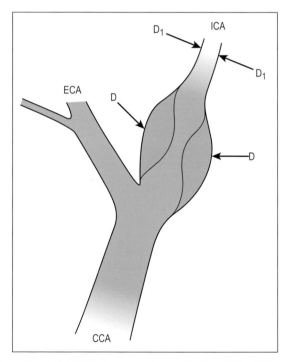

**Fig. 14.30** ■ NASCET criteria. NASCET % stenosis = [1 − (D/D1)] × 100%. CCA, common carotid artery; ECA, external carotid artery; ICA, internal carotid artery.

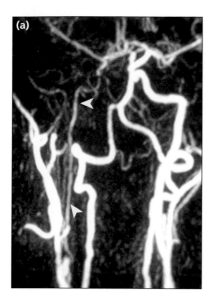 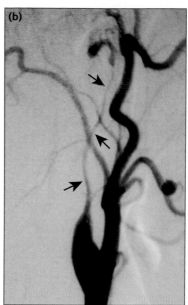

**Fig. 14.31** ■ Typical 'string-like' appearance of carotid dissection. (A) MRA: the right internal carotid artery (ICA) is dissected (arrowheads). (B) Lateral view from a selective carotid angiogram showing IAC dissection (arrows). (Image (B) courtesy of Dr P Turner.)

# Troubleshooting

### Catheter 'jumps' around the aortic arch

- This is usually a consequence of the catheter being held under tension in the aortic arch (Fig. 14.32). Turn the catheter to face appropriately and pull it back slowly, trying not to 'bridge' the catheter. Occasionally, it may be necessary to use a larger-calibre catheter, particularly if initial attempts were with a 4Fr. A reverse curve catheter such as the Sidewinder can be useful in this situation.

### Unable to catheterize an arch vessel

- Perform a run in the LAO 30° projection and use this to confirm the anatomy and exclude an origin stenosis. Choose an appropriately-shaped catheter.

### Unable to advance catheter into arch vessel

- Once again, this is usually a consequence of the catheter being held under tension in the aortic arch. Try advancing more wire into the artery to increase stability, perform a run to establish the anatomy and avoid passing the wire up the internal carotid artery. Make use of the subclavian and axillary arteries to get 'a good purchase'. It is rarely necessary to resort to using a larger catheter or a guide-catheter. If you are in trouble, pull the catheter back into the descending aorta and get help!

### The external carotid artery superimposes on the internal carotid artery This is fairly common on the AP projection. Try a 15° ipsilateral anterior oblique projection. Another common problem is for fillings to project over the ICA. This can also be solved by a suitable oblique projection.

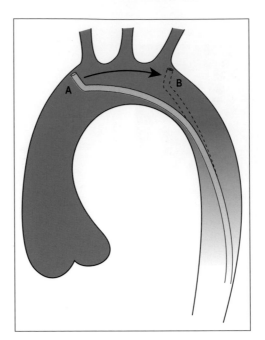

**Fig. 14.32** ■ In position A, the catheter is under tension against the inner curve of the aortic arch. As it is withdrawn, it suddenly springs, making controlled catheterization impossible.

# Vascular measurement

It is necessary to know the size of vessels to choose appropriately-sized angioplasty balloons, stents and stent-grafts. There are several methods for making these measurements, mostly using software incorporated into angiographic units. Some will make estimates based on the size of the angiographic catheter in the vessel. In other circumstances, an external calibration such as a coin of known diameter is placed adjacent to the vessel, e.g. during carotid stenting (Fig. 14.33). Most angiographers have a rough idea of what vessel size to expect for most vessels in general peripheral arterial intervention (see Chapter 15, Angioplasty and Stenting).

A variety of accurate measurements of vessel diameters and lengths are required to choose the correct size stent-graft for endovascular aneurysm repair and transjugular intrahepatic portosystemic shunt (TIPS). Most measurements can be made using contemporary CT and MR software packages. Where this is not available, angiography can be performed using a special catheter with calibrated markings along the shaft. Simply use these to calibrate the angiographic image.

**Alarm:** For measurement to be accurate, the catheter ideally should be in the vessel being measured or at least in the same horizontal plane. If this is not the case, large magnification effects can drastically affect measurement accuracy!

The measurements necessary to size aortic stent grafts are described in detail in Chapter 17.

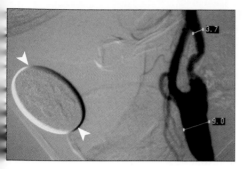

**Fig. 14.33** ■ Lateral view from a selective carotid angiogram. A 26-mm diameter metal disk (2p coin) is taped on the ipsilateral mandible (white arrowheads). This is used to calibrate the angiography machine for accurate measurement of the carotid artery for sizing the appropriate protection device and stent.

**Table 14.17** Trauma vascular imaging depends on the clinical scenario

| Scenario | Modality |
| --- | --- |
| **Always acute!** | |
| Penetrating injury (knife/bullet etc) | CT or DSA to show nature of vessel injury. CT is extremely helpful in the chest and abdomen to show additional visceral injury |
| **Blunt trauma** | |
| Focal, e.g. limb injury | Ultrasound may be used in the emergency room to diagnose focal injury, e.g. occlusion. Angiographic imaging is needed for more detail of the distal circulation and DSA may be required in the operating theatre |
| Major trauma | Head to foot CT scan is needed to assess all injuries: bony, solid organ, bowel, vascular etc. DSA is used for intervention |

# Trauma vascular diagnosis

Trauma includes a wide range of physical insults, from penetrating wounds to massive blunt injury. Trauma has become increasingly important to the interventional radiologist with the recognition of the importance of rapid control of bleeding before the onset of cooling and coagulopathy. Interventional radiologists are involved in:

- Diagnosis: from the CT scan!
- Stopping bleeding
- Embolization
- Stent-grafting
- Balloon arterial occlusion (endovascular tourniquet)
- Demonstration and management of arterial injury (Table 14.17).

The most important consideration is the patient's condition. The patient must be adequately triaged by an experienced clinician. Do not waste time performing angiography when the patient needs emergency surgery. Major life-threatening injuries must be dealt with before attending to less severe problems. You cannot perform angiography and resuscitate the patient at the same time. Make sure that there is adequate clinical support to manage potentially unstable patients. For any of this to be effective, interventional radiology must be integrated into the trauma pathway. Interventional radiology is most effective to rapidly resolve a single life-threatening bleed. There is no time for embolization in the presence of multiple sites of bleeding but rapid placement of an intra-aortic occlusion balloon can be lifesaving.

Once the decision to perform angiography has been made, establish the objectives of the study and discuss them with the referring clinician. Plan the study so that the important information is obtained as quickly as possible. Look at the major targets first and do not be distracted by minor abnormalities. You can always return to these later if they are relevant. You may be asked to 'Just look at … while you're here.' This is inappropriate unless it is of immediate clinical relevance.

We are principally concerned with the diagnosis and management of arterial injury but do not forget that veins are thinner walled and more easily damaged than arteries. The angiographic signs of arterial injury are discussed below. The abnormality depends on the mechanism of injury, the severity of the injury, the general condition of the vessel and the condition of the patient. In essence, vessels are either damaged by penetrating injury or by stretching and tearing. The injury may affect the full thickness of the vessel wall or just one of the component layers.

## Signs of vascular injury

**Penetrating injury** This is usually manifest by contrast extravasation or false aneurysm. Occasionally, there will be a significant adventitial and medial tear in the absence of intimal injury and the result is an almost normal angiogram. Sometimes, bleeding will have stopped. Look out for spasm (truncated vessels) and the presence of vascular deviation caused by haematoma.

**Blunt injury** The mechanisms of injury are vascular compression and stretching. These actions can tear the intima, media or adventitia and may lead to the formation of intramural haematoma. Minor injury causes spasm; more severe injuries are manifest as dissections of increasing severity leading ultimately to occlusion or rupture. It is essential to demonstrate the distal run-off to allow planning of any surgical reconstruction. As smaller muscular arteries commonly go into spasm when injured, consider giving an antispasmodic drug to reveal the true condition of the underlying vessel.

**Blunt aortic injury** Aortic trauma is a life-threatening injury and the majority of patients with significant ascending aortic injury die at the scene of the accident. The aorta is injured either by direct compression and rupture (usually fatal) or because of shearing forces during injuries to the upper chest. CT should be performed on patients with a suitable mechanism of injury. Spiral or multislice CT with 3D reconstruction and MRI give more information about other injuries and will rarely miss an aortic abnormality. Angiography is required if the CT is positive for significant aortic injury, as stent-graft repair has become the first-choice treatment.

**Hepatic and splenic injury** Blunt hepatic and splenic trauma is usually diagnosed on CT and if intervention is required it will usually be for active hepatic arterial bleeding or splenic false aneurysms. Angiography may be requested to investigate persistent post-operative bleeding. Start with a flush aortogram to ensure that there is no other obvious bleeding source and then perform selective hepatic and splenic arteriograms and portal vein studies. If an arterial bleeding source is identified, embolization is often the treatment of choice.

**Renal injury** Renal trauma is usually diagnosed on CT, so angiography is not usually performed in the acute setting. Occasionally, angiography is necessary when there is persistent

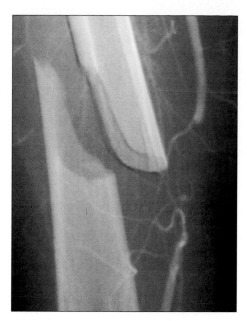

**Fig. 14.34** ▪ Acute occlusion of the superficial femoral artery secondary to femoral fracture. At surgery, there was extensive dissection causing the obstruction; the patient made an uneventful recovery after a short jump graft was inserted.

haematuria after blunt injury. Selective arterial embolization may allow treatment of a focal arterial injury without loss of the affected kidney.

**Pelvic injury** Major pelvic fractures are invariably associated with massive blood loss, often from venous injury and from the bone ends. If CT demonstrates arterial bleeding, then embolization should come before operative fixation of the fractures. Bleeding can occur at any of the pelvic arteries but the lateral sacral artery seems particularly prone to injury. These lesions can most often be readily treated by embolization.

**Peripheral vascular injury** Blunt traumatic injury can occur as the result of direct trauma or dislocation, e.g. the popliteal artery. Angiography may demonstrate dissection, disruption or occlusion (Fig. 14.34). Penetrating wounds – either human-made or fracture fragments – may cause acute bleeding with extravasation or pseudoaneurysm formation. Selective embolization may be appropriate if the injured vessel is not vital.

# Suggestions for further reading

Standards of Practice Committee, Society of Cardiovascular and Interventional Radiology. Standard for diagnostic arteriography in adults. J Vasc Intervent Radiol 1993;4:385–395.

**Renal**

Wijesinghe LD, Scott DJA, Kessel D. Analysis of renal artery geometry may assist in the design of new stents for endovascular aortic aneurysm repair. Br J Surg 1997;84:797–799.

The position of renal arteries as demonstrated in a cadaver study.

**Mesenteric**

Bakal CW, Sprayregen S, Wolf EI. Radiology in intestinal ischaemia: angiographic diagnosis and management. Surg Clin North Am 1992;72:125–139.

Laing CL, Tobias T, Rosenblum DI, et al. Acute gastrointestinal bleeding: emerging role of multidetector CT angiography and review of current imaging techniques. Radiographics 2007;27:1055–1070.

Rollins ES, Picus D, Hicks ME, et al. Angiography is useful in detecting the source of chronic gastrointestinal bleeding of obscure origin. AJR Am J Roentgenol 1991;156:385–388.
Confirms that the best angiography will reveal a source of bleeding in about 50% of cases. Some required repeat angiography.

Rosen RJ, Sanchez G. Angiographic diagnosis and management of gastrointestinal hemorrhage. Radiol Clin North Am 1994;32:951–967.

Tew K, Davies RP, Jadun CK, et al. MDCT of acute lower gastrointestinal bleeding. AJR Am J Roentgenol 2004;182:427–430.

Yoon W, Jeong YY, Shin SS, et al. Acute massive gastrointestinal bleeding: detection and localization with arterial phase multi–detector row Helical CT. Radiology 2006;239:160–167.

### Hepatic

Catalano OA, Singh AH, Uppot RN, et al. Vascular and biliary variants in the liver: implications for liver surgery. Radiographics 2008;28:359–378.

Soulen MC. Angiographic evaluation of focal liver masses. Semin Roentgenol 1995;30:362–374.
A beautiful pictorial review.

### Pulmonary

Grollman JH. Pulmonary arteriography. Cardiovasc Intervent Radiol 1992;15:166–170.

Knows so much about the subject they named a catheter after him! Describes the use of angled pigtail catheters.

Hudson ER, Smith TP, McDermott VG, et al. Pulmonary angiography performed with iopamidol: complications in 1434 patients. Radiology 1996;198:61–65.

### Carotid angiography

Fox AJ. How to measure carotid stenosis. Radiology 1993;186:316–318.

### Calibrated angiography

Thurnhur SA, Dorffner R, Thurnher MM, et al. Evaluation of abdominal aortic aneurysm for stent graft placement: Comparison of Gadolinium enhanced MR angiography versus helical CT angiography and digital subtraction angiography. Radiology 1997;205:341–352.
Describes the techniques for imaging of AAA and demonstrates the measurements required.

### Trauma

Laing CL, Tobias T, Rosenblum DI, et al. Acute gastrointestinal bleeding: emerging role of multidetector CT angiography and review of current imaging techniques. Radiographics 2007;27:1055–1070.

# 15

# Angioplasty and stenting

Angioplasty and stenting are cornerstone techniques in interventional radiology and have widespread non-vascular and vascular applications. The key skills and equipment choices remain largely the same, regardless of the site.

## Basic principles

Atherosclerotic plaque is incompressible. Concentric plaque splits during balloon angioplasty and the intima and media stretch and tear (Fig. 15.1). When there is eccentric plaque, the tears occur at the interface between the plaque and the adjacent normal artery (Fig. 15.2). This often causes deep clefts and occasionally results in distal embolization of the plaque. Balloon dilation stimulates nerve fibres in the adventitia, causing discomfort. Severe pain usually indicates that the vessel is being excessively dilated and at risk of rupture. Luminal gain occurs because progressive dilation irreversibly stretches the adventitia. Over a period of weeks, the damaged intima undergoes a period of 'remodelling'. This involves neointimal hyperplasia, which restores the smooth intimal surface.

## Equipment

Over the years, changes in materials have led to a decrease in both the size of the catheter shaft and the physical bulk of the angioplasty balloon. This allows angioplasty to be performed through smaller sheaths, and in some cases higher balloon inflation pressures are possible. In general peripheral angioplasty, most centres will continue to use 'over the wire' balloons for everyday applications.

Monorail ('rapid exchange') systems are typified by cardiology angioplasty balloons and stents. In a monorail system, the guidewire channel does not run the length of the catheter; instead it exits after about 15 cm (Fig. 15.3). This allows the use of shorter guidewires and can improve control. Remember, you will need a guide-catheter or sheath to perform angiography, as the catheter does not have a lumen. In practice, they are most useful for specialist applications such as carotid angioplasty and stenting. Monorail systems simplify introducing and withdrawing the catheter as the wire is controlled very close to the sheath. To remove a monorail system the guidewire is fixed, and the catheter can then be pulled back until it stops at the point at which the wire channel exits. After this, the last portion is handled in the same way as usual.

Angioplasty catheters are available in a range of diameters from 2 mm to over 25 mm and in lengths from 60 cm to 120 cm. Variations in balloon materials, coatings and catheter construction give a range of catheters, from everyday workhorses (Fig. 15.4) for SFA angioplasty to thoroughbreds that are capable of negotiating the most tortuous circulation. Cutting balloons even have miniature blades embedded in their walls.

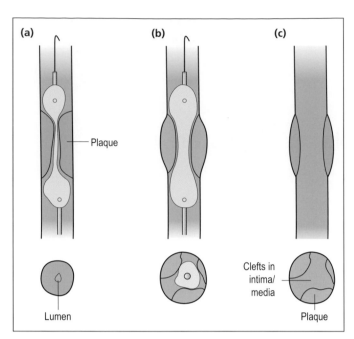

**Fig. 15.1** ▪ Angioplasty of concentric plaque. (A) Balloon 'waisting' in stenosis before plaque rupture. (B) Balloon dilation – the plaque is ruptured but the plaque volume unchanged. (C) Balloon deflation – the luminal area is increased because of stretching of the media/adventitia and intimal clefts.

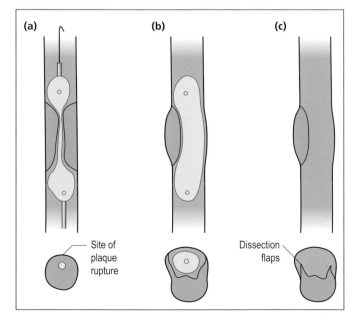

**Fig. 15.2** ▪ Angioplasty of eccentric plaques. (A) Balloon 'waisting' in stenosis before plaque rupture. (B) Plaque has ruptured at its thinnest point – eccentric media/adventitia stretching. (C) Post-angioplasty dissection flaps in eccentric lumen. Plaque volume is unchanged.

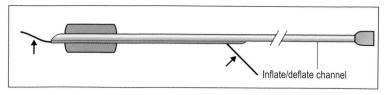

**Fig. 15.3** ■ Schematic view of a monorail angioplasty balloon. The guidewire (arrows) enters the catheter at the tip and exits after about 15 cm. The remainder of the catheter shaft is the inflate/deflate channel (chevron).

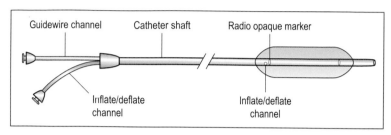

**Fig. 15.4** ■ Typical angioplasty balloon construction. Note the balloon length refers to the distance between the markers over which the balloon is of its rated diameter. The catheter shaft comprises the guidewire lumen and the inflation channel. Smaller shaft sizes can be achieved with thinner materials and smaller inflate/deflate channels.

**Table 15.1** Rough guide to balloon and stent diameters

| Aorta | 10–15 mm |
|---|---|
| Common iliac | 8 mm |
| External iliac | 7 mm |
| CFA, proximal SFA | 6 mm |
| Distal SFA | 5 mm |
| Popliteal | 4 mm |
| Crural | 2–3 mm |

In day-to-day practice, balloon choice is dictated by a few simple concepts.

**Balloon diameter** The diameter of the arterial segment immediately adjacent to the lesion should be measured on the pretreatment angiogram. Always be careful to avoid measuring an area of post-stenotic dilation. In practice, most operators use an approximate guide (Table 15.1).

Scale the balloon size up or down to suit the patient, e.g. a small elderly woman is likely to have smaller vessels than a large, muscular man.

**Balloon length** To minimize intimal damage to the adjacent vessel wall, choose the shortest balloon length that allows treatment of the diseased segment. An exception to this principle is when a short balloon cannot be held in a stable position during inflation. This phenomenon is akin to what happens when you pinch a lemon pip between your fingers and it shoots out. In these circumstances a longer balloon length will add stability.

**Tip:** To minimize this balloon migration, ask your assistant to inflate the balloon while you hold the catheter and wire to maintain the balloon in the correct position. This is an active process performed under fluoroscopic control.

*Shaft lengths* The shaft length of an angioplasty balloon is always longer than the 'working' length. The presence of the side-arm for balloon inflation means the balloon cannot be inserted up to the hub. The bulk of work in the iliac or femoral circulation can be reached with a 75-cm balloon shaft. For other sites and approaches, consider the height of the patient and lengths of balloon catheter and guidewire that you will need. Remember to ensure the guidewire is long enough to allow catheter exchange.

*Sheaths* Always use angioplasty balloons through a sheath; the balloon profile is lovely when it goes in but even the best balloon has 'wings' when deflated that will cause an irregular arteriotomy on removal. The manufacturer records the appropriate sheath size on the balloon packet, so it is always worth checking. The sheath size will always be larger than the shaft diameter to accommodate the balloon flaps. It may be possible to squeeze a virgin balloon through a smaller sheath but it will be a devil to remove through the same sheath later.

**Tip:** When removing balloons and catheters, always keep an eye on the sheath to make sure that it is not heading for an early and bloody exit. If it is moving with the catheter, ask your assistant to hold it in place while you concentrate on the catheter and wire.

**Under pressure** A consequence of the wide variety of balloon materials available is that balloons vary in their **compliance**. A balloon rated as 6 mm will be 6 mm at the recommended inflation pressure (another piece of information on that discarded packet). As the pressure is increased, a compliant balloon will progressively expand; this is intended to allow precise tailoring of some cardiology balloons. The majority of modern balloons have a limited compliance range, but occasionally, particularly with the latex balloons provided with stent-grafts, compliance can be a problem.

Angioplasty balloons have a maximum-rated inflation pressure. If this is not exceeded, the manufacturer has 95% confidence that 99.9% of their balloons will not burst. Balloons may rupture in stents and very tight calcified stenoses. As the balloon is designed to tear longitudinally, this rarely has any significant sequel (Fig. 15.5). Less than 1% of balloons will tear circumferentially (Fig. 15.6). This does pose a problem during withdrawal through the sheath, akin to backing through a doorway with an open umbrella!

**Inflation** The only way to be certain a balloon is being used at the correct pressure is to use an inflation handle with a pressure gauge (Fig. 15.7). The syringe barrel in this device has a thread and the syringe plunger is screwed into the barrel with a progressive and controlled increase in the balloon pressure.

Use approximately one-third strength contrast to inflate the balloon. Manual inflation using a standard syringe was favoured by the founding fathers of intervention, but even the strong will find it impossible to exert a sustained pressure. In addition, it hurts the delicate skilled hand and may result in a hernia. Certainly for small-vessel balloons and for lesions likely to require prolonged or high-pressure inflation, an inflation handle and gauge are recommended.

The dilating force is related to the diameter of the balloon; therefore, for the same pressure, a larger balloon will apply a greater force on the vessel wall. In practice, 3-mm balloons are often inflated to 12 atm while 15-mm balloons only require a pressure of 4–6 atm.

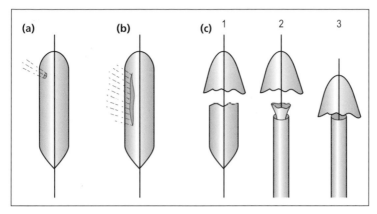

**Fig. 15.5** ■ Burst angioplasty balloons. (A) 'Pin-hole' tear: common and of no significance.
(B) 'Longitudinal' tear: rare, but seldom a problem. (C) 'Circumferential' tear: very rare, but serious as
balloon will impact in sheath when it is withdrawn.

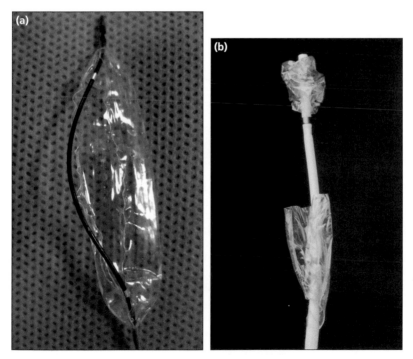

**Fig. 15.6** ■ Examples of (A) longitudinal and (B) circumferential balloon tears. Balloons with longitudinal
tears are easily removed. With a circumferential tear (B), the distal balloon crumpled up and wedged in
place as it was pulled into an 8Fr-reinforced sheath, and surgical removal was required.

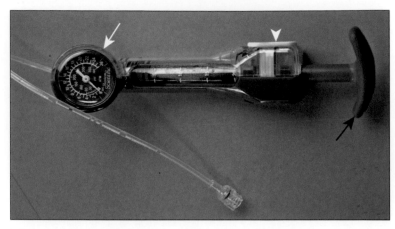

**Fig. 15.7** ■ Inflation handle. The balloon is inflated by screwing the handle (black arrow) clockwise until the gauge (white arrow) shows the appropriate pressure. Pressing the button (arrowhead) releases the screw thread; the handle can then be pulled back to deflate the balloon. Further aspiration with an empty 20 mL syringe may be needed to empty the balloon completely.

Fluoroscope during balloon inflation – check the balloon remains in position and that the balloon has completely 'de-waisted'. Try to feel how much pressure you are applying with the inflation device and regularly check the pressure gauge to ensure that you do not exceed the recommended pressures.

 **Alarm:** Don't try this at home. Inflating an angioplasty balloon with saline and air until it bursts makes an impressive bang, and gives an idea of the damage it could cause in a blood vessel.

The duration of inflation varies from operator to operator (depending on their attention span) and between lesions. There is no real science here but we recommend:
- For a stenosis, inflate for 1 minute.
- For a resistant stenosis, keep topping up the balloon to sustain the inflation pressure until the stenosis yields or you give in and get a cutting balloon.
- For an occlusion, allow 2–3 minutes.
- For a dissection flap, allow 3–5 minutes at low pressure.

**Deflation** Contrast is viscous and can be slow to aspirate from the balloon; the inflation handle will not always deflate the balloon completely. Before removal, aspirate the balloon as completely as possible using an empty 20 mL syringe. Clockwise rotation of the balloon during withdrawal will help wrap the balloon wings onto the catheter shaft and reduce the profile. If the balloon is reluctant to come out of the sheath – **STOP** – do not impact the balloon as it will cause the sheath to concertina. Try to aspirate the balloon again, if necessary with a 50 mL syringe, and confirm on fluoroscopy that the balloon is deflated. Very rarely, a balloon will not deflate. Do not panic but simply puncture the balloon with a Chiba needle.

## Procedure

There are four stages to angioplasty and stenting:
- Vascular access
- Crossing the lesion

- Dilating the lesion
- Completion angiography.

**Vascular access**  As always, plan the procedure before starting. Use the preintervention angiogram to determine the best point of access; a good rule is to use the shortest, straightest route possible. The fewer curves the angioplasty balloon has to negotiate, the better. As always there are occasions when it is better to seek an alternative approach, such as when there is a local problem at the optimal access site or when there are lesions above and below the CFA that require treatment, e.g. combined iliac and SFA disease. Improvements in equipment allow angioplasty and stenting across the iliac bifurcation and thus treatment of bilateral lesions via a single puncture. The contralateral approach reduces your ability to 'push' through a very tight lesion. If necessary, simply make an antegrade puncture.

**Crossing the lesion**  Angioplasty can be used to treat both stenoses and occlusions.

A **stenosis** has to narrow the lumen by 50% before it becomes haemodynamically significant; a 50% diameter reduction results in a 75% reduction in the luminal cross-sectional area. Even the tightest stenosis can be negotiated with patience, a little skill and the right tools. Simple stenoses are readily negotiated with a guidewire alone: either a curved hydrophilic wire or a Bentson wire (Fig. 15.8).

More complex stenoses can be a challenge, and the key is to steer through the narrow segment, using a shaped catheter and a curved hydrophilic wire. A pin-vice is invaluable to turn the wire in the correct direction. **Take your time and never use force**. If the wire starts to buckle, there is a good chance it will cause a dissection. If the wire starts to spiral down

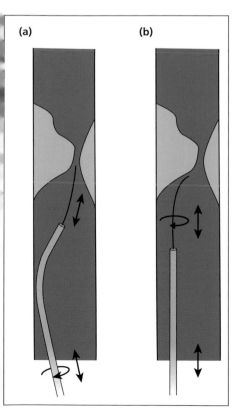

**(a)**          **(b)**

**Fig. 15.8** ▪ Crossing a stenosis. Obtain a decent angiogram to use as a 'route map'. Use fluoroscopy fade or roadmap if available. (A) Straight wire and curved catheter. Turn the catheter to direct the wire through the stenosis. (B) Angled hydrophilic wire and straight catheter. Turn the wire, giving the wire space to rotate outside the catheter. You can practise this by trying to catheterize the nozzle of a syringe using different catheter/wire combinations.

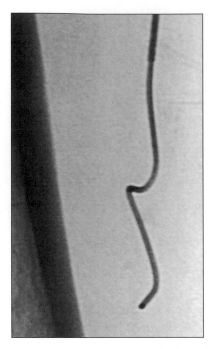

**Fig. 15.9** ■ Typical spiral appearance of a guidewire that is dissecting.

the artery, it is dissecting! (Fig. 15.9). Hydrophilic wires are great for crossing the lesion and equally easy to pull out; exchanging for a conventional wire after negotiating the lesion is infinitely safer. To exchange the wire, pass a catheter through the lesion, inject contrast to confirm intraluminal position and then put in a suitable wire such as a 3-mm J wire.

 **Tip:** Use a pin-vice to help steer the hydrophilic wire. If you have not got one, then dry the wire to allow you to grip it. Be careful! A dry wire will stick to your gloves and is easily pulled out!

Crossing **occlusions** is more complex and requires a little more patience. It is vital to get a high-quality angiogram at the start. Look at the shape of the vessel at the point of occlusion. The artery often tapers to a point – this is your target. Start with a straight wire and use a Cobra catheter to direct it to the apex of the occlusion (Fig. 15.10). The wire will often pass straight through the occlusion with minimal resistance. If there is no obvious point to enter the occlusion, gently probe it with a straight wire, using a shaped catheter to direct it. Once the wire enters the occlusion, proceed as above.

When the guidewire has crossed the lesion, treat it with care and respect; keep a wire across the lesion until the end of the procedure. This will allow rescue if the wheels come off. Always take the opportunity to perform an angiogram to prove you are in the target vessel. It is possible to be fooled by a wire position in a small collateral vessel behind the target vessel, with disastrous results. The choice of support wire depends on the anatomy but, as a rule, the more curves to negotiate, the stiffer the wire required, e.g. for a standard SFA a 3-mm J wire is fine but for a tortuous iliac segment an Amplatz wire may be necessary. J wires are the safest support wires, as the end of the wire inevitably moves during catheter exchanges.

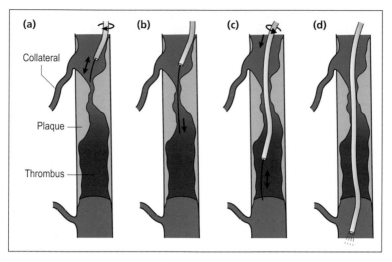

**Fig. 15.10** ■ Crossing an occlusion (see also Fig. 15.11). Occlusions occur where there is thrombus at the site of a stenosis. The thrombus propagates to the next collateral. (A) Gently probe the 'apex' of the occlusion with a straight wire, using a curved catheter to steer. (B) Typically, the wire will enter the thrombosed lumen with a slight give in resistance. (C) Advance the catheter into the occlusion to support and steer the wire through. (D) Perform an angiogram to confirm intraluminal position.

Make sure that the tip of the wire is always visible to avoid damaging the distal vessels! After crossing the lesion, give a bolus of heparin, usually 3000–5000 units.

**Dilating the lesion** There are a variety of different techniques used to mark the area for angioplasty: if you are lucky, there is an obvious bony landmark at the site of the lesion, although this is rarely the case in the SFA.

- On modern X-ray machines, use the roadmap or fluoroscopy fade facility to position the balloon. Roadmaps need a cooperative patient and operator and it is essential that no movement occurs unless your machine is capable of remasking the image.
- Inject contrast during fluoroscopy and position sponge forceps to mark the stenosis; either apply a metallic marker to the thigh or use a chinagraph pencil to mark the position on the screen. Confirm this is in the correct position with another angiogram. **Do not move the table after marking.**

Use an appropriate balloon size for the target vessel. The balloon length may be shorter than the target length and overlapping dilations will be necessary. It does not matter whether this is started proximally or distally.

**Completion angiography** Post angioplasty, remove the balloon catheter but remember you haven't finished yet. Always leave the wire through the lesion in case a bail-out procedure is necessary (remember how long it took you to cross the lesion in the first place!). A completion angiogram should be performed to assess the treated segment and the distal run-off. Look for:

- Residual stenosis: less than 30% residual stenosis is the aim
- Dissection flaps: most angioplasty sites will have a minor dissection which appears as a small linear defect; this will heal in time. Occasionally, the intimal/medial interface has been very disrupted and a flap extends into the lumen that reduces flow distally

- Venous filling: venous opacification sometimes occurs extending from the angioplasty site into the adjacent vein. This is rarely of any consequence and can safely be left alone
- Run-off: final angiograms must include the circulation distal to the angioplasty site. Compare with the preintervention angiogram, looking particularly for distal embolization.

**Tip:** A useful technique that allows you to preserve guidewire access across a contralateral lesion is to inject around a 0.018-inch guidewire using a Tuohy–Borst adaptor and 0.035-inch lumen catheter when performing completion angiography.

**Subintimal angioplasty** is a technique best avoided in the early stages of an interventional career. It would more appropriately be called extraluminal angioplasty or even 'who knows where you are angioplasty'. It is likely that many occlusions are traversed extraluminally without the operator knowing. In an occlusion, it is difficult to know what plane you are in within the artery wall. There are two distinct strategies to extraluminal angioplasty.

1. Most commonly, an attempt is made to traverse the occlusion in the standard way but the guidewire does not make progress. If this happens, reach for your friend the Terumo wire and advance it until it forms a loop beyond the catheter tip (Fig. 15.11). If the loop can now be advanced with relatively little resistance, this is fine. Only go as far as the point where the artery re-forms. Now comes the clever bit, re-entering the true lumen of the vessel! Frequently the wire drops spontaneously straight back in; if not, this can take a considerable time using a shaped catheter and wire.
2. The alternative is to deliberately enter the vessel wall above the occlusion. You will usually need a straight wire and a shaped catheter such as the Berenstein to do this. Sometimes it is necessary to use the 'wrong end' of the wire to manage this. Do this with great care, as the alternative is transmural angioplasty. Extraluminal position can be confirmed by injecting a small amount of contrast into the wall. Once this has been achieved, a hydrophilic wire is advanced in a loop as above.

The outcome of extraluminal angioplasty is akin to the false lumen in an aortic dissection. The channel communicates with the true lumen via tears at the entry and re-entry sites.

There are a few caveats to 'extraluminal angioplasty':

- 'Extraluminal angioplasty' is seldom successful in heavily calcified vessels.
- Closely observe the diameter of the guidewire loop. If it starts to exceed the expected vessel diameter, you are at best 'subadventitial' and will not succeed. STOP – you can always try again another day.
- Don't propagate the false lumen far beyond the point at which the vessel reconstitutes, you will only occlude it.
- Consider using a stiff/supportive guidewire, e.g. the stiff Terumo, to help the catheter overcome friction when it is advanced.
- Consider using a low-profile angioplasty balloon catheter. They are excellent for dilating the lesion and can also be used to cross the lesion when a conventional catheter has failed.

Supporters of the extraluminal approach claim better long-term patency rates, particularly for long segment disease, because of the smooth subintimal lining. The downside of the technique: it can be very difficult to re-enter; there is a higher incidence of vessel perforation and collaterals are occluded – important if the subintimal tract fails.

**Angioplasty consent issues** Angioplasty consent issues: immediate and long-term outcomes, symptom relief, recurrent stenosis.

**Complications**
- The 3Bs of arterial access: bruising, bleeding and blockage at the puncture site.

- Generic angioplasty related: vessel occlusion, rupture or dissection, usually fixed by stent or stent graft, distal embolization 1–4%, often of no clinical importance. About 1% of patients will require surgery.
- Site-specific: obviously emboli to the brain or the kidney are going to be much more important.

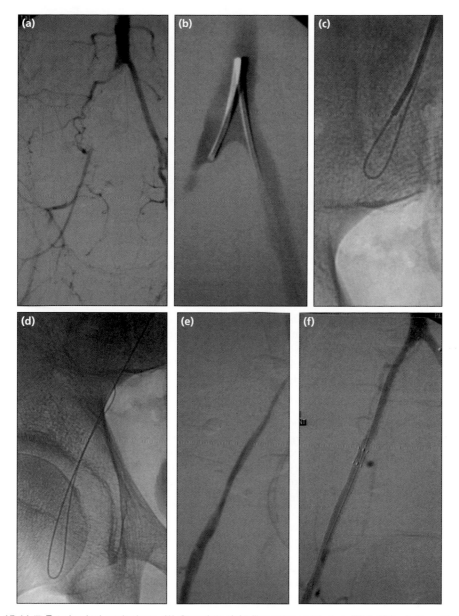

**Fig. 15.11** ▪ Extraluminal angioplasty. (A) Complete right iliac artery occlusion. (B) A Sidewinder catheter is used to engage the origin of the CIA. (C) A loop has been formed in a hydrophilic wire and is advanced through the occlusion. (D) The loop has re-entered the arterial lumen in the CFA. (E) Injection around a 0.018 inch guidewire shows the extraluminal tract. (F) Completion angiogram following stenting.

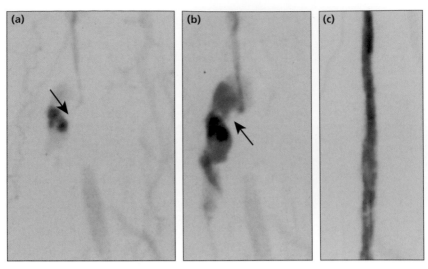

**Fig. 15.12** ■ (A, B) Guidewire perforation (arrow) of the SFA. (C) The extravasation resolved following satisfactory angioplasty.

## Troubleshooting

*Unable to cross the lesion* It may sound obvious, but vary your approach and technique. Try different catheters and wires. Consider whether it might be possible to cross it coming from the other side of the lesion, e.g. with a contralateral or a popliteal puncture.

*Unable to cross the lesion despite exhaustive efforts* Stop! In most situations, it is possible to come back on another day and sometimes the lesion seems effortless on the second attempt.

*A guidewire perforation occurs* This is likely to settle spontaneously. Simply pull back and repeat the angiogram after waiting for a couple of minutes to ensure there is no persistent extravasation (Fig. 15.12).

*The wire crosses the lesion but the catheter will not follow* This is particularly likely in heavily calcified lesions. Hold the guidewire as taut as possible and try to advance the catheter through the stenosis by rotating from side to side as you push. If this fails, use the lowest-profile catheter available; sometimes using a microcatheter is the only way, though. Rarely, it may be necessary to cross the lesion with a 0.018-inch guidewire; a low-profile angioplasty balloon can be used to predilate the lesion to 3 mm.

 **Tip:** Sometimes it is impossible to get a catheter to follow the 0.035-inch wire through a lesion. In these circumstances there is no option but to withdraw the wire and exchange for a more supportive wire or a low-profile 0.018-inch wire. Quite often a stiff hydrophilic wire will pass through the lesion, leaving you wondering what all the fuss was about. Supportive 0.018-inch wires cannot be steered but may surprise you by making it across; you then have the advantage of being able to move immediately to angioplasty with a low-profile balloon!

*A dissection flap is seen post angioplasty* Most angioplasty sites show angiographic evidence of dissection after angioplasty. A dissection is only significant if it impedes distal flow

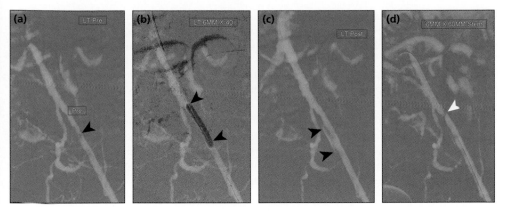

**Fig. 15.13** ■ Managing flow-limiting dissection. (A) External iliac stenosis (arrowhead). (B) Inflation of appropriately sized balloon (arrowheads). (C) Very deep dissection cleft post angioplasty (arrowheads) did not settle with prolonged balloon inflation. (D) Appearance following placement of a self-expanding stent (arrowhead).

(Fig. 15.13); in the iliac segment, this can be assessed with pressure measurements. If a flow-limiting dissection is present, then:

- First try a low-pressure balloon inflation for 3–5 minutes across the dissection flap. This often 'tacks' the flap back into position. If you restore brisk flow you have succeeded.
- Persistent dissections can be readily treated by stenting across the flap.

*There is a greater than 30% residual stenosis* Residual stenosis can occur because the lesion has been under-dilated, or secondary to elastic recoil. Measure the adjacent target artery and repeat the inflation with a balloon 1 mm larger than this vessel.

- If possible, measure the pressure gradient across the lesion. If no gradient is present, stop.
  - Many stenoses will remodel after angioplasty and if there is a 30–50% residual stenosis in a non-critical vessel, it may be appropriate to leave it.
  - If elastic recoil occurs (the angioplasty balloon completely expands but the lesion recoils on deflation), then arterial stenting is indicated. Do not stent lesions that it has not been possible to 'de-waist' during angioplasty as you simply line a stenosis with a stent.
- The balloon waist cannot be abolished. This occurs in tough lesions – most commonly in dialysis access and in grafts. **Do not** be tempted to just increase the inflation pressure; it is likely to burst the balloon, and the resulting explosion will probably damage the vessel. Instead, either use a high-pressure balloon to overcome the stenosis, or use a cutting balloon.

Consider using a **Cutting angioplasty balloon**. These are balloons developed for treating restenosis in coronary arteries. They have mini-razor blades incorporated into the wall, which make small cuts in the fibrous tissue, allowing dilation. Cutting balloons should be sized according to the diameter of the stenosed lumen rather than the adjacent normal vessel, e.g. you may only need a 3-mm cutting balloon in an 8-mm fistula vein; follow this with a regular 8mm angioplasty. Using a small balloon has two advantages: there is a marked reduction in sheath size and less risk of contrast extravasation.

*Distal embolization occurs* Obtain good quality angiograms to assess the run-off and the presence of any collaterals.

- Assess the clinical status of the limb. If the limb is well perfused and the embolus is into a non-critical branch vessel, then further intervention is inappropriate.
- Obtain ipsilateral access and perform clot aspiration (see Thrombo-suction, Fig. 19.4; p. 235).

*Extravasation occurs post angioplasty* Extravasation indicates disruption of all layers of the arterial wall and prompt action is essential. Brisk haemorrhage can occur, particularly in the iliac segment and aggressive resuscitation may be required.

- Reintroduce the balloon and perform a low-pressure inflation proximal to the rupture to tamponade the bleeding. Sometimes this is sufficient to allow a small hole to seal.
- Contact a friendly vascular surgeon and warn them you may need their skills.
- Put in a large drip and set up a saline infusion. Monitor the patient's pulse, BP and oxygen saturation. Take blood for a coagulation screen and cross-match.
- Wait for 5 minutes, then repeat the angiogram. If extravasation persists, reinflate the balloon to maintain haemostatic control.
- If expertise and equipment permit, a stent-graft can be inserted (Fig. 15.14). This will not only rescue the situation but also prolong your increasingly tenuous friendship with the vascular surgeon. If nothing works, the patient will need immediate surgical intervention!

# Angioplasty and stenting of specific sites

This section outlines the clinical and technical steps for successful angioplasty/stenting for the most common indications. The key determinants of success of angioplasty are:

- Arterial inflow and outflow
- Lesion morphology: stenosis or occlusion, length, calcification, plaque distribution
- Net lumen gain: a balance between vessel diameter and elastic recoil.

As a general rule, you can expect a good outcome for a focal stenosis in a large vessel with good inflow and run-off and a poor result in a long occlusion of a small, blind-ending vessel. Many of the complications are common to all angioplasty procedures:

- Puncture site haematoma: 2–3%; commoner with larger sheaths, obesity and hypertension
- Distal embolization: overall ~2%
- Angioplasty site thrombosis: overall ~1%.

Unless particularly relevant, these will not be discussed for each site.

## Aorta

Focal aortic stenoses and coarctation are ideal for angioplasty and have a technical success rate exceeding 95%, with excellent 5-year patency rates. Stents can be reserved for cases of elastic recoil, flow limiting dissection and recurrent stenoses. Pressure measurements are essential in the initial assessment of these lesions. Frequently, apparently severe stenoses on angiography do not produce a significant pressure drop. As a generalization, if the catheter and wire pass through without a struggle, there is no significant pressure drop.

### Procedure

*Access* Bilateral femoral access is needed for lesions that involve the aortic bifurcation, which should be treated with bilateral simultaneous common iliac balloons extending into the aortic bifurcation (Fig. 15.15). If a lesion is in the distal infrarenal aorta, either use a balloon with a short taper or use kissing balloons. The taper on some 15–18-mm

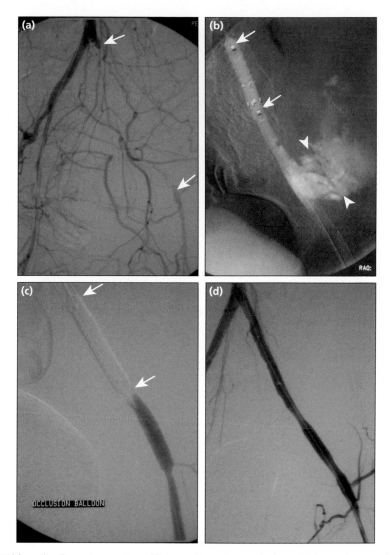

**Fig. 15.14** ■ Managing iliac artery rupture. (A) Long iliac artery occlusion, which was traversed from the contralateral femoral artery. (B) Following stenting there was severe pain during EIA angioplasty. The balloon was immediately inflated in the CIA (arrows). Angiography demonstrated EIA rupture with extravasation (arrowheads). (C) Balloon inflated to tamponade the rupture site. Brisk extravasation persisted despite prolonged inflation. (D) A stent-graft has been deployed via the ipsilateral femoral artery. The occlusion balloon was pulled back to the CIA during deployment.

balloons extends 1–2 cm beyond the balloon marker and will wreak havoc if it is in an iliac artery!

*Catheterization*  These lesions always look easy to cross but in practice it can be quite tricky to negotiate a 1–2-mm channel in a 12-mm artery. **Safety first**: once you have traversed the stenosis with a hydrophilic guidewire, this should be exchanged for a stiffer wire, e.g. an Amplatz super-stiff, prior to balloon insertion.

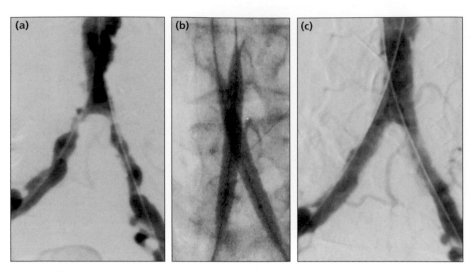

**Fig. 15.15** ■ (A) Stenosis involving the distal aorta and CIAs. (B) Kissing angioplasty balloons. (C) Completion angiography.

*Runs* Always perform AP and lateral runs to allow angiographic assessment before intervention. Identify the visceral vessels; infrarenal stenoses are typically just distal to the inferior mediastinal artery (IMA). In most patients, occlusion of the IMA during angioplasty will have no consequence; however, if the IMA is the dominant intestinal vessel, occlusion must be avoided. If necessary, angioplasty can be performed with a protection wire or balloon in the IMA from the brachial route.

*Complications* The principal risk is distal embolization secondary to treatment of a large atherosclerotic plaque. Iliac trauma from the balloon is an avoidable risk with good angiographic technique.

## Iliac arteries

Angioplasty is an effective treatment for symptomatic iliac atherosclerotic disease. Initial technical success rates of 90–95% are achievable in suitable patients, and 80–90% 5-year patency rates are achieved for stenoses <5 cm in length. Patency rates are lower for occlusions, heavily calcified lesions and stenotic disease that exceeds 10 cm in length, and primary stenting should be considered in these circumstances.

Iliac diameters are usually between 6 mm and 8 mm; however, take particular care in the external iliac artery in females, which can be small and is prone to dissection, spasm and rupture. Remember to measure the size of the target vessel before dilation. If the EIA is narrowed throughout its length, it may well be secondary to vasospasm (Fig. 15.16). Inject 100 mg of glyceryl trinitrate via the sheath and repeat the angiogram after a few minutes.

A single balloon is ineffective for lesions involving the distal aorta and impinging on the origin of the common iliac artery (Fig. 15.17). In this situation, simultaneous inflation of a balloon in each CIA origin ('kissing balloons') is needed. Kissing balloons are also used to prevent embolization of plaque into the contralateral iliac system. This is most likely to occur when using a balloon-expandable stent to treat a CIA occlusion.

The internal iliac artery may be occluded if angioplasty or stenting is performed across its origin. In a male patient with a unilateral internal iliac, this may cause impotence and you will not have done his buttock claudication any favours! Protect the internal iliac artery by

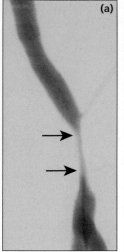
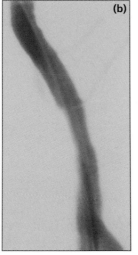

Fig. 15.16 ■ (A) Apparent stenosis of the CFA (arrows). Note the smooth outline characteristic of spasm. (B) Appearance following intra-arterial administration of GTN 200 µg.

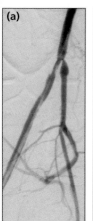
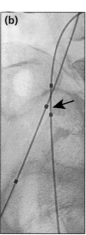
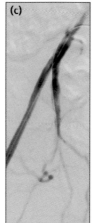

Fig. 15.17 ■ (A) Stenosis involving the EIA and the origin of the solitary internal iliac artery (IIA). (B) Angioplasty balloons in situ; the balloon artery (arrow) has been placed from the contralateral approach. (C) Completion angiography.

inserting a guidewire into it from the contralateral route. If the internal iliac artery origin is diseased, then angioplasty it as well (Fig. 15.17) – a male patient may be very grateful. If the internal iliac is at risk of occlusion, make sure you discuss the potential implications of this during consent.

Pressure measurements (Chapter 14, Angiographic Diagnosis) are invaluable for assessing the significance of iliac lesions. Pullback pressure measurements are particularly useful in multifocal disease.

## Procedure

*Access* Use the ipsilateral CFA whenever possible. If the common femoral is difficult to palpate, use an ultrasound-guided puncture to gain access. If the CFA is severely diseased, consider a combined procedure with CFA endarterectomy – this way you don't even need to obtain haemostasis.

*Catheterization* Sometimes it is impossible to negotiate a lesion from the retrograde approach. Use a Sidewinder or Sos catheter to manipulate over the bifurcation and try to cross the lesion from above (Fig. 15.11). If successful, the wire can either be snared or manipulated through the sheath (see Fig. 22.4) or permit ipsilateral passage of balloons.

*Runs* Initial angiograms from the aorta tend to overestimate the length of occlusions. Perform a run with simultaneous injections from both the aorta and the ipsilateral sheath. Always perform obliques and use the run that shows the lesion in profile during attempted catheterization.

## Complications

Complications are more frequent in occlusions than stenoses and are considerably more frequent in the external than the common iliac artery.

Distal embolization occurs more frequently in occlusions and is often impossible to treat by clot aspiration because of the pre-existing 6–7Fr retrograde puncture used to perform the angioplasty. Primary stent insertion minimizes the risk by trapping atheroma and thrombus against the vessel wall.

Iliac rupture (Fig. 15.14) can occur after angioplasty, particularly of the external iliac artery. Blood loss can be very rapid and prompt balloon tamponade is essential. It is now that you realize the importance of having a stent-graft available for 'endovascular rescue'. If this fails, seek immediate surgical assistance.

## Common femoral artery

CFA stenoses are often the result of large calcified eccentric plaques. As the CFA is superficial, lesions are often treated by endarterectomy rather than angioplasty. If the stenosis is post surgical try angioplasty instead. CFA angioplasty is sometimes performed in association with iliac/SFA intervention on the grounds that it will not preclude subsequent endarterectomy. If performing angioplasty, access often has to be from the contralateral groin or the arm; a protection balloon may be necessary if the lesion involves the profunda origin. Try to avoid stents in the CFA as they will be prone to repeated flexion (Fig. 15.18) and will preclude arterial access and complicate any future surgery.

## Superficial femoral artery

Angioplasty of the SFA for claudication is bread and butter for most radiologists. Angioplasty confers immediate benefit and appears to improve outcome in the mid-term compared with best medical therapy and exercise. Overall patency rates for SFA disease are around 50% at 3 years. As always, short non-calcified stenoses offer the best long-term results; 5-year patency is 70%. The results of angioplasty in stenoses or occlusions longer than 10 cm are much poorer but angioplasty may be appropriate if the patient is not a surgical candidate and has rest pain or tissue ischaemia. Stents are usually reserved for bail-out procedures and are best avoided in the popliteal artery (flexion again). Stent-grafts in the SFA remain largely unproven compared with endovascular and surgical alternatives.

Doppler ultrasound is very useful to identify whether stenoses are haemodynamically significant prior to angioplasty, particularly in multifocal disease, or to follow-up interventions.

## Procedure

*Access* The ipsilateral groin provides the shortest, straightest route. Perform an antegrade puncture using the guidelines given in Chapter 11, Vascular Access. Combined iliac and

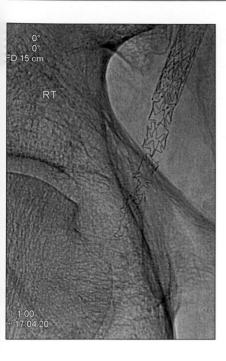

**Fig. 15.18** ■ Stent fracture due to repeated flexion of the distal EIA/CFA (courtesy Dr Sapna Puppala).

SFA lesions are best treated from the contralateral approach. Rarely, a lesion cannot be crossed from the antegrade route and a popliteal puncture may provide a more favourable route.

*Catheterization* Stenoses are usually negotiated with a hydrophilic guidewire. Occlusions may be more readily traversed with a straight wire and shaped catheter. Always perform a run after successfully crossing the lesion to confirm re-entry into the target vessel. Dilating a collateral will cause havoc and few things are more embarrassing than creating a 5-mm hole through the side of the SFA.

*Runs* In difficult lesions, manipulate a catheter and guidewire to the target lesion then perform a magnified view to optimize the chances of steering through the lesion. Choose the largest magnification that allows visualization of the lesion and the target run-off vessel, as this keeps the wire in view at all times.

## Complications

The most frequent complications are puncture site haematoma (2%), distal embolization (2–3%) and angioplasty site thrombosis (1%).
Vessel perforation occasionally occurs during femoro-popliteal angioplasty but seldom has clinical consequences. Anticoagulation should be reversed if necessary; balloon tamponade, stent-grafting or, rarely, coil embolization should be used if bleeding fails to settle.

## Tibial vessels

Tibial angioplasty is a useful technique to increase blood flow to allow for ulcer healing. Patency is poor; hence, it is less useful in patients with rest pain that will recur if there is restenosis. The durability and the risks make it inappropriate for the treatment of claudication.

**Fig. 15.19** ▪ Extraluminal angioplasty of the posterior tibial artery. (A) Diseased tibioperoneal trunk (white arrow) and posterior tibial artery (black arrow). (B) Following extraluminal recanalization of the posterior tibial artery, in line run-off is restored.

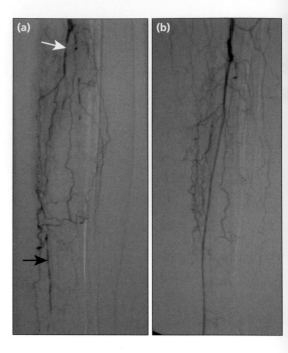

Small-calibre, low-profile balloons (2–4 mm) and 0.014–0.018-inch guidewires are required. These vessels are extremely prone to vasospasm and the use of antispasmodic agents is essential. As always, the elusive single focal non-calcified stenosis does best, but more diffuse disease can be successfully treated and may stay open long enough to permit ulcer healing. Extraluminal angioplasty can be particularly effective in crural vessel occlusion (Fig. 15.19).

## Renal artery

Renal artery angioplasty and stenting is a complex procedure; access can be difficult and when there is a problem, the consequences are rapid and serious – there may be renal loss even with immediately available surgical support. Renal angioplasty should only be attempted by angiographers who are already competent in all aspects of peripheral angioplasty.

**Renal angioplasty consent issues**
- Lack of evidence of benefit
- The 3Bs of arterial access
- Risk of CVA if using the arm approach
- General risks of angioplasty
- Specific to kidney – renal loss resulting in need for dialysis overall about 2% if treating entire renal mass.

Renal angioplasty is undertaken for the treatment of either ischaemic renal failure or hypertension. The clinical outcomes are poorly understood. The preliminary results from a large multicentre randomized trial (ASTRAL) suggest that revascularization confers no advantage compared with best medical therapy alone. Patients in the trial were those who were felt not to be disadvantaged by inclusion. In other words, they tended to have chronic renal impairment and hypertension. There are four groups of patients unlikely to be included in the study and they remain the clearest indications for renal angioplasty/stenting:

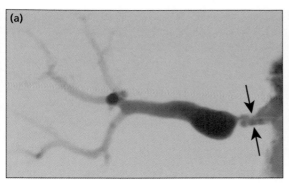
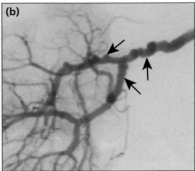

**Fig. 15.20** ■ (A) Atheromatous ostial renal artery stenosis (arrows) with post-stenotic dilation. (B) Typical beaded appearance of fibromuscular dysplasia (arrows) involving the distal renal artery and its branches.

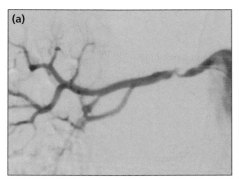
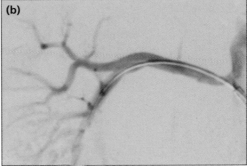

**Fig. 15.21** ■ Atheromatous stenosis in the mid-renal artery (A) before and (B) after angioplasty. Hypertension was cured but returned 2 years later and was again successfully treated.

- **Flash pulmonary oedema** – the aetiology of this condition is incompletely understood but treating the underlying renal artery stenosis is usually effective.
- **Hypertension refractory to treatment**. A few patients have hypertension which is poorly controlled despite maximal drug therapy, or malignant hypertension, or do not tolerate the antihypertensive medication. In these patients it is worth trying renal artery angioplasty and stenting, with the caveat that there will be no improvement in about a third of patients.
- **Hypertension in children** with fibromuscular dysplasia or neurofibromatosis.
- **Rapidly decreasing renal function with preserved renal size**. These patients are going to require renal replacement therapy in the near future and have nothing to lose. This group of patients is least likely to benefit from revascularization therapy.

The majority of renal stenoses are secondary to atherosclerotic lesions that tend to involve the proximal renal artery or its ostium (Fig. 15.20A). Fibromuscular dysplasia can affect any part of the renal artery and has a characteristic beaded appearance at angiography (Fig. 15.20B). Angioplasty success rates are highest with fibromuscular dysplasia, moderate with non-ostial atherosclerotic stenoses (Fig. 15.21) and poorest with ostial lesions. Ostial lesions are due to aortic wall atheroma and are prone to elastic recoil. Most angiographers will opt for a primary stent placement when dealing with an ostial lesion (Fig. 15.22).

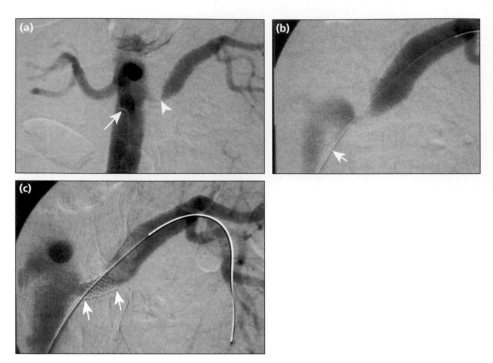

**Fig. 15.22** ■ Renal artery stenting for severe hypertension. (A) $CO_2$ angiogram using a Cobra catheter in the aorta (arrow), high-grade ostial stenosis (arrowhead) with poststenotic dilatation affecting the entire renal artery. (B) The stenosis has been crossed, angiography performed by injection through the Cobra catheter (arrow) around an 0.018-inch guidewire. (C) Completion angiogram obtained as (B). Note that the stent (arrows) has been dilated to 6 mm to match the diameter of the contralateral renal artery.

## Intervention in renovascular disease

Ischaemic nephropathy is only likely to be relevant when the stenosis affects the whole functional renal mass. In patients with two kidneys, impaired renal function in the presence of unilateral renal artery stenosis (RAS) indicates another renal pathology. Frequently, one of the renal arteries is already occluded, with a significant stenosis in the contralateral artery. The risk of progression to renal occlusion is about 10% within 2 years, and the rationale for treatment is prevention of dialysis. Preintervention assessment must include creatinine clearance and ultrasound assessment of renal length. When the creatinine is greater than 300 μmol, the damage is seldom reversible. Similarly, a kidney smaller than 8.5 cm is unlikely to develop useful function in response to angioplasty.

Primary technical success rates for renal artery angioplasty exceed 90% in most series; clinical success is considerably poorer, as shown by the ASTRAL trial. It is difficult to predict which patients with hypertension will benefit from angioplasty; 'suck it and see' is often the only answer. Typically, young patients with fibromuscular hyperplasia respond well and patients with unilateral disease do better than those with bilateral disease. Hypertensive patients are only 'cured' in 15–20% of cases, although blood pressure control is often improved. The results for ischaemic nephropathy indicate that in appropriately selected patients (i.e. reasonable renal function at the time of percutaneous transluminal angioplasty), approximately 30% improve renal function, with a further 20% stabilizing renal function. It is worth noting that without revascularization only about 1 in 6 patients will ever need dialysis; many more will succumb to other complications of cardiovascular and cerebrovascular disease.

## Equipment

- Basic angiography set.
  - Cobra, RDC and Sidewinder catheters from the CFA approach. Berenstein or Multipurpose catheters from the arm.
  - 4–5Fr sheath – almost all renal artery stenting can be performed through a 5Fr sheath using low-profile balloons and stents; some can be treated using 4Fr systems.
- Low-profile 5–7-mm × 2-cm angioplasty balloons (make sure that they are long enough if you are using the brachial or radial approach).
- Supportive guidewire – the authors' favourite is the 0.018-inch Platinum Plus wire with a 3-cm floppy tip. This allows positioning angiography to be performed around the guidewire.
  - Renal stent: 15–18 mm long × 5 or 6-mm diameter for most patients, used by most operators as the primary treatment for ostial disease and essential for a bail-out procedure.
- Antispasmodic agents: nifedipine, GTN.
- Protection wire systems are advocated by some authors but remain unproven. Most systems were designed for the carotid artery and are not suitable for all patients with RAS.

## Procedure

Review the aortogram and plan the access and optimal angiographic projection. Patients with a steeply angled renal artery or with severe aorto-iliac disease may require treatment from a brachial or radial approach. If the aorta has gross atherosclerotic plaque, then plan to do the procedure through a guide-catheter to minimize the risk of cholesterol embolization.

*Access* Tailor this according to the renal artery geometry. Use the arm approach for caudally angulated vessels, in the presence of abdominal aortic aneurysm or severe aortoiliac disease.

 **Tip:** It is often best to approach the renal artery from the contralateral CFA.

*Catheterization* The stenosis is crossed with a hydrophilic wire. This is subsequently exchanged for a supportive wire such as the Platinum Plus. When learning the procedure, it is helpful to be able to image whilst the balloon/stent is being positioned. This can be achieved in three ways:

- Injection around a guidewire using a Tuohy–Borst adaptor. This works best when using $CO_2$ or when using a balloon with a 0.035-inch lumen in combination with a 0.018-inch wire (Fig. 15.22).
- Bilateral access – this has several advantages, including the ability to position the balloon and perform postangioplasty images from a contralateral pigtail catheter.
- Use a guide-catheter/sheath to permit per-procedural imaging.

*Dilation* Always measure the required balloon size, taking care not to include an area of post-stenotic dilation. If the entire renal artery is dilated, measure the contralateral renal artery. In practice, most males require a 6-mm balloon, with small female patients needing 5-mm dilation. Warn the patient that it is normal to experience mild loin pain during angioplasty. Ask the patient to let you know when discomfort is felt and be careful if dilating more than this.

## Complications

- **Transient renal insufficiency**: prevention is better than cure. Pre-hydrate the patient, give *N*-acetylcysteine; use carbon dioxide or iso-osmolar non-ionic contrast (Iodixanol) and minimize contrast volume; perform diagnostic and therapeutic examinations separately.

- **Flow-limiting dissection**: readily treated with stent insertion.
- **Vasospasm**: use oral nifedipine 10 mg as a pretreatment and intra-arterial GTN 100-mg aliquots.
- **Intrarenal embolization**: thrombus may be treated with in situ thrombolysis.
- **Renal artery rupture**: either secondary to overdilation or subintimal balloon passage. Reinflate the balloon within the renal artery to tamponade the hole. Sometimes this is sufficient to allow a small defect to close. When this fails, reach for your friend the stent-graft and deploy it over the defect. If this doesn't work, leave the balloon inflated. It is good to have a strategy for this rare eventuality worked out before starting the procedure. Either embolize the kidney or call your ex-friend, the vascular surgeon. The warm ischaemia time for a kidney is fairly short (approximately 40 min) and therefore renal loss is likely.
- **Aortic dissection**: has been described. By this time your nerves will be jangling. Call for backup and if the dissection is symptomatic or flow limiting, it should be treated with a stent.

## Supra-aortic angioplasty and stenting

Roughly speaking, supra-aortic angioplasty and stenting can be divided into treatment of upper limb ischaemia and treatment of cerebral embolic disease and occasionally flow-limiting ischaemia (carotid and vertebral arteries). Both carry a risk of stroke. This is advanced intervention and should not be attempted without proper training and supervision.

### Supra-aortic angioplasty consent issues

- The 3Bs of arterial access
- General risks of angioplasty
- Specific to supra-aortic – risk of causing CVA; approximately 5% for carotid angioplasty and stenting. Probably less for arm ischaemia. As with carotid endarterectomy, the patient may prefer medical treatment alone.

### Upper limb angioplasty

Subclavian stenoses and occlusions can be successfully treated in 90% of patients and over 80% of patients have sustained clinical improvement at 3 years. Occlusions are best approached from the brachial route and are frequently stented to minimize the risk of cerebral embolization. Patients with subclavian steal usually have retrograde flow in the vertebral artery, which might confer some degree of protection against cerebral embolization, at least until the lesion is treated. Patients with antegrade vertebral flow can still undergo subclavian angioplasty. Some angiographers opt to protect the vertebral circulation with an additional balloon but there is no evidence for or against this practice.

## Carotid angioplasty

Carotid angioplasty and stenting are being used increasingly as an alternative to surgery for symptomatic carotid artery stenosis. Patients should be assessed in conjunction with a neurologist and carefully worked-up. The risk of stroke is around 5% and this must be discussed in advance. Patients should be started on clopidogrel (75 mg/day), a week before the procedure.

Remember that carotid intervention is of the greatest benefit in those patients with recently symptomatic stenosis (within 2 weeks); clearly these patients also have the greatest risk of embolic events. Patients with crescendo transient ischaemic attack (TIA) or with visible thrombus are not suitable for carotid artery intervention.

Evidence is still emerging regarding outcomes of carotid stenting compared to carotid endarterectomy and it is safe to say that the jury is still out. In these circumstances it is essential to regard the two approaches as complementary to each other. Carotid stenting probably has the advantage when there is a 'hostile neck' due to surgery, local pathology or radiotherapy.

The key to success is obtaining a stable position in the common carotid artery. Before starting, obtain an MRA or CTA to assess the aortic arch and carotid arteries. If the aorta is unfolded and the carotid arteries are tortuous, seek expert guidance as not all carotids can be treated by endovascular means. The technique of carotid artery stenting is rapidly evolving. Low-profile monorail (rapid exchange) angioplasty balloons and stents are used. Cerebral protection devices are becoming popular but, although attractive, remain unproven. These devices have different properties and discussion of their use is beyond the scope of this book. The basic principles of carotid angioplasty and stenting are set out below.

### Ten key steps to carotid intervention

1.  Obtain CFA access, fully heparinize the patient.
2.  Catheterize the symptomatic common carotid artery and perform a lateral carotid angiogram.
3.  Catheterize the distal external carotid artery and introduce a 260 cm length Amplatz wire (1-cm tip).
4.  Introduce an 80-cm guide-catheter or reinforced sheath into the common carotid artery (CCA) and perfuse this from a bag of pressurized, heparinized saline, which is run slowly.
5.  Place a coin of known diameter over the ipsilateral mandible close to but not obscuring the ICA. This is used to measure the diameter of the carotid artery. Perform another lateral carotid angiogram and measure the diameters of the ICA and CCA and the length of the diseased segment.
6.  Give atropine 1.2 mg into the sheath. This will cause the ipsilateral pupil to dilate. Warn the patient and ward staff that this is not a cause for concern.
7.  Cross the stenosis with a steerable 0.014- or 0.018-inch guidewire. This may be part of the cerebral protection device if one is being used. Use a 3-mm balloon to predilate lesions with a very tight stenosis.
8.  Pass the stent across the lesion and deploy it and dilate to an appropriate diameter, usually 4–6 mm.
9.  Perform a check angiogram to demonstrate the treatment site; carefully remove the cerebral protection device if one was used.
10. Use a closure device at the common femoral artery puncture site. This is a prime indication to use a closure device; large sheath, heparinized patient, clopidogrel.

## Cerebral protection devices

The concept behind cerebral protection is simple: prevention of cerebral emboli should prevent brain damage. A variety of cerebral protection devices exist, but all conform to two principal mechanisms for protecting the distal brain.

**Filter wires** These are steerable wires that incorporate a fine pore filter, which is deployed through the stenosis in a collapsed state and then opened like an umbrella when beyond the stenosis. Micropores allow flow throughout the procedure but the device will catch any embolic debris larger than the pore size. Following stent deployment, the filter is collapsed, removed and traditionally inspected to see what it contains.

**Flow reversal systems** The principle behind these devices is simple: the common carotid and external carotid arteries are occluded with balloons. A sheath in the CCA can then be

**Table 15.2** Cerebral protection devices: pros and cons

| Technique | Pros | Cons |
|---|---|---|
| Filter wire | Flow preserved throughout unless the filter becomes clogged, in which case it has done its job! | No protection until the lesion is crossed with the device and it is fully deployed |
| | Simple to deploy | Needs to be appropriate size for the vessel |
| | | Will still allow small emboli |
| | | Can snag on the stent during retrieval, causing anxiety all round |
| Flow reversal | Actively prevents emboli travelling forward up the ICA to the brain | Requires intact circle of Willis (at least anterior communicating artery). This should be assessed on pre-procedure imaging |
| | | Not tolerated by all patients; test occlusion of the ICA gives an indication of which patients may be suitable |
| | | Cumbersome to deploy |
| | | Requires increased sheath size |

aspirated or connected to the femoral vein and returned into the circulation. Flow in the ICA reverses and no emboli can pass to the brain.

Simply using an occlusion balloon in the ICA and then flushing and aspirating is the worst of both worlds (Table 15.2).

 **Alarm:** There is no evidence that cerebral protection devices improve outcome in carotid artery stenting.

# Vertebral artery intervention

The majority of symptomatic carotid artery disease is due to embolic phenomena; hence the need for primary stenting and cerebral protection. Vertebrobasilar insufficiency is usually a flow-related phenomenon. The lesions are typically short and focal; the proximal vertebral artery is by far the commonest site for disease, but occasionally stenoses are seen in the mid vertebral or basilar arteries. Angioplasty alone may be sufficient. Short balloon-expandable stents are indicated when there is recoil or restenosis. Low-profile coronary artery stents are ideal, as the vertebral artery origin is often fairly tortuous. Coronary stents are designed to conform to the curve of the vessel rather than straightening the vessel in the fashion of more rigid stents, such as those used in the renal arteries.

 **Alarm:** MIP images from carotid MRA tend to overcall vertebral artery stenosis, due to the orientation of the vessel orthogonal to the scan plane (check the next few you look at if you don't believe us). Always review the source images, which are much more reliable.

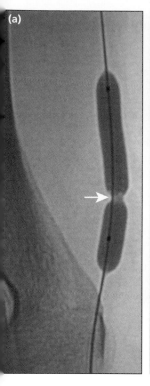
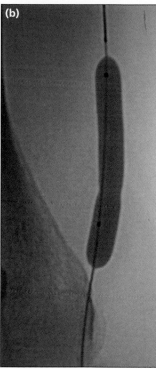

**Fig. 15.23** ■ High-pressure inflation to treat basilic vein stenosis. (A) Persistent waist (arrow) in conventional angioplasty balloon at 8 atm. (B) Following use of a high-pressure balloon inflated to 20 atm, the stenosis is abolished. Remember, do not exceed the rated pressure for the balloon or it will rupture.

# Venous angioplasty

Venous angioplasty has been used extensively in the treatment of central venous stenoses and dialysis outflow lesions. Recurrence is much more frequent in the venous system. Dialysis stenoses are particularly resistant and may require high-inflation pressures with a suitably strong balloon or the use of a cutting balloon (Fig. 15.23 and Fig. 21.5).

# Suggestions for further reading

**Peripheral angioplasty**

Bradbury AW, Ruckley CV. Angioplasty for lower limb ischaemia: Time for randomised controlled trials. Lancet 1996;347:277–278.
A thought-provoking surgical perspective.

Casteneda-Zuniga WR, Formanek A, Tadavarthy M, et al. The mechanism of balloon angioplasty. Radiology 1980;135:565–571.
How angioplasty actually works demonstrated in an experimental model. Shows the importance of plaque rupture and wall stretching.

Chetter IC, Spark JI, Kent PJ, et al. Percutaneous transluminal angioplasty for intermittent claudication: evidence on which to base the medicine. Eur J Vasc Endovasc Surg 1998;16:477–484.

Outcomes of angioplasty from the patient's perspective based on quality of life parameters. Provokes thought on patient selection.

Dotter CT, Judkins MP. Transluminal treatment of arteriosclerotic obstruction: Description of a new technique and a preliminary report of its application. Circulation 1964;30:654–670.
The start of an era, pioneer work, a must for historians.

Houghton AD, Todd C, Pardy B, et al. Percutaneous angioplasty for infrainguinal graft related stenoses. Eur J Vasc Endovasc Surg 1997;14:380–385.
Angioplasty seems to be the treatment of choice for short vein graft stenoses.

Johnston KW. Femoral and popliteal arteries: Reanalysis of results of balloon angioplasty. Radiology 1992;183:767–771.

Johnston KW. Iliac arteries: Reanalysis of results of balloon angioplasty. Radiology 1993;186:207–212.

Still the best studies of outcome in angioplasty. Honesty, clear follow-up and defined outcome measures.

Pentecost MJ, Criqui MH, Dorros G, et al. Guidelines for peripheral transluminal angioplasty in the abdominal aorta and lower extremity vessels. Circulation 1994;89:511–531.

Tonnesen KH, Bulow J, Holstein P, et al. Comparison of efficacy in crossing femoro-popliteal artery occlusions with movable core and hydrophilic guidewires. Cardiovasc Intervent Radiol 1994;17:319–322.

Do not use hydrophilic wires as your first choice.

Weitz JI, Byrne J, Clagett P, et al. Diagnosis and treatment of chronic arterial insufficiency of the lower extremities: A critical review. Circulation 1996;94:3026–3049.

### Upper limb angioplasty

McNamara TO, Greaser LE, Fischer JR, et al. Initial and long-term results of treatment of brachiocephalic arterial stenoses and occlusions with balloon angioplasty, thrombolysis and stents. J Invas Cardiol 1997;9:372–382.

A useful overview of the technique and outcomes.

### Renal angioplasty

Pohl MA. Natural history of renal artery stenosis: When to intervene. J Vasc Intervent Radiol 1999;10 (Suppl 2):144–150.

Most of what you need to know regarding patient selection for renal angioplasty and stenting, extensively referenced.

### Complications of angioplasty and stenting

Belli A-M, Cumberland DC, Knox AM, et al. The complication rate of percutaneous peripheral balloon angioplasty. Clin Radiol 1990;41:380–383.

Kobayashi K, Censullo ML, Rossman LL, et al. Interventional radiologic management renal transplant limitations, and technical considerations. Radiographics 2007;27:1109–1130.

Matsi PJ, Manninen HI. Complications of lower limb percutaneous transluminal angioplasty: A prospective analysis of 410 procedures on 295 consecutive patients. Cardiovasc Intervent Radiol 1998;21:361–366.

These articles help to set standards for acceptable practice.

# 16

# Stents and stent-grafts

## Stents

Stents are scaffolds used to support a vessel wall, and most are made from metal alloys. They are introduced in a compressed state and then expanded to line the vessel. Stent-grafts are stents covered with graft material and function as vascular conduits. Stents are used to treat stenotic and occlusive disease and stent-grafts are used to treat aneurysms and arterial rupture.

### Indications for stenting

A procedure may be undertaken with the intention of deploying a stent, so-called **primary stenting**. Iliac artery occlusions are often primarily stented to reduce the incidence of distal embolization (Fig. 16.1). Most angiographers will primarily stent ostial RAS without trying angioplasty because of the inevitability of elastic recoil.

A stent may be deployed to salvage an unsuccessful procedure. This is **secondary stenting** and it is the commonest reason to use a stent. The most frequent indication is failed iliac angioplasty with residual pressure gradient, stenosis or flow-limiting dissection (Table 16.1).

Most catheter laboratories will keep a selection of stents of different types and sizes on the shelf. This allows the operator a choice for different circumstances; in most cases the exact stent chosen is less important than selecting the correct size and deploying it accurately. Choice of which stent to keep on the shelf is influenced by several factors:

- Evidence of superior effectiveness: the immediate and long-term technical and clinical effectiveness should be the most important factors. Unfortunately, in a rapidly evolving market no manufacturer ever has any long-term data to support their product. Until they do, you have to assume that the device is indeed a stent.
- Ease of use: there is not much point in a device that is complicated or unreliable in its deployment.
- Profile: the expansion ratio of stents is improving all the time, meaning that larger devices can be delivered through smaller sheaths. In practice, most stents up to about 12 mm will pass through a 6Fr sheath, some will even pass through a 5Fr sheath and a few smaller stents pass through a 4Fr sheath.
- Trackability and flexibility: the ability of a stent to reach its target site and to conform to the vessel anatomy. Some stents pass readily over the aortic bifurcation and can be deployed in the contralateral iliac system; others don't manage this even with a stiff wire (Fig. 16.1).
- Cost: in many circumstances a specific stent type is not required. In this case, the choice of stent is pragmatic and the cheapest may well be the best.

**Fig. 16.1** ■ (A) Typical long iliac occlusion. (B) Two overlapping stents have been deployed from the contralateral approach. Note the proximal stent position at the iliac bifurcation (arrow) and the distal at the inguinal ligament. Unilateral stents can be used to treat these patients, provided the stents are accurately deployed and do not cover the contralateral iliac artery origin.

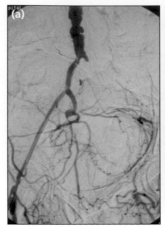 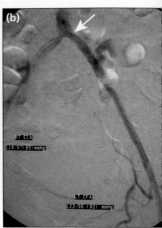

**Table 16.1** Indications for arterial stenting

| Indication | Primary | Secondary |
| --- | --- | --- |
| Failed angioplasty | ✗ | ✓ |
| Risk of embolization | ✓ | ✗ |
| Iliac occlusion | ✓ | ✗ |
| Ostial RAS | ✓ | ✗ |
| Restenosis | ✓ | ✗ |
| Carotid artery | ✓ | ✗ |

# Stent terminology

There are many stents in a crowded market. A few descriptors will help you understand what the company representative is talking about.

*Balloon-mounted* No prizes for guessing what this means. Most come ready attached to the balloon; very few now have to be crimped in place by the operator.

*Self-expanding* These have inherent radial force leading them to tend to expand to their rated diameter. In practice, angioplasty is also necessary.

*Material* Most balloon expandable stents and the Wallstent are made of alloys of stainless steel, and virtually all new self-expanding stents are made of nickel titanium alloys (Nitinol). Nitinol has a 'thermal memory' and expands to a preset diameter at body temperature.

*Additional properties* The stent surface can have different finishes or coatings or properties such as drug elution or radioactivity. Although there is evidence regarding their use in the coronary arteries, the value of these is unproven in the peripheral circulation.

*Lattice or mesh* This is formed by stent struts or by overlapping braided wires.

*Open or closed cell structure* This refers to how stent rings are interlinked. Closed cell designs have links between each element, whereas open cell stents have fewer links. This affects stent flexibility and radial force. Open cell designs are the most flexible and closed cell stents have the greatest radial strength. Open cell designs have greater gaps in surface coverage, which is sometimes a disadvantage, as plaque can prolapse through the gap.

*Markers* Markers may be on the stent, the delivery system or both. They show the stent position, orientation (in stent-grafts) and degree of deployment. Markers are also used to indicate degree of overlap between components. As Nitinol is not very radio-opaque, many stents have platinum or tantalum markers on the stent crowns.

 **Alarm:** Positioning and significance of markers on stents and stent-grafts is specific to each device and may have important implications for successful deployment, especially in complex cases where multiple devices are used. Make sure you are familiar with the system you are using before starting.

Some stents, such as the Wallstent and some balloon expandable stents, shorten during deployment. This has largely been overcome on newer stent designs and modern self-expanding stents can be deployed very precisely.

In practice, everyone has their own favourite stents, but in reality, within individual stent groups and particularly for Nitinol stents, there is not a great deal to choose between manufacturers. There are circumstances, however, which need strength and those which require flexibility either to reach their destination or to conform to vessel curvature.

# Balloon-mounted stents

Most balloon-mounted stents are made of stainless steel; balloon dilation is necessary to expand them to their working diameter. Once deployed, most have high radial strength. There is usually some shortening during deployment but this is very predictable unless the stent is expanded beyond its recommended working range, in which case marked shortening will occur. Balloon-mounted stents tend to be less flexible than their self-expanding counterparts and are less suited for use in tortuous vessels or at points of flexion. Stents are typically oversized by 1 mm to ensure secure fixation when deployed. Balloon expandable stents can be 'flared' within their rated range of diameter by using balloons of different size to deploy them; if this is important, start with the smaller diameter.

Balloon-mounted stents may be purchased separately and manually crimped onto an appropriately-sized balloon at the time of the procedure. This is becoming unpopular, as such stents are never as well gripped as a factory crimped stent and it only takes one to go walkabout to persuade most operators to carry a greater stock of devices to cater for different diameters and lengths. A properly mounted stent grips securely on the balloon; this is essential to prevent migration. If the stent slides on the balloon, STOP. Do not attempt to deploy it or both you and the stent will 'come unstuck'.

Some stents require an introducer to pass through the sheath's haemostatic valve. Failure to do so will result in the stent dislodging from the balloon before it is in the patient. This may also occur during the stent's passage to and across the deployment site, and is one of the reasons for using guide-catheters.

 **Tip:** Many angioplasty balloons have a hydrophilic coating to help them pass through tight strictures. This virtually guarantees that the stent will not stay in place. Try inflating and deflating the balloon before crimping the stent in place. Increased friction is obtained at the price of a slight loss of profile.

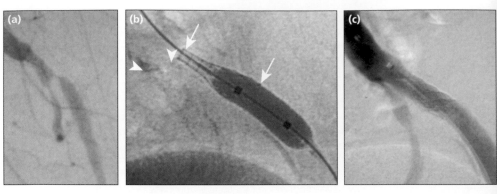

**Fig. 16.2** ■ (A) High-grade calcified EIA stenosis prior to femoropopliteal grafting. (B) During deployment the balloon has 'been pushed out' of the stent (arrows); note the stent has not moved and remains perfectly placed in relation to the origin of the IIA (chevrons). In this case the balloon was deflated and repositioned to deploy the remainder of the stent. (C) Completion angiogram.

## Troubleshooting

There are some well-known potential pitfalls with balloon-mounted stents, which can sometimes be prevented or salvaged if recognized early. When things do go wrong, try to keep the situation in perspective. Remember not to cause more harm than necessary. It is often best to summon a more senior colleague or obtain surgical help.

**The stent moves proximal or distal to the balloon markers prior to deployment (Fig. 16.2)** Do not attempt deployment if either end of the stent has moved outside the balloon markers. If there has been significant stent movement, asymmetrical balloon inflation will push the stent off the balloon.

   **If the whole stent remains on the balloon**:
- Partially inflate the balloon with contrast as this helps the stent to grip the balloon.
- Attempt to reposition the stent over the stenosis.
- If the stent begins to migrate, deflate the balloon and gently try to recapture the stent. If this fails, then it is probably best to deploy this stent either where it is or, even better, at a safe site such as the CIA.
- If repositioning is successful, slowly inflate the balloon. Deploy the stent as normal if it remains in position.

   **If the stent has come off the balloon**:
- Find the stent! It is usually on the catheter shaft or in the groin sheath. Some stents are poorly opaque and it may be necessary to take spot radiographs to locate them.
- Withdraw the stent into the sheath, then remove sheath and catheter and insert a new sheath (use one that you have prepared earlier). Do not forget to crimp the stent on this time when you reuse it.
- If you are unlucky, the stent will come completely off the balloon but will still be on the wire. This is much harder! Pass a 4Fr straight catheter through the stent and exchange for a 0.018-inch wire. Try to capture the stent with a small profile angioplasty balloon. Alternatively, pass a gooseneck snare alongside the guidewire and snare the stent by lassoing the wire.

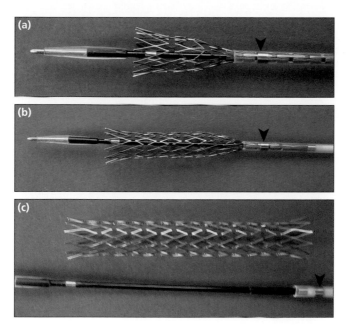

**Fig. 16.3** ■ A self-expanding stent opening as the outer sheath is retracted. Note that the distal marker (arrowheads) moves back with the sheath but the stent remains in the original position.

# Self-expanding stents and stent-grafts

In their compressed state, these devices are constrained by a sheath or membrane that prevents them from expanding. This acts as the delivery catheter to take the stent to the target. The stent automatically expands as it is progressively uncovered by withdrawing the sheath (Fig. 16.3).

## Deploying self-expanding stents

All of the current systems deploy in one of the following ways; none is complicated once the basic principles have been grasped. Each is just a method for removing the stent covering while leaving the stent correctly positioned at the target site.

*Pusher and sheath system* This was the original technique and variations on the theme are the basis for most systems. Some aortic stent grafts and IVC filters also function in this way.

1. A long sheath is placed at the target deployment site.
2. The 'device' comes separate from the delivery sheath. It is typically held in a cartridge and introduced into the delivery sheath using a 'pusher'; this is just a blunt ended dilator.
3. The pusher is used to advance the stent to the end of the sheath.
4. The action now reverses; the pusher is held completely still to maintain the position of the stent and the sheath is retracted, progressively releasing the stent as it is exposed (Fig. 16.4).

*Pusher and sheath incorporated into a single delivery catheter* This is the most common contemporary mechanism and is the basis for deploying many stents and stent-grafts. To deploy the stent, the central component of the catheter is fixed in position and the outer sheath manually pulled back (Fig. 16.5).

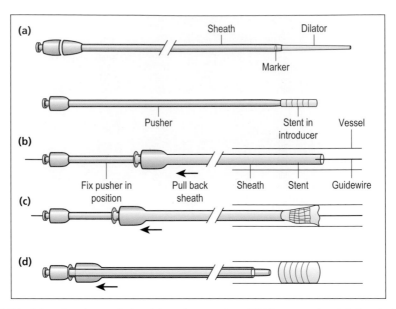

**Fig. 16.4** ■ Principles of pusher and sheath introducer system. (A) The outer sheath is inserted just beyond the target site using a tapering dilator. The dilator is removed and the pusher used to introduce the stent into the sheath. (B) The pusher is advanced until the stent is at the target site. The pusher is then fixed in position and the sheath pulled back. (C) Continue pulling back the sheath to progressively deploy the stent. (D) When the sheath is fully retracted, the stent is deployed.

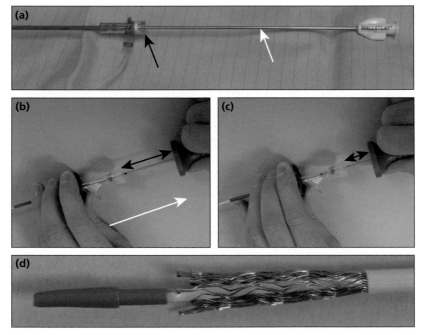

**Fig. 16.5** ■ Deploying a stent using an integrated pusher and sheath delivery system. (A) Delivery sheath (black arrow) and pusher (white arrow). (B, C) The pusher is fixed and the sheath pulled back (white arrow) until the stent is deployed. (D) Stent opening as it is unsheathed.

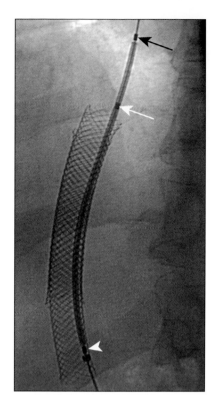

**Fig. 16.6** ▪ Wallstent markers shown during a TIPS revision. The distal marker (white arrowhead), the proximal marker (black arrow) and the 'critical marker' (white arrow) which indicates roughly the point to which the stent will shorten and the limit of deployment for resheathing.

**A note on using the Wallstent** Its braided construction allows it to conform to different diameters but also results in significant shortening during deployment. Because of this, it is best restricted to situations where precise positioning is not critical. The deployed length of the Wallstent depends on the final diameter. A chart on the back of the packaging helps you predict how long the stent will be, e.g. a 10 × 68-mm long Wallstent is roughly 95 mm long when constrained, and it will shorten to 83 mm long at its minimum recommended diameter of 7 mm. It is 77 mm long at 8 mm and 69 mm at 9 mm. The markers at the end of the Wallstent delivery catheter bear little relation to the final position of the stent (Fig. 16.6). The critical marker lies closer to the proximal end; this indicates the limit to which the stent may be deployed and still resheathed, and roughly where the proximal end of the unconstrained stent will shorten to. Because the constrained length of the Wallstent is so much greater than the deployed length, it is not suitable for use in situations where there is little space beyond the target.

**Tip:** It is common practice to start with the distal end of the Wallstent well beyond the target site. When the stent has partially opened, it can be pulled back until the 'critical' marker is in position. This is fine in TIPS or in superior vena cava obstruction (SVCO), but is best avoided in an occluded iliac artery unless you are intending to embolize the run-off.

*'Trigger' and 'screw' systems* All these systems are a modification of the pusher and sheath and incorporate either a trigger mechanism or a screw mechanism to gradually unsheath the stent. Trigger systems can be operated one-handed, and less coordination is required to deploy them.

*Ripcord system* This is currently exclusive to stent-grafts manufactured by Gore and is employed on devices used in aortic aneurysm, peripheral circulation and TIPS. The stent is held constrained by a fabric cover rather than a sheath. Pulling the ripcord undoes the seam and releases the stent-graft.

 **Alarm:** The positioning markers are different in different systems! On some systems the markers are on the stent, on some they are on the delivery catheter and on others a combination of both. Check that you are familiar with the device you have chosen, especially if the markers do not correspond to the final position of the stent. Failure to appreciate this will lead to malpositioning.

## Choosing that stent

Basically, you will use what your boss likes, but there are some factors that influence whether you reach for a balloon expandable or self-expanding stent. The check box lists the factors that should be considered in individual cases (Fig. 16.7).

- **Strength of the stent** – balloon expandable stents tend to exert the greatest radial force; this can be advantageous in calcified lesions.
- **Precise positioning** – the Wallstent is probably best avoided in these circumstances as it can shorten unpredictably even in experienced hands. In the past, critical positioning was an indication to choose a balloon-mounted stent. This is no longer the case; most self-expanding stents can be deployed as accurately as their balloon-mounted counterparts (Fig. 16.1). The reasons for this are enhanced visibility of the stent and near elimination of shortening on modern designs.
- **Conformability** – in general, self-expanding stents are better at conforming to the vessel wall, particularly where there are changes in calibre or there is tortuosity. However, newer open cell balloon expandable stents tend to be less rigid. Balloon expandable stents can be dilated to different diameters (obviously this requires more than one balloon) but as the smallest balloon is used first, the potential for migration is greater.

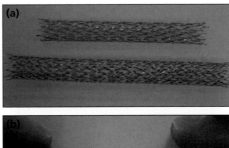
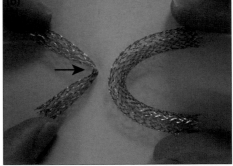

**Fig. 16.7** ■ Differences in stent properties: the shorter stent (Sinus-Repo, OptiMed) has higher radial force and can be resheathed but is more prone to kinking (arrow). The longer stent is more flexible (Sinus-SuperFlex, OptiMed).

- **Risk of compression post deployment** – avoid balloon expandable stents and think hard whether you really want a stent at all. There have been several reports of balloon expandable stents being deformed by external compression, e.g. in the carotid, subclavian and popliteal arteries. In these circumstances, a self-expanding stent is better but even this may be damaged by repeated compression.
- **Future imaging** – if MRA is part of your plan for follow-up, stick with Nitinol; the latest designs will cause minimal artefact. Forget about using a stainless steel stent, the susceptibility artefact will obscure all the vascular detail.
- **Might need to resheath the stent** – the only stents currently available that can be resheathed when partially deployed are the Wallstent and the SuperFlex.

 **Alarm:** Nitinol stents must be accurately sized. Unlike balloon-mounted stents, they cannot be overexpanded; they will recoil back to their nominal diameter. A Nitinol stent needs to be 1–2 mm larger in diameter than the target vessel.

## Guide to safe stenting

Stenting is usually a straightforward procedure.

- Obtain the best possible angiogram centred over the deployment site.
- Use fluoroscopy fade or bony landmarks to identify the deployment site. A useful technique is to ask an assistant to mark important landmarks on the monitor with a chinagraph pencil. The stent can then be deployed relative to these; remember to stand in the same position to avoid parallax.
- **Never** move the table or image intensifier once in position. Parallax will affect the landmarks.
- Consider the implications of incorrect positioning, in particular the effects of covering vital vessels! If necessary protect these with guidewires or balloons.
- Measure the lesion length and the diameters of the normal vessel proximal and distal to it. Choose the correct size stent. Most modern angiography equipment has the facility to make measurements. If this is not available, then use either a calibrated catheter or balloon or an external ruler.
- Position the stent.
- Perform a check angiogram to confirm the position of the stent and markers before deployment – this is the time to be sure that you know the significance of each marker (Fig. 16.8).
- Use continuous fluoroscopy while deploying the stent. Take your time!
- Screen during withdrawal of the delivery system.
- Use angioplasty to 'tailor' the stent to the vessel wall. All stents, including self-expanding stents, need a balloon for complete deployment.
- Perform completion angiography and pressure measurements and check run-off vessels for distal embolization.

## Troubleshooting

### Ooops, I didn't size the diameter correctly, my stent looks too small and looks as though it will migrate

*Balloon deployed stent* Okay – this can be easily rescued. Use a 50-mL syringe to deflate the balloon as much as possible. Continue to apply suction to maintain a low profile, then carefully withdraw the balloon from the stent. Screen during removal of the balloon if the stent isn't opposed to the wall. It is all too easy to accidentally displace the stent. Make sure you keep the guidewire access in situ. Now insert an appropriately-sized balloon and dilate the stent up.

**Fig. 16.8** ■ Stent positioning and deployment in iliac stenosis. (A) Angiogram from the contralateral iliac, stent markers (white arrowheads). (B) Post deployment and angioplasty, stent position (white arrowheads).

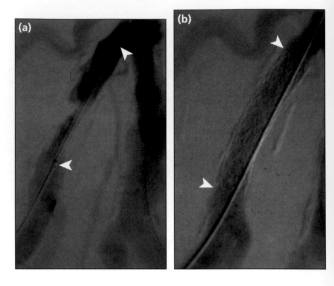

*Self-expanding stent* Hmmm, a little trickier. You have two options, depending on how much space you have on either side of the stent. If you have space, you can deploy an overlapping larger diameter self-expanding stent; this will secure the smaller stent, but the second stent seldom has enough strength to open out the initial Nitinol stent further. If there is no space, then an alternative possibility is to insert a balloon expandable stent within the self-expanding; the second stent will be strong enough to oppose the Nitinol stent to the wall. It's best to pick a similar length of stent.

# Stent-grafts

Besides EVAR, one of the most important indications for using stent-grafts is the treatment of vessel rupture during angioplasty. **All catheter laboratories should keep one or two stent-grafts in reserve specifically to treat this eventuality**. Your patient and their lawyer will expect you to know how to use it!

Covered stents reline the vessel and hence treat ruptures, exclude aneurysms and may prevent restenosis (Fig. 16.9). They are an attractive concept but are still in evolution.

Various stent coverings are available, with the most common being Dacron (polyester) and ePTFE (polytetrafluoroethylene). Polycarbonate, woven Nitinol and autologous vein have also been used. In order to reduce the profile of the delivery catheters, the graft material is thin-walled compared with conventional surgical grafts, and in the long term their durability is uncertain. The proximal and distal portions of the device are often uncovered to improve anchorage.

## Stent-graft terminology

*Straight* Straight grafts are most commonly used in iliac artery aneurysm or to repair post-traumatic false aneurysm or arterial rupture.

*Tapered* Tapered grafts are needed when there is discrepancy between vessel diameters at the proximal and distal anchorage sites, e.g. in aorto uni-iliac grafts.

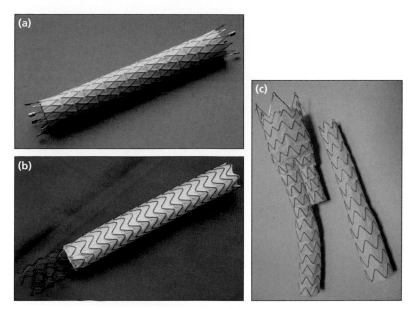

**Fig. 16.9** ■ Three different types of stent-graft: (A) peripheral – Fluency (Bard); (B) TIPS – Viator (Gore); and (C) aortic – Endurant (Medtronic).

*Birfucated* Bifurcated stent-grafts are used to repair abdominal aortic aneurysms that extend into the common iliac vessels. They divide into two limbs: the ipsilateral limb is typically combined with the larger diameter body (like a tapered graft) and the contralateral limb plugs into a socket in the body.

*Fenestrated* Fenestrated grafts are custom-made and have notches fabricated in the sides corresponding to the position of branch vessels that need to be preserved, e.g. the renal arteries. Fenestrated grafts are suitable in aneurysms in which the neck is short but of normal calibre.

*Branched* This is the next step in the evolution from fenestrated grafts intended for use in ectatic and aneurysmal necks. Here, the branches are used to bridge the gap between the stent-graft and the vessel to be preserved.

# Stent-grafting – basic rules

Stent grafting is not dissimilar to stenting but the margins for error are fewer. For a stent-graft to be effective, it must fit precisely within the target vessel. An undersized graft will allow blood to flow between it and the vessel wall. Oversized devices will have creases in the graft material which may adversely affect flow, lead to endoleaks and promote thrombosis. **Calibrated angiography** and CT are usually used to measure the target vessel dimensions. In general, the stent-graft diameter should be 10–20% greater than the diameter of the implantation site. Length is also important; too long a covered stent may occlude important branch vessels.

**Spontaneous and iatrogenic arterial rupture** Use similar principles to choosing a stent for occlusive disease. Choose a device that is long enough to cover the defect in the artery wall and is an appropriate diameter (i.e. oversized by at least 1 mm). Remember that it may be

**Fig. 16.10** ■ The great escape: (A) A 13.5Fr dialysis catheter has been placed in the right common carotid artery. The low puncture (arrow) would necessitate a thoracotomy to repair surgically. (B) Following placement of a Wallgraft (Boston Scientific), the dialysis catheter was removed without bleeding after the graft was placed. Note the end of the graft (arrow) overhangs the origin of the subclavian artery. Covering the hole was much more important than the potential for arm ischaemia.

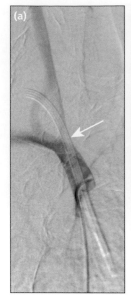
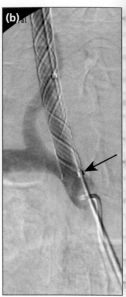

necessary to increase the size of your arterial sheath; most stent-grafts require at least an 8Fr sheath. Choose the stent-graft that is simplest to use and most likely to do the job effectively.

**Three devices to 'Get out of jail free':** You must have the equivalent of at least one of these on your shelf and know how to use it, unless you want to support a lawyer.

- **Balloon deployable** (e.g. Jostent, Abbott Vascular) – a simple PTFE stent graft that is crimped onto an angioplasty balloon and deployed as a conventional balloon-mounted stent. Advantage is that a single device can treat a range of diameters (4–9 mm); the disadvantages are that it is less flexible, will be more difficult to get around tortuous vessels and will not conform as well to variation in arterial calibre as a self-expanding graft.
- **Wallgraft** – a variation of the Wallstent – if you can use the Wallstent you can use this. Tends to shorten like the Wallstent. Not the number one choice if working close to critical branch vessels (Fig. 16.10).
- **Self-expanding** (e.g. Fluency, Bard) – effectively like deploying a Nitinol stent with similar shortening and other characteristics. Remember, if it is Nitinol-based you really need to make sure you deploy the correct size as you can't simply balloon it up – the Nitinol recoils (See above for troubleshooting solution).

**Occlusive disease** Stent-grafts are currently being evaluated for use in occlusive disease in situations where angioplasty and stenting are ineffective. The principal goal is the treatment of long segment stenosis or occlusion of the superficial femoral and popliteal arteries. There is no current evidence to suggest that stent-grafts are more effective than uncovered stents in the iliac arteries.

# Suggestions for further reading

Nosher JL, Chung J, Brevetti LS, **et al**. Visceral and renal artery aneurysms: a pictorial essay on endovascular therapy. Radiographics 2006;26:1687–1704.

# 17

# Endovascular aneurysm repair (EVAR)

Interest in endovascular treatment of aortic and other aneurysms is increasing. The technique and technology continue to evolve and improve. Delivery systems are simpler and lower profile, and grafts are more durable and much more readily available, in a vast range of lengths and diameters. There is no financial advantage in using stent-grafting to treat AAA. The patient benefits are in terms of reduced physiological stress during the procedure (no aortic cross-clamping, less peripheral ischaemia, reduced blood loss) and also a shorter convalescence (no abdominal wound). Large randomized trials show that operative mortality in 'fit' patients undergoing EVAR is roughly a third of that in patients treated by open operative repair. The price is a greater need for long-term surveillance and repeat intervention.

There is not enough space to cover the nuances of every clinical scenario and each device, so the emphasis here is on generic aspects of terminology, assessment for stent-grafting and basic principles of deployment of devices.

## EVAR terminology

**Endovascular abdominal aortic aneurysm repair (EVAR)** With conventional bifurcated and aorto uni-iliac (or AUI as the cool operators term them) devices, roughly a third of patients with AAAs will be straightforward to treat. Another third will be untreatable, mainly owing to lack of suitable implantation sites, awkward angulations or difficulty with access. The remainder may be treatable but would be expected to be more challenging and higher risk.

AUI systems are most frequently used when the CIAs are so aneurysmal that a seal is not possible within the artery with a bifurcated device. The uni-iliac limb is deployed within the EIA and the contralateral iliac artery is occluded, followed by a fem-fem cross-over. AUI devices are also favoured by some in emergency EVAR as they allow more rapid control of the leaking AAA (Fig. 17.1).

**Aneurysm exclusion with a straight stent-graft** Less than 10% of AAA will be suited to a tube graft. The main use for tube grafts will be the treatment of thoracic aortic pathologies, arterial rupture, iliac aneurysm and false aneurysm repair (Fig. 17.2). If you can accurately deploy a stent, then you should have no difficulty deploying a straight stent-graft. If not, the best place to learn is to insert the contralateral iliac limb during a bifurcated stent-graft.

**Endovascular thoracic aortic aneurysm repair (TEVAR)** The greatest advantage of endovascular repair is likely to be in patients with thoracic aortic aneurysm (TAA), acute aortic dissection with ischaemic sequelae and in traumatic aortic rupture. TEVAR is increasingly used in aortic syndromes such as penetrating ulcer and intramural haematoma.

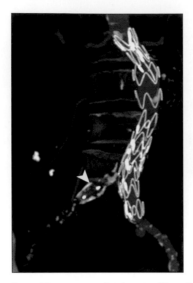

**Fig. 17.1** ■ AUI stent graft in a patient with a narrow distal aorta. Note the Amplatzer plug in the contralateral CIA (yellow arrowhead). A left to right cross-over graft supplies the right leg.

Avoiding a thoracotomy substantially reduces morbidity and mortality compared with surgical repair. TEVAR should be performed on an installation that allows 30–60° LAO angulation.

 **Alarm:** The feared complication of TEVAR is paraplegia due to spinal ischaemia. This is most likely if there is extensive coverage of the dorsal aorta and previous AAA repair. If there is any sign of paraplegia developing, cerebrospinal fluid (CSF) drainage should be instituted.

**Emergency endovascular abdominal aortic aneurysm repair (E-EVAR)** This is the repair of ruptured aneurysms, and traumatic aortic injury is a specialist service requiring a team of interventional radiologists, surgeons and anaesthetists, a suitable environment with high-quality imaging and a cupboard full of stent-grafts. E-EVAR is only practicable in centres where these are readily and rapidly available and in certain centres this might be logistically possible during the day but not out of hours.

# Assessment for endovascular stent-grafting

Endovascular aneurysm repair requires far more detailed assessment than is necessary for surgery.

- **Computed tomography with multiplanar reformats** is currently the method of choice and has largely replaced angiography using calibrated catheters. CT is able to accurately measure the diameters, lengths and angulation of the aneurysm, its neck and the iliac arteries (Fig. 17.3).

 **Tip:** Use suitably wide windows when reviewing the images to allow you to distinguish between calcification in the vessel wall and contrast enhancement in the lumen.

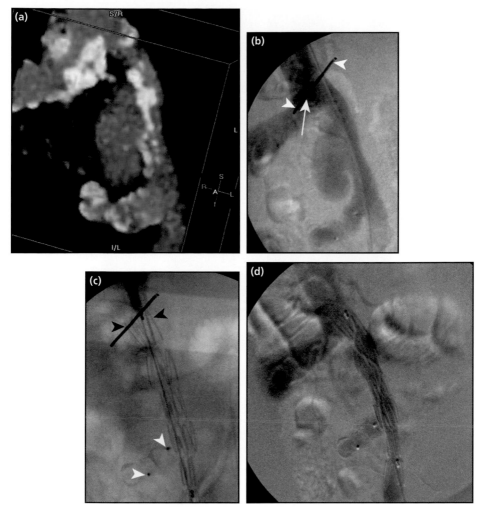

**Fig. 17.2** ■ Endovascular repair of left CIA aneurysm using a tapered graft. (A) CT reformat shows morphology, allows accurate sizing and appropriate view. (B, C) Photographs of the angiographic display showing chinagraph pencil (white arrowheads) marking the target drop zone; the proximal CIA is shown by the yellow arrow. (C) Stent-graft has been deployed according to the marker. Note the Amplatzer device (yellow arrowheads) occluding the IIA. (D) Completion angiogram showing exclusion of the aneurysm. Note that the graft is flush with the origin of the CIA and only appears to overlap the contralateral CIA.

- **MRI** is not widely used to assess AAA due to limited availability. It can offer similar information to CT but with the disadvantage that calcification is not as readily appreciated. Remember that MRA only shows the flowing lumen and other sequences are required to assess the true extent of the aneurysm and the vessel wall.
- **Ultrasound** can be used to assess peripheral arteries for tube graft repair, as only simple diameter and length measurements are needed. Ultrasound does not provide sufficient information for EVAR.
- **Calibrated angiography** is only needed when CT/MRI with reformats is not available (see Chapter 16, Stents and Stent-Grafts) (Fig. 17.4).

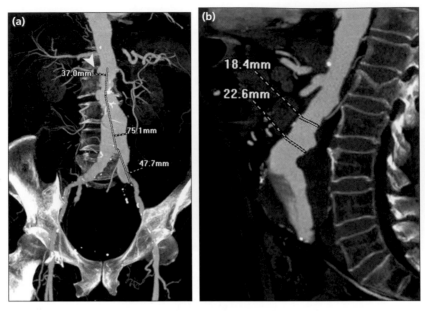

**Fig. 17.3** ■ Use of CT to assess AAA suitability for EVAR. (A) Coronal MIP allowing lengths to be assessed. Yellow arrowhead indicates level of the renal arteries. (B) Sagittal MIP showing angulation of the neck.

**Fig. 17.4** ■ CT reformat (A) and calibrated angiogram (B) of a patient with AAA.

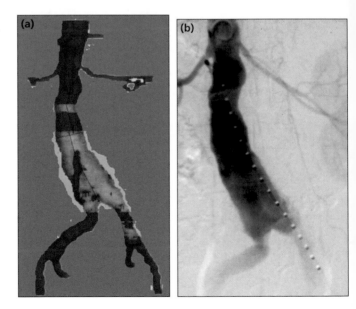

**What to look for** There are three As of aneurysm repair to assess.

## Access: The common femoral and iliac arteries

Currently available devices are introduced via 18–28Fr (6–9 mm) sheaths. If the access vessels are too small, diseased or tortuous, you will be unable to insert the delivery system.

## Contraindications

- **Technical challenge**: more than one ≥90° angulation, especially if there is heavy vascular calcification, which makes the arteries rigid.
- **Too narrow**: iliac artery diameter <7 mm. Another access issue occurs when the distal aorta is too small; this can prevent access for a contralateral iliac limb.

## Solutions

- Inadequate access can be remedied by providing alternative routes, such as cutdown onto the iliac arteries and placement of a temporary conduit. In some cases angioplasty will suffice to treat a focal stenosis.
- Distal aorta too small: in this case use an AUI graft and femoro-femoral cross-over graft, but don't forget to occlude the contralateral side as otherwise the aneurysm sac will be perfused (Type II endoleak) via retrograde flow.

 **Alarm:** Take great care that a delivery catheter does not jam in the iliac arteries during insertion or removal as it is quite possible to avulse the iliac artery during over-zealous manoeuvres. This is fatal unless you have a swift and decisive surgeon or have anticipated the situation with an aortic balloon in place and ready to inflate. In either case, the procedure is likely to convert to open repair, defeating the whole object of EVAR.

# Anchorage sites

These are the points at which the stent graft makes a seal with the arterial wall. These must be of suitable diameter and length for the proximal and distal stents.

## Contraindications

- **Technical challenge**: the following make the procedure more difficult and more likely to go wrong: proximal neck length less than 10 mm, proximal neck angulation ≥60°, conical neck (especially if enlarging distally).
- **Suboptimal surface**: extensive thrombus or atheroma within the neck makes achieving a seal less likely and migration more likely.

## Solutions

- In theory, all issues with the proximal neck can be remedied by the use of grafts with suprarenal fixation (Fig. 17.5) or fenestrated grafts which have a greater contact with the wall or branched grafts which anchor proximally in the 'normal' aorta. In practice, consider whether this will be better for the patient than an open repair.

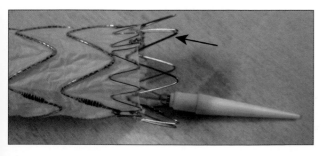

**Fig. 17.5** ■ Graft with anchor stent (arrow) proximal to graft material.

**Tip:** If the neck is short and angulated, then use reformats to assess the optimal obliquity to use for positioning angiography during graft deployment.

## Adequate visceral blood supply

Branch vessels have important implications for stent-grafting and must be assessed on the pre-procedural angiograms. The stent-graft must not cover vital arteries to the intestine, kidneys or brain, etc.

### Contraindications

- **Aberrant vessels**: low renal artery origin. Aberrant branch vessels from the aortic arch.
- **Essential vessels**: the inferior mesenteric artery (IMA) will be covered during stent-grafting; if the SMA is severely diseased, bowel infarction is likely.
- **Unwanted vessels**: branch vessels may adversely affect aneurysm exclusion, e.g. when treating an iliac artery aneurysm, retrograde flow through a patent IIA would leave the aneurysm perfused.

### Solutions

- **Aberrant vessels**: simply decide if the vessel can be sacrificed e.g. a small accessory renal artery.
- **Essential vessels**: some aneurysms can be made suitable for EVAR by performing extra anatomical grafting to prevent ischaemia, e.g. femoro-femoral cross-over. In other cases, the length of the anchorage site can be increased by more complex surgery, e.g. carotid subclavian bypass grafts, mesenteric/renal bypass or anastomosis of the carotid and subclavian arteries to a graft from the ascending aorta. Others can be treated with fenestrated or branched grafts.
- **Unwanted vessels**: in these circumstances, the artery should be embolized prior to deployment of the stent-graft to prevent type II endoleak, e.g. IIA. The same applies when the left subclavian artery is covered during TEVAR. The IMA and large lumbar arteries may be embolized pre-procedure.

## Deployment of a modular bifurcated stent-graft (Fig. 17.6)

This is a complex practical procedure that requires a well-integrated team of vascular surgeons and radiologists and cannot be learnt from a book. Training usually commences on a simulated aneurysm before performing in vivo deployment. The general concept of graft deployment will be considered but details of individual devices will not be included.

## Stent-graft deployment: a step-by-step guide
### Phase 1: surgical pause

1. Check that everyone involved knows the plan for deployment, approach, choice of graft/s, anticipated difficulties and any arteries that will be preserved (usually the lowest renal) or sacrificed, e.g. small accessory renal, lumbar, IMA.
2. Check everyone knows their roles.

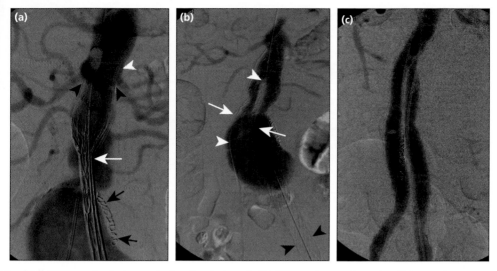

**Fig. 17.6** ■ Stages in deployment of aortic stent graft. (A) $CO_2$ angiogram through a Cobra catheter positioned just above the renal arteries (white arrowhead). The graft is partly open, the upper stent crowns (black arrowheads) are immediately below the renal arteries and the graft has been deployed as far as the white arrow. Note coils in the IMA (black arrows). (B) Angiogram following deployment of the body and ipsilateral limb (black arrowheads). The catheter (arrowheads) has been pulled back and used to cannulate the contralateral limb (white arrows) of the stent graft. (C) Completion angiogram showing aneurysm exclusion.

3. Check that you have all the kit you anticipate needing and any back-up equipment – balloons, wires, snares, stents, catheters and additional stent-grafts/extensions.
4. Use fluoroscopy to demonstrate the graft markers and ensure that it is correctly oriented before you place it in the patient – it can be almost impossible to rotate the delivery system once it is in the patient!

## Troubleshooting

If there is a problem at this stage that cannot be resolved – don't start the case.

## Phase 2: access

5. Surgical cutdown* to access the CFA to allow introducer placement. Vascular slings are placed around the upper CFA, the SFA and PFA, as well as any large branches. Tightening these maintains haemostasis.
6. A 6Fr sheath is inserted into each CFA. Puncture the vessel in its mid-portion away from any obvious large plaque. **Ensure that there is room for you to hold the artery between two fingers above the puncture**. This will allow you to support the vessel during graft insertion and compress it during exchanges.
7. A catheter is passed from the ipsilateral CFA into the thoracic aorta; negotiating out of the aneurysm can be harder than you might expect.
8. A highly supportive 260-cm guidewire is passed into the thoracic aorta just distal to the arch (note the position of the end of the wire on the drapes as this will give you an

*EVAR can be performed percutaneously using a suture device to 'pre-close' the artery.

indication that the tip remains in the correct place); this wire will be used to insert the stent-graft.

# Troubleshooting

*Insufficient space to control the artery* This is not a time for compromise; extend the incision and if necessary divide the inguinal ligament.

*Severely diseased common femoral arteries* This should not be a surprise, as they were included in the assessment. If necessary, perform endarterectomies or consider access via the external iliac artery or a temporary conduit.

## Phase 3: Positioning

**EITHER** (useful if the proximal neck is short)

9.  Catheterize the lower renal artery from the contralateral CFA and insert a supportive 0.018-inch wire well into the artery. Bring the catheter back to the proximal artery. This marks the position of the renal artery for stent-graft deployment. Check whether the catheter runs along the upper or lower border of the artery (go to 11). If you use a Tuohy–Borst adaptor you can perform positioning angiography around the wire; with the catheter in the proximal artery, contrast will reflux into the aorta.

**OR** (used in the majority of cases)

10.  Place a pigtail catheter at the level of the renal arteries from the contralateral groin.
11.  Perform initial angiography to demonstrate the neck and renal arteries. Use the optimal oblique projection; this was assessed from the pre operative CT.
12.  Check the graft orientation and then insert the delivery system until the top of the graft (covered stent) is just above the renal arteries.
13.  Perform a magnified angiogram to demonstrate the position of the renal arteries. The table is locked in position and the exact level of the lowest renal artery is marked on the monitor using a suitable pen or chinagraph pencil (check with a friendly radiographer before using an indelible marker on the screen!).

# Troubleshooting

*Unable to catheterize the renal artery* Go back to basic principles of catheterization: use the correct catheter wire combination.

*Cannot see renal arteries* Try repositioning the catheter and trying alternative projection.

*Contrast does not reflux from the renal artery into the aorta* Pull back the catheter to the arterial ostium.

## Phase 4 Deployment of the body

14.  Using continuous fluoroscopy, start deployment of the stent-graft just above the renal arteries.
15.  As the graft starts to open, perform fine positioning so that deployment will be immediately caudal to the lowest artery you are intending to preserve (almost invariably the renal that you have marked!).

16. Perform additional runs as needed, to confirm position. Remember you can still do this if you are using the catheter and wire in the renal artery.
17. Fully deploy** the aortic component of the graft, which, depending on the device, may include the ipsilateral iliac arterial limb.
18. Resheath the nose cone of the delivery device in accordance with the manufacturer's instructions!
19. Remove the initial introducer system, either leaving a sheath in position or immediately insert a secondary device if required. Remember, haemostasis can be achieved by tightening the arterial sling.

# Troubleshooting

*The device starts to migrate cranially during deployment* It is important to recognize this early, before there is extensive wall apposition. Under fluoroscopy, simply apply steady downward traction and the device will normally move down in a controlled fashion. If the device will not move, you will realize the value of a protection wire in the renal artery that you have just covered!

*The device starts to migrate caudally during deployment* Keep calm, you cannot advance the device once it is in apposition with the vessel wall. If the neck is sufficiently long, deploy as normal, bearing in mind that you are likely to end up more distal than intended and might cover an IIA. If the neck is short, the device is likely to migrate into the sac if it slips further; this is very bad! Deploy the contralateral limb and then use the introducer to hold the device in position. Catheterize the contralateral limb from below and deploy an aortic cuff to fix the device in place.

*The nose cone will not resheath* Use fluoroscopy to try to identify the problem. Do not just tug it backwards as this may well cause the graft to migrate. Usually the delivery system can be advanced to a different position and then you can try again. If this fails, you are in trouble. Sometimes the nosecone can be controlled by snaring it from the arm, on other occasions conversion to an open repair is needed.

## Phase 5 Deployment of the contralateral limb

20. The contralateral iliac limb stump must now be catheterized.
21. Insert another stiff wire the same distance as the first one.
22. If you are intending to preserve the IIA, now is the time to check where it is by performing a suitably angulated angiogram. After wiping off the marker for the renal artery, you can mark the IIA's position on the intensifier screen.
23. Insert the contralateral limb deployment system and line up markers to ensure sufficient overlap with the body of the graft and avoid covering the IIA.
24. Deploy the contralateral iliac limb.

# Troubleshooting

*Direct catheterization of the contralateral limb from the iliac artery can be difficult in a large aneurysm* Usually a forward-facing catheter such as a Berenstein will do the job; if this fails,

---

**Some operators prefer to only deploy the graft until the contralateral limb is open in order to preserve an element of stability if the graft position is 'tenuous'.

try a USL shape. The tip forms in the aneurysm sac and can angle perfectly to catheterize the contralateral limb. An alternative is to approach from over the neobifurcation using a reverse curve catheter such as a Sos Ommi or USL. In this case, the wire is snared in the aneurysm sac from the contralateral groin; this is usually much harder than you would think.

Rarely, a brachial puncture is required and a wire manipulated through the contralateral limb and snared into the sheath via the contralateral access.

## Phase 6 Completion angiography (sometimes a misnomer as this is the start of all the trouble!)

25. Place a pigtail above the graft and perform angiography in AP and oblique projections to look for position, perigraft leak, perfusion of important vessels.

# Troubleshooting

*Flow through the graft is very slow* This may be because we are blocking the outflow with large sheaths. The easiest trick here is to simply attach a 20-mL syringe to the side-arm of the sheaths and aspirate during the contrast injection.

*Contrast seen outside the graft within the sac* Decide whether it is:

- **Type I**: around the graft anchorage points (not a snug fit!). If the graft is in the correct position, try inflating a moulding balloon in the neck until its sides are parallel with the graft wall (this is not angioplasty!). If leak persists, try again and then try a large stent to improve anchorage. If the graft is too low, then an extension cuff will probably be needed to create a seal (it is one of the items you checked at the start of the case). If the leak persists, try the moulding balloon/stent again. If it remains more than a tiny amount after this, consider converting to open repair. Very small leaks will sometimes seal if left for the anticoagulation to wear off.
- **Type II**: via collateral vessels, lumbar arteries and IMA. Ignore unless they subsequently lead to sac expansion.
- **Type III**: limb dislocation. Insert another limb to bridge the gap.
- **Type IV**: leakage through the graft material due to porosity; this will settle when the heparin wears off.

# Suggestions for further reading

NCEPOD report into aortic aneurysm. 2005.
  Available at: www.ncepod.org.uk/2005report2/
  aneurysm_repair.html.

# 18

# Embolization

Embolotherapy is the deliberate blockage of blood vessels; it is usually performed to stop haemorrhage and may be lifesaving. Embolization is sometimes used as an adjunct to surgery and in the treatment of a variety of benign and malignant tumours. Many embolic agents are available to block vessels of different sizes, from arteries to capillaries. Some embolic agents are temporary and others permanent. The choice of the agent used depends on the individual circumstances of the case.

## General principles

The aim of embolization is to block the target vessel or territory as selectively as possible to minimize 'collateral damage' to non-target structures. Good-quality pre-embolization imaging is essential.

*The target anatomy* A thorough knowledge of the vascular anatomy is essential before embarking on a procedure. Arterial variants are common and must be considered before opening fire. Anastomoses between arterial territories are particularly important for two reasons:

- Outflow and inflow vessels must be blocked. This situation is typified in the case of a gastroduodenal artery aneurysm, which will receive supply from both the hepatic artery and the SMA via the pancreaticoduodenal arcade (Fig. 18.1).
- Blockage may affect adjacent arterial territory, sometimes with disastrous results, e.g. bronchial and spinal arterial anastomoses.

*Level to block* Occlusion can be achieved at any level from main artery to capillary level, depending on the agent. Decide at the outset whether you need to block a feeding vessel or an entire vascular bed. In general, to treat bleeding only the source vessel needs to be blocked but to treat a tumour the entire tumour circulation should be occluded.

 **Consent issue** Always consider the potential adverse consequences of blocking the target vessel(s) and of collateral damage, especially to end organs. Post embolization syndrome (pain, fever and sickness) is common when embolizing tumour and solid organs. This should be discussed with the patient and referring clinician and documented in the notes prior to attempting the procedure.

*Which embolic agent* Ask the following questions:
1. Will temporary occlusion do the job? Most trauma cases can be satisfactorily treated with temporary occlusion, using Gelfoam. Gelfoam occlusion lasts for between a few days and

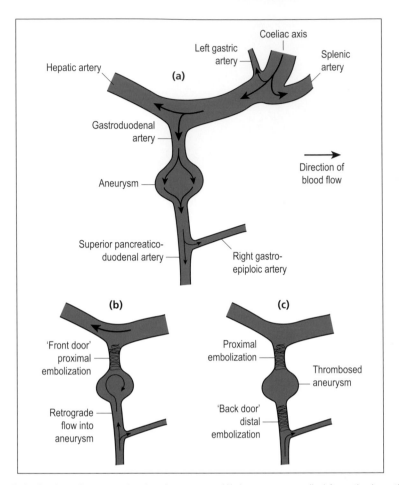

**Fig. 18.1** ■ Embolization of a gastroduodenal aneurysm. (A) Aneurysm supplied from the hepatic artery via the gastroduodenal artery. (B) Proximal embolization only closes the 'front door'. The aneurysm is perfused retrogradely via the pancreaticoduodenal arcade. (C) Proximal and distal embolization closes the 'front and back doors'. The aneurysm is no longer perfused and will thrombose.

    a few weeks and gives the vessel a chance to heal. Gelfoam is readily available, easy to use and prepare and is fairly safe.
2. What level of occlusion is required? If a permanent agent is needed, then determine the size of the target vessel; coils are used to occlude medium-to-small arteries; polyvinyl alcohol (PVA) particles are used to occlude multiple small arteries, arterioles and capillaries. Unless you are expert, avoid the use of liquid embolic agents.
3. Are adjuncts such as chemotherapy or radiotherapy needed, e.g. liver tumours?
4. Will repeat access ever be required? Generally for tumours or inflammatory conditions, blocking the parent vessel with a bunch of coils is less than helpful if re-treatment is required, e.g. bronchial embolization.

*Safety* Use separate trolleys when dealing with particulate or liquid embolic agents to prevent contamination of the remaining equipment. Use either different size syringes or marked syringes to handle these agents. **Discard any contrast, saline or syringes if there is any possibility that they might have mixed with the embolic agent.**

*Pain control* Where the procedure is anticipated to be painful, e.g. fibroid embolization, prescribe premedication and ensure suitable post-operative pain relief.

## Key steps for safe embolization

- Good-quality preliminary angiography.
- Think carefully about collateral pathways.
- Use the shortest, straightest approach, particularly if coils are involved.
- Always use endhole-only catheters.
- Test stability of the catheter position with the guidewire if using coils or test injections of contrast if using particulate agents. If the catheter moves during testing, there is little chance of it remaining in place during treatment.
- Use non-heparinized saline to flush catheters and dilute contrast; thrombosis is the aim.
- Use continuous fluoroscopy during embolization. There is no point in a low radiation dose if it results in non-target embolization.
- Monitor the flow. This will be obvious when using particles suspended in contrast. When using coils, perform intermittent runs.

# Embolic agents

In broad terms, there are two types of embolic agent: those intended to permanently occlude the target vessel and those that only induce temporary blockage. Embolic agents may be further divided into:

- Mechanical occlusion devices: coils and vascular plugs
- Particulate agents: PVA, Gelfoam and autologous blood clot
- Liquid agents: sclerosants and adhesives.

## Coils and plugs

Coils and plugs are permanent embolic agents and are used when you need to block a few feeding vessels or to pack small aneurysms. They have three effects:

- They damage the intima leading to release of thrombogenic agents.
- They provide a large thrombogenic surface.
- They cause mechanical occlusion of the lumen.

The first two factors are the most important; even the tightest packed coils will not effectively block a vessel without thrombus. The coils resemble short segments of guidewire but do not have a central mandrel. The coil is pushed through the catheter and extruded at its distal end. Friction between the coil and the lumen of the catheter progressively damages the lining and this can cause considerable problems when multiple coils are required. If you notice increasing resistance to coil introduction, change the catheter before it blocks!

 **Alarm:** Coils can cause havoc with subsequent imaging, e.g. beam hardening and star artefact on CT. Not all coils are MRI compatible. Stainless steel coils cause most problems. Check the manufacturer's guidelines.

*Coil types* All embolization coils are intended to block vessels but there are various types available with different properties. Unless you are performing a specific task such as coiling a cerebral aneurysm, conventional coils and microcoils compatible with your catheter are all you need. It is worth being aware of a few concepts to impress your boss and in case you come across a particularly challenging patient.

**Fig. 18.2** ■ A typical fibred embolization coil.

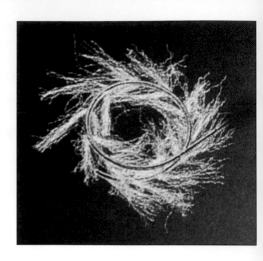

*Coil material* This effects visibility and strength. Most coils are made of stainless steel or platinum. Platinum coils are more radio-opaque, steel exerts the greatest radial force. Soft/liquid coils exert virtually no radial force and are very soft and forgiving during deployment. They tend to come in long lengths that can be packed very tightly, even by non-experts.

 **Tip:** When using soft/liquid coils it helps to deploy a conventional coil first to act as a scaffold for the 'floppy' coil to form against.

*Fibred coils* Most standard coils have fibres attached to promote thrombosis (Fig. 18.2).

*Coil shapes* There is a range of shapes: conventional circles, straight, pyramidal and diamond, to name but a few. Pyramidal and diamond-shaped coils promote rapid thrombosis as they fill the lumen more easily.

*Coatings* Can be used to increase thrombogenicity.

*Detachable coils* Remain attached to the pusher wire until released. This allows test deployment to ensure appropriate size and placement. A variety of mechanisms exist for this, including screw threads, electrolysis and simple interlock. Very useful in high-flow positions, e.g. arteriovenous (AV) malformations.

*Hydrogel coils* Have a hydrophilic coating; this swells and increases the cross-sectional area of the coil.

*Liquid coils* These very soft metal coils are designed to be injected down microcatheters into sites that are awkward to reach.

## What size coil?

There are many types of coil available; all have three size parameters:

*Diameter of the coil wire* This is equivalent to guidewire diameter and varies from 0.014 inch to 0.038 inch. Use a coil that is the correct diameter for your delivery catheter – too big and it will not fit; too small and it may jam with the pusher in the catheter.

**Fig. 18.3** ■ Embolization of a vertebral artery for renal metastasis. The effect of coil size: 3-mm coils (arrowheads) have packed tightly but a 4-mm coil has remained straight (arrows).

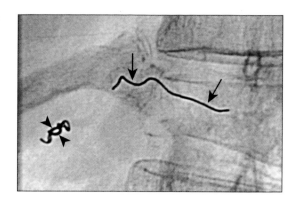

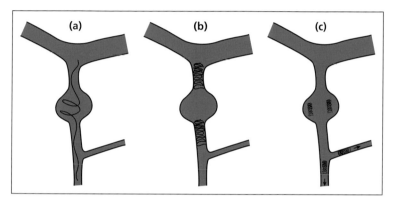

**Fig. 18.4** ■ Importance of coil size. (A) Oversized – does not pack down and may not thrombose. (B) Correctly sized – packs tightly in the vessel. (C) Undersized – migrated distally, non-target embolization.

*Unconstrained length* This varies with the type of coil but, in general, increases with the coiled diameter. Shorter coils are much easier to manage. Very floppy coils often come in very long lengths due to their ability to pack very tightly into just about any shaped space.

*Diameter of the formed coil* Coils come in a large range of diameters from 2 mm to over 20 mm. There are even 'straight' coils for blocking tiny vessels, e.g. in the colonic mesentery. Coils should be slightly oversized relative to the diameter of the target vessel as this allows them to grip the vessel wall and to be closely packed (Fig. 18.3). Grossly oversized coils tend to behave like a guidewire and pass along the vessel rather than coiling up. Undersized coils do not lodge and will migrate downstream. For example, on Cook coils, a coil labelled 35-5-10 will pass through a catheter that will accept a 0.035-inch guidewire; the total extended length of the coil will be 5 cm and the unconstrained coil diameter will be 10 mm. Note that not all coils use this shorthand on the label!

**Tip:** Coils that form perfect loops are undersized. Correctly sized coils are slightly compressed and have an irregular contour (Fig. 18.4).

## Using coils

*Position the catheter* Before even opening that coil, confirm that the catheter position is stable by passing the coil pusher/guidewire to its tip. If the catheter dislodges during this manoeuvre, it will definitely displace if you try to deploy a coil through it!

*Introducing coils into the catheter* Coils are held straight in a short cartridge which is discarded after the coil has been pushed into the catheter. The tip of the cartridge is placed into the hub of the catheter and the coil is pushed into the catheter using the provided pusher or the stiff end of a straight guidewire. Make sure that you hold the cartridge and the catheter tightly together if you do not want the coil to deploy in the catheter hub!

 **Tip:** Many coils come in opaque metal cartridges. Bend these and dispose of them as soon as they are used to avoid sham deployment.

*Standard coil pushers* Once the coil is in the catheter, it is normal to use the reverse end of the guidewire to advance it 10–20 cm along the catheter. Coils can be pushed with conventional straight guidewires, microcoils require special pusher wires.

*Microcatheter coil pushers* The guidewires supplied with microcatheters cannot be used to deliver coils. Special microcoil pushers have a flexible plastic fibre tip on a stiff metal shaft. They are packaged separately and have to be requested! Use the back end of the wire until the coil is at least 30 cm into the catheter.

*Extruding coils* This is the stage when things are most likely to go wrong. Be careful to hold the catheter in position as the coil is pushed to its tip. Slowly start to push the coil out of the catheter; you may feel slight resistance as it starts to coil. Make sure that the catheter is not pushed back out of the target vessel. Continue slowly until the whole coil is out of the catheter.

 **Tip:** If you cannot tell where the coil ends and the pusher starts, back the pusher off a few millimetres and look for the gap on the fluoroscopy image.

Problems are usually associated with:

- Incorrect sizing of the first coil. If you are concerned about the stability of the first coil a trick is to anchor the first portion in a small branch vessel just beyond the target site. The coil will deploy straight and as the catheter is pushed back will anchor it in position.
- The temptation to place 'just one last coil'; we know from bitter personal experience that whimsical last coil is almost certain to back out of the target vessel and cover a vital territory. A key to success in intervention is to know when you have done enough. If you must succumb to the 'just one more coil', minimize the risk by using smaller, shorter coils towards the end of the procedure.

*Packing coils* To be effective, coils should be tightly packed together (Fig. 18.5). This can only be achieved if the catheter is in a stable position and the coils are correctly sized. Following placement of the first coil, the catheter may have to be pulled back a few millimetres to allow subsequent coils to be deployed.

 **Tip:** Note how much of the pusher remains outside the catheter when the coil is about 15 cm from deployment. For subsequent coils, do not screen until you reach this stage.

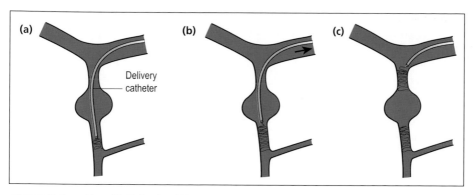

**Fig. 18.5** ■ Coil packing. (A) Coils should be tightly packed together in 'nests' starting with the most distal. (B) The catheter should be withdrawn slightly with each coil. (C) Make sure that you leave enough space for the last coil to form in the target vessel.

After multiple coils have been deployed, it can be difficult to be certain the last coil has been completely deployed and is clear of the catheter; always use the guidewire against the coil to back the catheter off.

*Completion angiography* After a few coils have been deployed, perform an angiogram to assess flow. It is helpful to pull the catheter back a little and to inject gently in order not to dislodge newly formed clot. When the flow is very slow, wait for a couple of minutes to see if the vessel thromboses. If there is still brisk flow, then more coils are needed. If the flow has stopped, you can usually stop too.

## Troubleshooting

**Unable to obtain selective catheter position** Go back to basic principles. Try different catheter shapes and angiographic projections. Try using a hydrophilic catheter or a microcatheter. Guide-catheters can be useful in tortuous or aneurysmal vessels. If the optimal position is not obtainable, consider more proximal embolization but remember that the collateral damage will increase.

**Unable to obtain a stable catheter position** There are several possible solutions. Make sure that the catheter is the optimal shape for the vessel. Try a more supportive catheter (larger French size or a guide-catheter to support the catheter). Consider an alternative approach, e.g. from the arm rather than the leg.

**The delivery catheter is pushed back during coil deployment** Concentrate on holding the catheter in position. It is often helpful to get assistance from a colleague, particularly when using co-axial systems. A reasonably long coil that has had less than 25% extruded can sometimes be withdrawn along with the catheter with great care. This clearly risks the coil being lost and embolizing elsewhere. This has to be balanced against the risk of deploying the coil where it is.

 **Tip:** If only a short amount of coil remains it can usually be deployed and will often surprise by shortening back into the target vessel or lying flat against the parent artery wall.

**A coil is misplaced** This usually occurs when the catheter position is not stable, the coil is incorrectly sized or when deployment is attempted in too short a vessel segment. Only attempt retrieval if the coil is likely to occlude a significant vessel, otherwise you will probably cause more harm than good. Coils can be retrieved using a snare or endovascular forceps.

**A coil jams in the delivery catheter** This occurs when the coil is the wrong size for the catheter, when there is a tight bend or kink in the catheter or when the catheter has been damaged by previous coils or particulate agents. Fluoroscope to determine the position of the coil. First try to free the coil by flushing with saline; use a 1-mL syringe as this gives the highest pressure. If this fails, try using the stiff end of the guidewire/pusher; unfortunately, this seldom works. If the coil is in the catheter *outside* the patient, then cut off the end of the catheter including the coil. Pass a guidewire through the catheter and exchange it for a new one. If the coil is in the catheter *inside* the patient, there is no option but to remove the catheter with loss of the position.

 **Tip:** Do not jeopardize a hard-won position; exchange the delivery catheter before it fails, if you feel that there is increasing resistance to coil passage. Consider changing the delivery catheter if using coils after PVA particles.

## Amplatzer vascular plug (AVP)

The AVP is a self-expanding Nitinol wire mesh with one or three segments (Fig. 18.6). The AVP is mounted on a delivery wire by a screw thread; this allows test deployment to check position and size to be checked before the device is released. The AVP shortens considerably as it expands from its constrained state: the minimum final length of the device is 10–15 mm. AVP are sized in 2-mm increments from 4 to 16 mm. The AVP is particularly useful in high-flow situations where there is a single large vessel to occlude; occlusion is more rapid and safer than the deployment of multiple coils.

## Using the AVP

*Assess the target* As with all embolization, imaging is the key. The size and length of the target vessel must be assessed. If the site is suitable, a device is chosen which is 30–50% larger than the target vessel diameter.

*Suitability* The AVP must be delivered to the target site in a guide-catheter or long sheath – this is a limitation as it cannot be used in very tortuous vessels.

*Access* Choose a sheath size appropriate to the AVP/guide-catheter needed. Suggested guide-catheter sizes are 4–8-mm 5Fr, 10–12-mm 6Fr and 14–16-mm 8F.

*Catheterization* The vessel should be catheterized in the usual way. Once a catheter is in place, a supportive wire should be used to allow the guide-catheter to be advanced into position *across* the target deployment site.

*Deployment* The AVP comes constrained in a cheater to allow introduction into the delivery catheter. Feel free to push it out of the cheater to see how it expands as it is readily pulled back in. Simply pop the cheater through the haemostatic valve and use the delivery wire to push the plug to its destination. Once in place, the sheath is pulled back to allow the AVP to expand. Applying forward pressure will allow the device to compress.

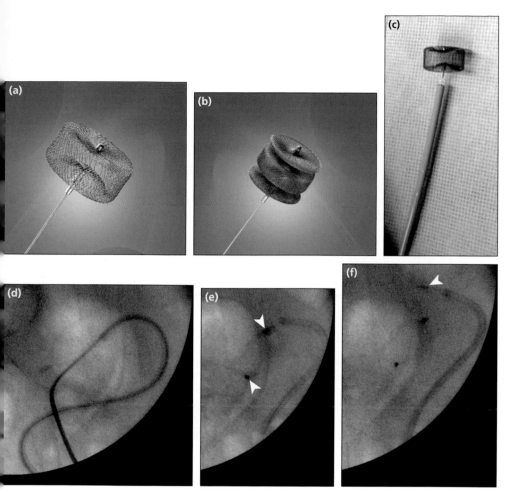

**Fig. 18.6** ■ Amplatzer vascular plug (A) Amplatzer I. (B) Amplatzer II. (C) With guide-catheter. (D) Guide catheter advanced deep into the target vessel. (E) The AVP is advanced to the target site (white arrowheads) and the guide-catheter pulled back to deploy it. (F) When happy with position, the delivery wire is rotated anticlockwise to release (white arrowhead). (Images (A) and (B) courtesy of AGA Medical.)

*Check angiogram* Perform a check angiogram to confirm position of the device. If it is in the correct place, then simply turn the delivery wire anticlockwise to unscrew and release the AVP. You should wait 5–10 minutes before performing another check angiogram to confirm occlusion.

## Particulate embolic agents

Particulate embolic agents are used when blockage of multiple vessels is desired, e.g. fibroid and tumour embolization. Particulate agents can be considered according to the duration of action:

- **Temporary occlusion**: e.g. Gelfoam, autologous blood clot
- **Permanent occlusion**: polymers e.g. PVA.

When using particulate material, stop embolization when there is slow 'to and fro' flow in the vessel. If you continue until flow stops, you are left with a loaded catheter and any further injection or flushing will lead to reflux! When flushing the catheter, remember that it contains residual embolic material; careless flushing causes non-target embolization! Flush slowly and carefully with non-heparinized saline until no further contrast emerges; it is then safe to perform angiography.

## Gelfoam

Gelfoam comes in different forms with completely different uses:

- **Gelfoam powder** comprises small particles (40–60 μm); vessel occlusion occurs at the capillary level; hence tissue necrosis is likely.
- **Gelfoam sheet** is cut into 'pledgets' 1–2 mm in size, or larger 'torpedoes' 1–2 × 10– 15 mm; these are used to block larger vessels; tissue infarction is rare.

*Gelfoam pledgets* Simply prepared using sharp scissors to make parallel cuts about 1 mm wide across the Gelfoam sheet until it resembles a comb (Fig. 18.7). This is then trimmed at right angles to this to make 1 × 1 mm pieces. The pledgets are soaked in about 20 mL contrast for a few minutes to allow the Gelfoam to soften. Syringing the Gelfoam back and forwards in the gallipot will help soften the particles. When the pledgets become soft and slightly translucent, they are ready to use.

*Using Gelfoam pledgets* The soft pledgets can be drawn up into a 20-mL syringe. This should be connected to a 5-mL syringe via a 3-way tap. The 20-mL syringe is the reservoir and the 5-mL used to inject the pledgets. Pledgets can be injected through conventional angiographic catheters and guide-catheters. Microcatheters will tend to block. Gelfoam floats in contrast and therefore injection should be made with the syringe nozzle pointing upwards. Injection is made under continuous fluoroscopic guidance and continued until the flow in the target

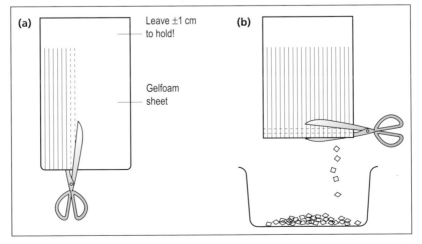

**Fig. 18.7** ■ The Gelfoam comb. (A) Cut 1 mm longitudinal strips into the Gelfoam sheet. (B) Cut transversely across the Gelfoam comb. Do not forget to catch the pledgets in a gallipot.

vessel is almost at a standstill. Check angiography shows a characteristic pruned appearance, with the main vessel and proximal portions of branches filling.

## Gelfoam torpedoes

These are made from the same Gelfoam sheet but cut into larger squares.

*Using Gelfoam torpedoes* 5 × 5 mm stamps can be rolled and injected like large pledgets; use only with a very stable catheter position. 10 × 10 mm stamps are used dry and rolled tightly, then can be pushed into a catheter or sheath; in this form they are excellent for plugging tracts (refer to Chapter 25, Biopsy and Drainage).

## Polyvinyl alcohol

PVA comes in a range of particle sizes, 150–1000 μm. The particles wedge in vessels of the corresponding diameter, where they cause thrombosis and fibrosis. Particles in the range 300–500 μm are suitable for most purposes.

*Preparing PVA* One vial of PVA is suspended in 10–20 mL of full strength contrast. The contrast allows the injection to be visualized on fluoroscopy. The suspension is mixed with a syringe.

*Using PVA* Aliquots of the suspension are injected slowly in small pulses under fluoroscopic control. Some PVA preparations tend to form clumps of particles, others rapidly 'float' to the top of the suspension; frequent mixing is required in either case. Check continually for reflux of the suspension. When there is slow flow, make a test injection with contrast to determine a safe rate of injection.

 **Tip:** When using PVA, use a 20-mL syringe as a reservoir connected via a 3-way tap to a 5-mL syringe to inject the suspension (Fig. 18.8). This greatly simplifies mixing the PVA to avoid aggregation and separation of the suspension.

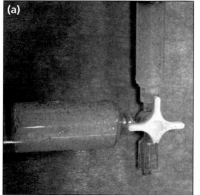 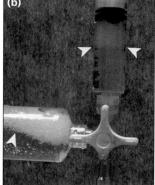

**Fig. 18.8** ◼ Mixing PVA. (A) Shows the PVA particles evenly suspended in the contrast; this suspension is ready to use. (B) After about 30 seconds the PVA begins to float to the surface of the contrast (arrowheads). The suspension requires further mixing before it is used.

*Alternative permanent agents* There are an increasing number of available preparations of PVA and other agents (e.g. tris-acryl) and also alternative particulate agents intended to augment the embolization procedure, e.g. drug-eluting particles, radioactive particles.

 **Alarm:** Do not assume that particles of the same size are directly interchangeable with conventional PVA. Many of the new agents are much more uniform in size, compressible or do not clump together; this can result in more distal embolization than intended or even flow through microvascular shunts, with disastrous consequences. As always, learn the kit but in principle use a larger size.

## Autologous blood clot

This is rarely used and is reserved for situations in which a short duration of occlusion is desirable, e.g. post-traumatic high-flow priapism. A sample of the patient's blood is withdrawn at the start of the procedure and allowed to clot in a gallipot. The clot can be macerated and aspirated into a syringe for injection into the target vessel.

 **Tip:** If the blood does not clot in a reasonable time (when you have achieved your highly selective position) then add a small amount of calcium or thrombin.

# Liquid embolic agents

Liquid agents divide into two main categories: sclerosants and glues. The former includes absolute alcohol and sodium tetradecyl sulphate (SDS). The use of tissue adhesives such as cyanoacrylate and Ethibloc has also been described but these products are not readily available and are not licensed for intravascular use in many countries. The final category of agent is Onyx, a polymer which is injected dissolved in dimethyl sulphoxide (DMSO). The Onyx sets into an inert cast as the solvent elutes.

Liquid agents are certainly the most difficult of the embolic agents to control and are the least forgiving. Their use is best restricted to expert hands and, therefore, only limited discussion is given.

 **Tip:** Consider using an occlusion balloon catheter to prevent unwanted reflux of liquid agents during embolization.

## Absolute alcohol

Absolute alcohol causes cell death by dehydration. It will damage any tissue it contacts. Extravasation will cause local tissue necrosis. Because alcohol is not visible fluoroscopically, it is mixed 1:1 with contrast. Safe injection rates, which do not cause reflux or extravasation, are determined by making test injections of contrast. Frequent check angiography is mandatory to ensure that the situation does not change as thrombosis occurs. As absolute alcohol injection is often very painful, suitable sedation and analgesia must be used. Alcohol is one of the ultimate permanent embolic agents and is principally used to treat vascular malformations and tumours.

## Sodium tetradecyl sulphate

SDS is commonly used in venous sclerotherapy, low flow malformations and as an adjunct to coil embolization during the treatment of varicocoele. There are two techniques for using SDS:

- A few millilitres of SDS are injected after the initial coils have been deployed. Take particular care to avoid spill of SDS into the epididymal veins as this will cause epididymitis. It is not as powerful a sclerosant as absolute ethanol but should still be used with caution.
- The SDS is made into a foam by mixing with air (Tessari method). Simply use a 3-way tap connect a syringe with 1 mL of SDS to another with 2 mL of room air. Inject backwards and forwards until a foam is formed. SDS foam is injected in a similar fashion to liquid but floats and tends to travel further … therefore use with care.

# Clinical scenarios

## Varicocoele

Embolization of varicocoele is requested in symptomatic and subfertile patients. It is an elective procedure and very straightforward. It is therefore an ideal case on which to learn coil embolization; whether it has any therapeutic benefit for the subfertile is open to debate!

## Equipment

- Basic angiography set.
- Hydrophilic guidewire.
- Hydrophilic Cobra II and Sidewinder II catheters.
- Embolization coils and SDS.

## Procedure

*Access* The right CFV is often used, but the right IJV should be considered – the approach is in-line and there is no need for bedrest postprocedure.

*Catheterization* Most varicocoeles are left-sided; the spermatic vein joins the midpoint of the left renal vein (Fig. 18.9). Catheterize the renal vein with a hydrophilic Cobra II catheter. It may be necessary to use a Sidewinder to catheterize the right spermatic vein, which joins the anterior IVC just below the right renal vein.

*Runs* Perform a venogram to demonstrate reflux down the spermatic vein. Use a hydrophilic guidewire and the catheter to cannulate the vein. If possible, the catheter should be taken down to the level of the inguinal canal. Deploy coils here and demonstrate blockage of the vein. The catheter is withdrawn to the midpoint of the vein. A further venogram is performed to look for small collateral veins. These can be treated by further coil deployment, or some practitioners may use a liquid sclerosant such as SDS. Use with caution as the gonadal vein may communicate with important structures.

Make sure the coils are large enough to lodge in the spermatic vein or they will become effective pulmonary emboli.

## Troubleshooting

**No reflux is seen** You know there is reflux from the ultrasound. Occasionally there is a competent valve at the top of the spermatic vein and the source of the reflux is a renal capsular vein beyond.

**The spermatic vein goes into spasm** Relax! Explain to the patient that this is not uncommon and always self-limiting. Give a small dose of GTN (100 µg), wait 1 minute and

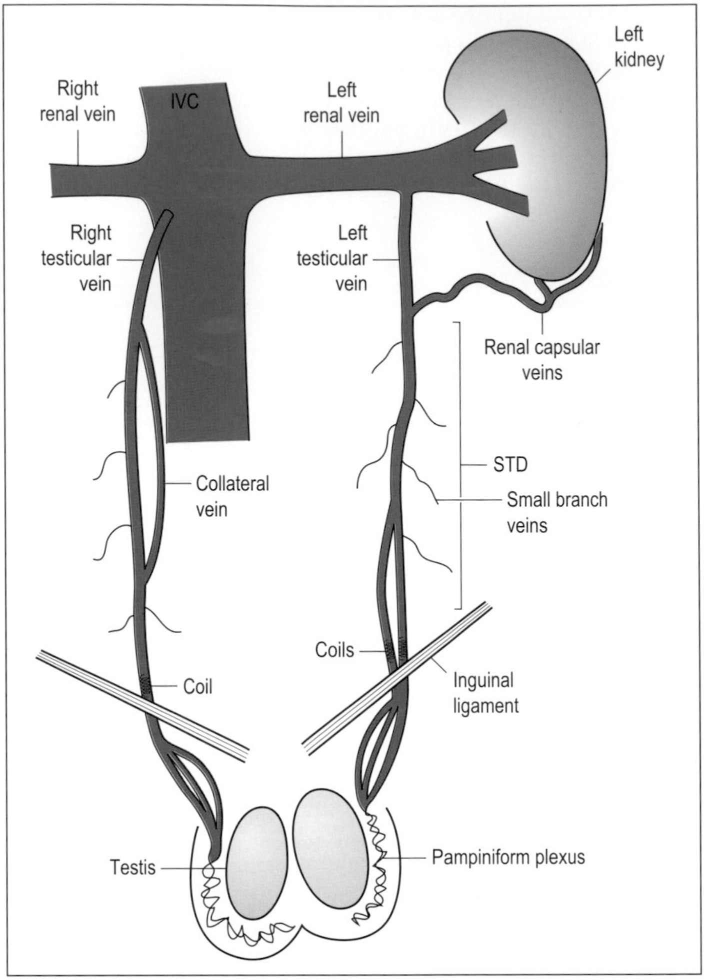

**Fig. 18.9** ■ Varicocoele anatomy. Coils are placed in the main veins just above the inguinal ligament. SDS may be used to sclerose small branch veins/potential collaterals. IVC, inferior vena cava.

then perform a gentle venogram. If the spasm has resolved, be gentle with the vein and this probably will not happen again. If spasm persists, give a further dose of GTN and then go and sit down for 5 minutes before looking again. The spasm will almost certainly have eased by now. If not, be patient. Give more GTN and go for a cup of tea before looking again. When the spasm does resolve, if you and the patient are feeling confident, continue as above.

## Uterine fibroid embolization (UFE)

This is a relatively new technique that has shown encouraging results in the treatment of symptomatic fibroid disease. The procedure in itself is not particularly technically demanding; however, there is a lot of work in developing and implementing appropriate protocols for assessment, procedural pain relief and post-procedural management. It is essential that the service is delivered in conjunction with a gynaecologist and in many countries there is a requirement that patients are included within a trial/registry.

## Assessment

Patients should have both gynaecological and imaging assessment. The minimum is a pelvic ultrasound but increasingly pelvic MR examination is used for assessment and follow-up. Fibroid embolization should not be used if the fibroids are pedunculated.

**Tip:** Gonadotrophin-releasing hormone (GnRH) analogues may be used in the medical treatment of fibroids. Delay embolization for 3 months after their use as the uterine arteries are small and extremely difficult to catheterize during treatment.

## Equipment

- Hydrophilic 4Fr catheter.
- Hydrophilic wire.
- Microcatheter.
- Particulate embolization: e.g. PVA or microspheres 500–1000 μm.

## Technique

Fibroid embolization is a painful procedure and patients generally have severe cramping pain for 12–24 hours, with some milder discomfort lasting for weeks. Analgesia is more effective if given before the onset of pain and at regular intervals. Pre-procedural analgesia usually includes an NSAID given by suppository, an intramuscular opiate and an anti-emetic.

Bilateral uterine artery embolization is usually required for adequate treatment. The uterine arteries are branches of the anterior division of the internal iliac artery. The internal iliac artery is selectively catheterized with a hydrophilic Cobra catheter. If the uterine artery is suitably large, the Cobra can often be advanced directly into the vessel. These vessels are prone to spasm so have a low threshold for using microcatheters. After selective catheterization has been achieved, embolization with permanent particles is performed, most typically PVA. The end point of embolization is to and fro flow within the uterine artery.

Intraprocedural analgesia should include an intravenous opiate; midazolam is often also given to alleviate anxiety.

**Alarm:** The ovaries are very radiation sensitive. Keep radiation to a minimum, use pulsed fluoroscopy if possible and avoid performing angiographic runs unless the anatomy cannot be resolved. Hence there are no figures in this section!

## Aftercare

Post-operative pain relief is best managed with a patient-controlled analgesia pump. The NSAID should be continued and an anti-emetic is required. Most patients can be discharged 24–36 hours post procedure on oral analgesia.

## Complications

Fibroid embolization carries significant risks but these should be balanced against the risks of a surgical procedure. It is essential that the patient receives both adequate information and an opportunity to discuss the potential complications (Table 18.1).

**Consent issue:** Patients undergoing UFE are relatively young; some are hoping to avoid hysterectomy in order to have children. Patients should be warned not only of the peri-procedural risks but also the possibility of premature menopause and infertility.

**Table 18.1** Complications of fibroid embolization

| | |
|---|---|
| Premature menopause | 2% |
| Fibroid expulsion | 2% |
| Sepsis | 1% |
| Hysterectomy | 1% |
| Death | <0.01% |

# Trauma

The role of imaging and intervention in trauma is changing rapidly. Whole body CT is becoming standard and the value of early embolization is increasingly recognized. Emphasis is on saving life and prevention of future morbidity. Early control of bleeding helps reduce transfusion and prevents coagulopathy and multiorgan failure.

 **Tip:** Make sure that angiography is alerted whenever a patient with major trauma is imminent/being scanned. That way everyone can prepare for action.

## Indication for embolization

- When the CT shows a focal bleeding source.

## Contraindication to embolization

- Severely unstable patient who requires immediate laparotomy; in these circumstances the only option you can offer is to place an occlusion balloon in the aorta. Only offer this if you are able to do it immediately without screening!
- When there are multiple bleeding sites in different vascular territories and embolization would be too slow.

Only undertake this type of treatment if you are confident in your technical ability to perform selective embolization. Make sure that the patient is suitably resuscitated and is stable enough to survive the procedure. Use the CT to plan the approach to embolization and the procedure you intend to perform. Aim straight for the likely bleeding vessel. If a bleeding source is identified, ask the following questions:

- Is the amount of extravasation responsible for the patient's condition? It is possible to overlook another more significant source of blood loss. Make sure that this is the only site of bleeding.
- Is the bleeding vessel supplied from a single territory? This has implications for treatment, as both the 'front and back doors' may need to be 'closed'.
- What would be the consequences of occlusion of the vessel? This must always be considered and is particularly important when dealing with end arteries. Don't think too long; at the end of the day it is better to be alive with a single kidney.
- Is embolization or surgery the appropriate intervention? Embolization is appropriate if it is likely to lead to prompt cessation of bleeding without causing significant collateral damage. Discuss the situation with a senior surgical colleague.
- Where preservation of flow is desirable, is it possible to use a stent-graft?

If the source is uncertain, perform initial angiograms to determine the source of the bleeding. Start with an overview of the target territory and proceed to selective catheterization as required.

Gelfoam can be particularly useful where there are multiple bleeding points in one vascular territory, e.g. liver trauma. Use coils to embolize larger proximal arterial injuries as selectively as possible and spare as much normal tissue as you can.

**Consent issue:** It is often impossible to obtain informed consent in the acute trauma patient, especially if they are ventilated and unconscious. Act in the patient's best interest and if possible inform relatives what is planned and detail the pros and cons of the procedure.

**Hepatic trauma** Embolization is indicated in the presence of false aneurysm or active extravasation.

**Blunt hepatic trauma** More commonly causes venous injury than arterial injury. Hepatic injury is often associated with pelvic trauma and other visceral injuries. Arterial bleeding is often focal and suitable for coil embolization. When the surface of the liver is bleeding from multiple points, use Gelfoam or particles. **Penetrating trauma** will either be due to stabbing by the public or by doctors. PTC, biliary drainage and hepatic biopsy are all good sources of referral. The typical iatrogenic injury is a small pseudoaneurysm and often requires meticulous angiography for detection. Hepatic arteries are not end arteries and there are multiple intrahepatic collaterals; if possible, start coil deployment distal to the lesion to prevent collateral 'back-door ' filling.

**Splenic trauma** Blunt injury is the commonest cause and embolization is indicated in the presence of false aneurysm or active extravasation; splenic laceration alone is not an indication for treatment. Unlike the liver, the spleen is an end organ, and vigorous embolization will lead to splenic infarction with the associated risks of hyposplenism. Two forms of splenic embolization should be considered:

- **Selective embolization** – this is the preferred option for any focal abnormality that can be readily catheterized.
- **Proximal embolization** – this is appropriate when there is diffuse injury, e.g. multiple bleeding sites that would take too long to embolize selectively. The splenic artery is occluded proximal to the short gastric arteries; the Amplatzer plug is good for this. The aim is to maintain perfusion while reducing perfusion pressure. This technique minimizes the risk of splenic infarction but does preclude further intervention if bleeding continues.

**Pelvic trauma** Major pelvic trauma is often accompanied by significant arterial and venous injury. Bleeding from bone and veins stops when the fracture is stabilized with a pelvic wrap. Arterial bleeding does not respond to this. If arterial bleeding is suspected, then embolization should come before fixation; the injured vessel almost inevitably lies over the fracture site. Remember, even relatively minor pelvic fractures can cause major arterial haemorrhage (Fig. 18.10).

**Renal trauma** This is often iatrogenic following biopsy and can usually be embolized highly selectively. Make sure that there are two kidneys before embolization of a large amount of renal tissue. Renal arteries are end arteries, therefore there is no need to worry about collaterals, just infarction.

**Tip:** Be pragmatic. If the patient is haemorrhaging and unstable, stop the bleeding and sacrifice the kidney; don't waste precious time trying to perform highly selective embolization (Fig. 18.11).

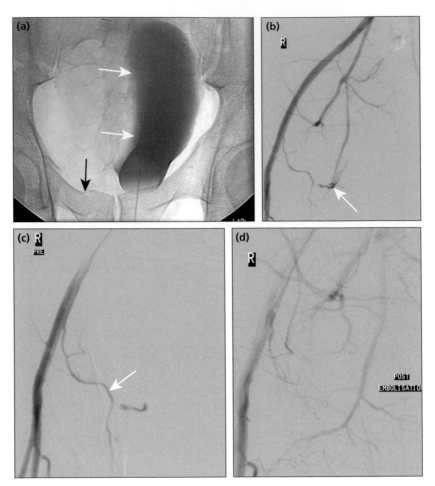

**Fig. 18.10** ■ Haemorrhage secondary to pubic ramus fracture. (A) Displacement of bladder by haematoma (white arrows), fracture (black arrow). (B) Initial angiogram suggesting extravasation (arrow) is from the IIA. (C) EIA angiogram showing bleeding from its corona mortis branch (arrow). (D) Post embolization the patient stabilized.

**Gastrointestinal bleeding** Embolotherapy has been described in the treatment of gastrointestinal bleeding in both the small and large bowel. Gastric and duodenal bleeding can be safely treated because of the extensive collateral supply. The classic scenario is the gastroduodenal artery aneurysm (Fig. 18.12). Bleeding sites beyond the ligament of Trietz can be embolized but the risk of infarction is much greater and embolization should only be undertaken if it can be performed highly selectively and with agreement by the surgical team to perform laparotomy if there is bowel infarction (Fig. 18.13).

 **Tip:** In simple terms, in lower gastrointestinal bleeding think CT and then embolization, and in upper gastrointestinal bleeding think endoscopy before embolization.

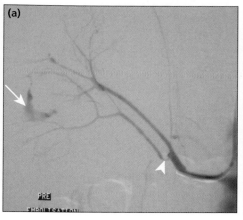
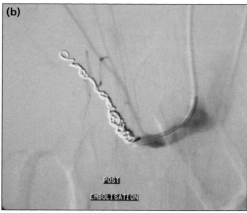

**Fig. 18.11** ■ Post biopsy haemorrhage. (A) Selective renal angiogram showing brisk extravasation (arrow) from a lower polar branch vessel with stenosis at its origin (arrowhead). The entire kidney is displaced upwards by the retroperitoneal haematoma. (B) Post non-selective embolization.

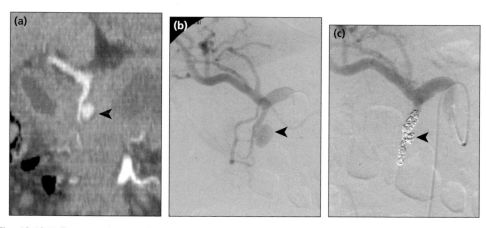

**Fig. 18.12** ■ Recurrent haemorrhage in a patient with pancreatitis. (A) Coronal CT reformat shows false aneurysm of the gastroduodenal artery (GDA) (arrowhead). (B) Selective hepatic artery angiogram showing near identical appearance. (C) Completion angiography showing aneurysm exclusion. Note that the coils extend beyond the aneurysm to 'close the back door' and also prolapse into the false aneurysm through the arterial defect (arrowhead).

# Complications

Embolotherapy has a high potential for complications and catastrophes. Obviously, all the standard complications of diagnostic angiography are present. Risks unique to embolization must be discussed pre procedure with the patient and include:

**Post-embolization syndrome** Post-embolization syndrome occurs as a consequence of tissue infarction, with subsequent release of vasoactive substances and other inflammatory mediators. It is most common with solid organ embolization, e.g. the liver, and broadly related to the extent of tissue infarction. After embolization, patients typically develop severe pain within hours, and over the next 24–72 hours have fever, nausea and vomiting, myalgia,

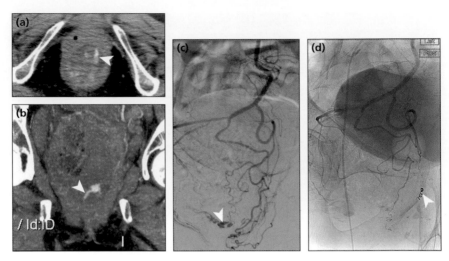

**Fig. 18.13** ■ Embolization for rectal bleeding. (A, B) Axial and coronal CT reformats showing contrast extravasation in the rectum (arrowhead). (C) Superior rectal artery angiogram showing extravasation (arrowhead). (D) following coil embolization (arrowhead) the patient stabilized with no ischaemic sequelae.

arthralgia and general debility. Affected patients need support with appropriate analgesia, intravenous fluids and nursing care. Symptoms tend to subside after ~72 hours but it can be a worrying time for both the patient and the clinician.

**Non-target embolization** As we explained earlier, it is usually possible to retrieve a misplaced coil with some skill and determination. Unfortunately, non-target embolization with permanent particulate or liquid agents is irretrievable. The consequences are dependent on the vascular bed affected but may be life-threatening. Clearly, great care to avoid this complication is the aim, but for each case you must be aware of the potential innocent bystanders, and prompt recognition and appropriate treatment, surgical or otherwise, may be lifesaving.

**Abscess formation** Ischaemic and infarcted tissue makes a great culture medium and prophylactic antibiotics are essential if a significant volume of tissue is embolized. If patients are persistently pyrexial after embolization, then blood cultures and appropriate imaging are needed.

**Tissue necrosis** Necrosis occurs when a tissue has been completely devitalized, usually by occlusion of the capillary bed. This can occur with physical occlusion with very small particle PVA or with absolute alcohol, which also causes perivascular necrosis. The result will be tissue infarction in solid organs or loss of overlying skin in more peripheral territories.

## Suggestions for further reading

There is no comprehensive review of embolotherapy so here are a variety of articles covering some important areas:

Aina R, Oliva VL, Therese E, et al. Arterial embolotherapy for upper gastrointestinal haemorrhage: outcome assessment. J Vasc Intervent Radiol 2001;12:195–200.

Bandi R, Shetty PC, Sharia RP, et al. Superselective arterial embolization for the treatment of lower gastrointestinal hemorrhage. J Vasc

Intervent Radiol 2001;12:1399–1405.

Drooz AT, Lewis CS, Allen TA, et al. Quality improvement guidelines for percutaneous transcatheter embolization. J Vasc Intervent Radiol 1997;8:889–895.
Standards for embolotherapy set by the SCVIR. Defines acceptable targets for success and failure.

Fenely MR, Pal MK, Nockler IB, et al. Retrograde embolization and causes of failure in the primary treatment of varicocoele. Br J Urol 1997;80:642–646.

Fernando HC, Stein M, Benfield JR, et al. Role of bronchial artery embolization in the management of hemoptysis. Arch Surg 1998;133:862–866.

Gomes AS. Embolization therapy of congenital arteriovenous malformations: Use of alternative approaches. Radiology 1994;190:191–198.

Hastings GS. Angiographic localization and transcatheter treatment of gastrointestinal bleeding. Radiographics 2000;20:1160–1168.

Kalva SP, Thabet A, Wicky S. Recent advances in transarterial therapy of primary and secondary liver malignancies. Radiographics 2008;28:101–117.

Katz MD, Teitelbaum GP, Pentecost MJ. Diagnostic arteriography and therapeutic embolization for post traumatic pelvic embolization. Semin Intervent Radiol 1992;9:4–12.
A clear overview.

Nicholson AA, Ettles DF, Hartley JE, et al. Transcatheter coil embolotherapy: A safe and effective option for major colonic haemorrhage. Gut 1998;43:79–84.
Embolize distally and with caution.

Pelage JP, Le Dref O, Mateo J, et al. Life-threatening primary postpartum hemorrhage: Treatment with emergency selective arterial embolzation. Radiology 1998;208:359–362.

Seppanen SK, Lepppanen MJ, Pimenoff G, et al. Microcatheter embolization of hemorrhages. Cardiovasc Intervent Radiol 1997;20:174–179.
Selective coil and PVA embolization in haemorrhage.

Sonomura T, Yamada R, Kishi K, et al. Dependency of tissue necrosis on gelatin sponge particle size after canine hepatic artery embolization. Cardiovasc Intervent Radiol 1997;20:50–53.
Size is important! Emphasizes the effect of particle size on target organ damage.

Worthington-Kirsch RL, Popky GL, Hutchins FL. Uterine arterial embolization for the management of leiomyomas: Quality of life assessment and clinical response. Radiology 1998;208:625–629.
Very topical currently.

# 19

# Thrombolysis and thrombectomy

## Thrombolysis

Arterial thrombosis, in native or graft vessels and dialysis fistula, is usually secondary to an underlying stenotic lesion. The aim of thrombolysis is to break down blood clot, restore perfusion, and reveal the vascular anatomy. The thrombolytic agent is delivered directly into the thrombus; systemic thrombolysis is much less effective for peripheral vascular thrombus.

When the vessel has been cleared, an underlying lesion should be carefully looked for and treated. Even partial clearing of the vessels may simplify any subsequent surgical procedure. The agents used for thrombolysis are discussed in Chapter 6, Drugs Used in Interventional Radiology. Only rt-PA is discussed in this chapter but the principles apply equally to the other agents.

### Indications and contraindications

This is about the only situation where the same condition, CVA, appears as both an indication and an absolute contraindication!

### Indications

It was hoped that thrombolytic therapy with fibrin-specific agents would be akin to a magic bullet and prevent patients requiring surgery. This has not proved to be the case and consequently thrombolysis is not as popular as a few years ago. The principal indications for thrombolysis are:

- Cardiac and acute stroke thrombolysis; though these are most often by intravenous bolus route.
- Dialysis access salvage.
- Acute or acute-on-chronic critical limb ischaemia (Table 19.1). Thrombolysis is not usually clinically indicated more than 6 weeks after the thrombotic event.
- Bypass graft thrombosis.
- Thrombosed popliteal aneurysm – the aim here is to clear the run-off vessels to allow bypass grafting.
- Peri-procedural thrombolysis – thrombosis may occur during interventional procedures and surgery. Acute thrombus is particularly likely to clear, and thrombolysis may salvage the procedure.
- Venous thrombosis, especially axillary vein and massive iliofemoral vein thrombosis.

### Contraindications

Thrombolysis is not without risk, particularly bleeding and CVA; the risk–benefit ratio is so unfavourable in some patients that thrombolysis is contraindicated.

**Table 19.1** Clinical categories of acute limb ischaemia

| Category | Description | Capillary return | Muscle paralysis | Sensory loss | Arterial Doppler signal | Venous Doppler signal |
|---|---|---|---|---|---|---|
| I Viable | Not immediately threatened | Intact | None | None | + | + |
| IIa Threatened | Salvageable, if promptly treated | Intact/slow | None | Partial | − | + |
| IIb Threatened | Salvageable, if immediately treated | Slow/absent | Partial | Partial | − | + |
| III Irreversible | Amputation regardless of treatment | Absent | Complete | Complete | − | − |

*Modified from the Consensus Report on Thrombolysis. J Intern Med 1996;240:343–355.*

- **Absolute contraindications**:
  - Irreversible ischaemia.
  - Major trauma, surgery or cardiopulmonary resuscitation within the past 2 weeks.
  - Stroke over 6 hours old and within the last 2 months. When the intention of treatment is not to regain cerebral function. Primary or secondary cerebral tumour. Risk of haemorrhage too high and no potential to regain function.
  - Bleeding diathesis: Any obvious potential bleeding source or bleeding problem, e.g. proven active ulceration, bladder tumour, recent surgery and haemorrhagic stroke.
  - Pregnancy.
- **Relative contraindications**:
  - Age >80 years; these patients have the highest risk of stroke and haemorrhagic complications.
  - The white limb – best treated by surgery.
  - Graft thrombosis within 4 weeks of surgery. Early graft failure is almost always due to a technical problem with the surgery, e.g. poor-quality vein, graft kinking.
  - Anticoagulation.
  - Knitted Dacron grafts – these rely on deposition of thrombus to be impermeable; hence they become porous during thrombolysis and marked extravasation may occur.
  - Vein graft – the vein relies on perfusion for its viability, and after about 3 days, the vein is irreversibly damaged. However, the run-off may be cleared, allowing subsequent regrafting.
  - Recent thrombolysis with no underlying cause demonstrable. Rethrombosis is very likely.
  - Thrombolysis with streptokinase within the previous 5 years. This is only relevant if using streptokinase, as antibodies persist for many years and limit the effectiveness of the treatment while increasing the risk of adverse reaction.
  - Cardiac emboli: thrombolysis may lead to further embolization.

# Equipment

There are different techniques for performing thrombolysis, and the equipment varies according to the strategy being used:

**Table 19.2** Guidelines for best arterial access

| Site of occlusion | Optimal arterial access |
|---|---|
| Iliac artery | Ipsilateral CFA if patent, otherwise contralateral CFA |
| CFA | Contralateral CFA or exceptionally brachial |
| SFA, PFA or femoropopliteal graft | Ipsilateral CFA |
| Femoro-femoral cross-over | Direct graft puncture or inflow CFA |
| Axillo-femoral graft | Consider surgery |

- Basic angiography set.
- Infusion catheters: a 4Fr straight catheter with sideholes is suitable in most cases.
- A pump suitable for arterial infusion.
- Co-axial systems or microcatheters may be helpful.
- Pulse spray techniques require special catheters and pumps.

## Procedure

*Access* The key to thrombolysis is knowing the vascular anatomy; this is obvious in native vessels but can be obscure in the presence of bypass grafts. Always clarify what grafts are in situ, look for operation notes and talk to the patient and a senior surgeon. **Before puncturing an artery, consider performing MRA or CTA to demonstrate the inflow anatomy and, with luck, the run-off vessels**.

The approach for thrombolysis can now be chosen. Make only a single arterial puncture (multiple punctures increase the risk of haemorrhage); the shortest most direct approach is usually the best as it affords the greatest scope for adjunctive intervention (Table 19.2).

When performing antegrade femoral artery puncture, use ultrasound to ensure safe femoral artery puncture, especially when puncturing a groin above or below an occluded graft. Use the contralateral approach in obese patients and when the femoral artery is occluded. If possible, avoid the brachial approach, as there is a risk of peri-catheter thrombus causing cerebral embolization.

Infra-inguinal grafts almost invariably arise from the anterior aspect of the CFA. Arterial puncture must be sufficiently proximal to allow manipulation of a shaped catheter (Cobra or RDC) to direct a straight guidewire toward the graft origin.

 **Tip:** To catheterize the graft origin, it is often helpful to obtain an angiogram in a steep oblique projection. Use roadmapping or fluoroscopy fade if these options are available.

*Direct prosthetic graft puncture* Is sometimes helpful, e.g. in femoro-femoral cross-over grafts. When the graft is palpable, fix it between forefinger and thumb and then perform a single wall puncture in the conventional manner. There is a very distinctive give and fall in resistance as the needle enters the graft lumen. Depending on the direction of catheterization, direct graft puncture will preclude accessing either the origin or the outflow. Retrograde lysis often occurs but sometimes it is necessary to make a second puncture from the other end of the graft – the 'crossed catheter technique'.

# Techniques and regimens

There are several different agents and methods for performing thrombolysis. All the techniques share a common principle: the delivery catheter is embedded in the thrombus. There is no evidence that any technique confers outcome benefit compared to the alternatives.

 **Alarm:** If a guidewire cannot be passed through the thrombus, it is probably organized and is much less likely to clear with thrombolysis.

The simplest technique is to infuse the lytic agent through a straight catheter. Variations on this theme have been proposed to accelerate the lytic process, but there is no evidence that this improves the clinical outcome and there are suggestions that complications such as bleeding and distal embolization may be more common. The dosages given below are for rt-PA. Heparin (250 IU/h) is usually administered via the sheath to minimize the risk of peri-catheter thrombosis.

- **Low dose infusion.** rt-PA is infused directly into the thrombus at a rate of 0.5 mg/h. (10 mg rt-PA in 500 mL of normal saline (0.02 mg/mL) run at 25 mL/h). The catheter tip is embedded into the proximal thrombus and the infusion started. Check angiography is performed every 6–8 hours and the catheter is repositioned distally as necessary. This form of thrombolysis often takes 24–72 hours.

 **Tip:** There is no need to perform check angiography overnight unless there is a clear clinical deterioration.

- **Bolus lacing followed by low-dose infusion.** The catheter is advanced to the distal portion of the clot and then 5 mg of rt-PA is injected at high concentration (rt-PA 1 mg/mL) as the catheter is pulled back through the proximal clot. A check angiogram is performed every 15–30 minutes. The bolus lacing is performed up to a total of three times (15 mg of rt-PA). If thrombus persists after this, a low-dose infusion is initiated as above.
- **Bolus lacing followed by high-dose infusion.** The technique is performed as above, but a high-dose infusion (rt-PA 10 mg in 100 mL, i.e. 0.1 mg/mL) is set up and run at 40 mL/h (4 mg/h) for up to 4 hours. Check angiography is performed every 60–90 minutes. After this, a low-dose infusion is used if indicated.
- **Pulse spray techniques.** These use special catheters with multiple sideholes or slits. The catheter endhole is occluded with a guidewire and the drug is injected in repeated 0.5 mL (0.05 mg rt-PA) high-pressure pulses every 30 seconds through the side-arm of a Tuohy–Borst adaptor. The theory is that this creates fissures in the clot, increasing the surface area exposed to the drug and therefore speeds up lysis. Manual injections are made using a 1-mL syringe; a tame registrar is essential for this, but if none is available, use a specialized pump.
- **Co-axial lysis.** When there is extensive thrombus, it is sometimes desirable to deliver the lytic agent at more than one site. Co-axial systems allow this. The simplest method is to infuse the drug through the arterial sheath into the proximal clot and through the catheter into the distal thrombus (Fig. 19.1). Microcatheters can be used to deliver the drug to the crural circulation.

# Procedural care

The patient must be looked after in a high-dependency area where their condition can be closely monitored. This can be on the vascular ward if staffing levels and experience permit.

**Fig. 19.1** ■ In the presence of extensive thrombus, the distal catheter is used to clear the run-off vessels while the sheath delivers the lytic agent to the graft. It is essential to secure the catheter and sheath. Failure to do so invariably leads to inadvertent removal, and the subsequent haemorrhage is extremely difficult to control.

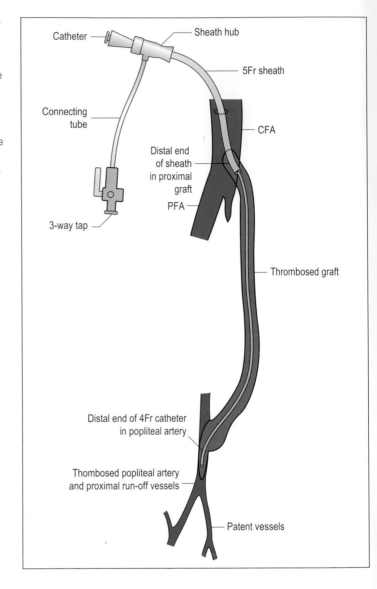

The patient is nursed in bed as flat as possible. The patient may have a light diet unless surgery is imminent. The following must be checked:

- Arterial puncture sites every 15 minutes, looking for bleeding/haematoma
- Limb viability – perfusion, pulses, Doppler signal, movement and sensation
- Urine output – the patient must be kept adequately hydrated. If necessary, IV fluids should be given and the patient catheterized
- Pulse, BP and temperature – 4-hourly
- Daily FBC, coagulation screen and fibrinogen, urea and electrolytes, glucose
- Analgesia should be regularly reviewed. **Intramuscular injections must not be given.**

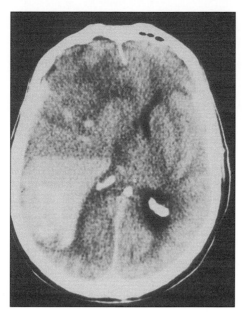

**Fig. 19.2** ■ Fatal acute haemorrhagic cerebral infarct during thrombolysis.

 **Tip:** It is essential to liaise closely with the surgical team. Keep the treatment plan under review and be alert to the need for surgical or radiological intervention.

## Endpoints

- If the patient's condition allows, thrombolysis is continued until the clot has cleared and flow has been restored. Try not to continue for more than 48 hours.
- Sometimes, there is no clearing of thrombus in between check angiograms. This is termed 'lytic stagnation' and is an indication to stop the procedure.
- Deterioration in the clinical status of the limb may necessitate urgent surgical revascularization.
- Bleeding occurs most commonly at the puncture site but can occur elsewhere; intracerebral (Fig. 19.2) and retroperitoneal bleeding may be fatal. If bleeding occurs, stop the infusion immediately. Confusion, agitation, tachycardia and hypotension indicate bleeding; if there is a change in the patient's mental state, the infusion should be stopped pending a thorough assessment.

## Adjunctive techniques

Successful thrombolysis usually reveals an underlying stenosis or occlusion. It is mandatory to correct these lesions by endovascular or surgical means. Failure to do so condemns the patient to re-thrombosis. Thrombolysis alone may not be sufficient to restore flow. The following techniques may be helpful:

- **Angioplasty and stenting** – used to treat stenoses and occlusions following thrombolysis. In high-risk patients it is worth considering directly stenting over thrombus. (Fig. 19.3)

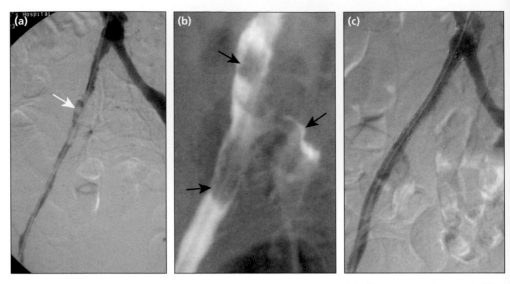

**Fig. 19.3** ■ (A) Acute critical limb ischaemia with near occlusion of the right iliac artery (white arrow). (B) Non-subtracted view clearly demonstrates saddle embolus (arrows) at the right iliac bifurcation. (C) The patient was warfarinized and had recently had a CVA, hence primary stenting was performed and a closure device used.

- **Thrombo-aspiration** – see below.
- **Surgical intervention** – embolectomy may be needed if there is distal embolization during thrombolysis. Fasciotomy is indicated if a compartment syndrome develops; this is most likely when there has been prolonged ischaemia and is recognized by painful swollen muscle, often with paralysis. If there is any suggestion of a compartment syndrome, make sure that the surgical team is aware and that they measure the compartment pressures. Bypass grafting or graft revisions are performed when thrombolysis reveals underlying disease that is not amenable to endovascular treatment.

## Complications

Unfortunately, complications of thrombolysis are not rare and may be life-threatening. Complications increase with the age of the patient, the duration of treatment and the dose of the lytic agent. Stop the infusion if a complication develops.

- CVA – can be thrombotic or haemorrhagic; overall incidence is 2–3%.
- Significant bleeding requiring transfusion or surgery – occurs in 7%. If there is any sign of bleeding, stop the infusion, check the clotting, transfuse the patient with blood and FFP. Consult a haematologist for advice if bleeding persists. Surgical intervention is often necessary. Try to intervene early before the patient becomes unstable.
- Distal embolization of thrombus – occurs in about 5% of patients; clinically, it is manifest as acute clinical deterioration with increased pain. Usually there are macroemboli, which will lyse spontaneously or can be aspirated. Microemboli are much more serious and may cause trash foot.
- Reperfusion syndrome – this is caused when there has been prolonged and severe ischaemia. Adult respiratory distress syndrome and renal failure are common sequelae and there is a high mortality.

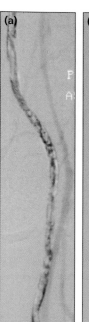
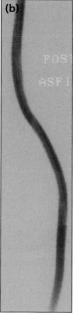
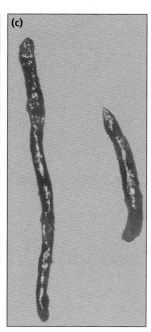

**Fig. 19.4** ■ (A) Thrombosed PTFE graft following (B) thrombosuction with an 8Fr catheter. (C) Some of the thrombus removed.

# Thrombosuction

Thrombus aspiration is the endovascular equivalent of balloon embolectomy. Large-bore catheters can be used to suck thrombus from grafts and occluded vessels. Typically, the technique is used as an adjunct to thrombolysis to accelerate reperfusion when there is a large volume of thrombus to clear. It also comes into its own when there has been a small distal embolus following angioplasty; in this case it is usually thrombo/atherosuction.

Thrombosuction is relatively safe in prosthetic grafts that have a large smooth lumen and do not collapse when they thrombose (Fig. 19.4). The catheter can be safely manipulated without a guidewire. The situation is different in diseased native vessels where repeated catheter passage is undesirable. The principal disadvantage of aspiration thrombectomy is the need for a large arterial puncture (7–8Fr) to permit passage of the catheter.

## Equipment

- Sheath with removable haemostatic valve is essential or the thrombus simply gets stripped off by the valve of the sheath during catheter removal.
- Large lumen catheters: typically 7Fr straight guide-catheter (6Fr lumen) for prosthetic graft and native SFA; 5Fr catheter (4Fr lumen) for native popliteal and crural vessels.
- 50-mL syringe.

## Procedure

*Access* Ipsilateral arterial access is essential.

*Catheterization* The vessel is catheterized in the conventional manner but a removable hub sheath is used.

*Technique* The aspiration catheter is embedded into the proximal occlusion and then the 50 mL syringe is attached. Pull back the syringe plunger to create a vacuum and advance the catheter until it occludes with thrombus. Maintain suction and withdraw the catheter. When the catheter reaches the sheath, the hub is removed; this prevents thrombus trapping on the haemostatic valve as the catheter is taken out. Brisk arterial backflow immediately follows, so quickly put a finger over the sheath until the valve is replaced. Flush the contents of the catheter/syringe through a gauze cloth to allow examination. The procedure is repeated as often as necessary until the vessel is clear.

## Troubleshooting

**Thrombus cannot be aspirated** There are two main causes:
- The thrombus is old; try again after a bolus of thrombolysis to soften the thrombus
- The catheter/sheath is kinked at the arterial puncture site: replace the sheath and try again, keeping it under slight tension as the catheter is pulled back.

**A central core of thrombus is removed but extensive thrombus remains** This is common in artificial grafts and is a limitation of the technique; use adjunctive thrombolysis to clear residual thrombus.

**Thrombus embolizes distally** This is a pitfall of the technique; advancing a large catheter can 'bulldoze' thrombus distally and may even impact it in a distal vessel. Try thrombolysis to clear the block and consider surgical embolectomy if necessary.

# Mechanical thrombectomy

Mechanical thrombectomy uses special catheters to macerate the thrombus. The residue is either small enough to pass through the distal circulation or is aspirated. The catheter has to be appropriately sized for the vessel and large sheaths may be necessary. These devices work best with fresh thrombus and small acute emboli.

## Equipment

There are several commercially available devices but only two modes of action:
- **Impeller-type devices** – typified by the Amplatz thrombectomy device (Fig. 19.5A). The impeller is driven by compressed air and rotates at up to 150 000 rpm. This creates a vortex, which draws thrombus into the impeller, where it is fragmented into tiny particles that pass through the distal circulation. The catheter is activated by a footswitch and is cooled/lubricated by perfusion with saline. The catheter should not be run for more than 60 seconds at a time.
- **Rheolytic catheters** (Fig. 19.5B). These devices utilize an injection pump to create a high-velocity saline jet which produces a zone of low pressure at the catheter tip. Thrombus is sucked into the jet and is broken up. The resultant slurry is cleared through the catheter into a drainage bag.

Some of these devices do not operate over a guidewire and hence they cannot be steered except with a guide-catheter. The smallest catheters of these types are 6Fr.

- **Fragmentation baskets**: these devices are essentially like a miniature egg whisk powered by battery, that breaks up thrombus. The basket is made of Nitinol and inserted collapsed within a covering catheter through a short 7Fr sheath over a 0.014-inch wire. The most

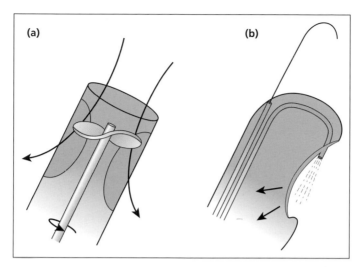

**Fig. 19.5** ■ Mechanical thrombectomy catheters. (A) The Amplatz thrombectomy device – the impeller draws in thrombus, which is macerated and expelled via the side ports. (B) A typical rheolytic catheter. A high-pressure jet creates a vortex, sucking in thrombus and removing the slurry via the exhaust port.

common application is in dialysis grafts. Use only in larger veins and be careful as vein size reduces, or near stents, etc., as these can easily get tangled up in the device with disappointing results.

# Procedure

*Access* Ipsilateral puncture is necessary.

*Catheterization* A standard vascular sheath is used.

*Technique* Rheolytic- and impeller-type devices are switched on just proximal to the thrombus and then advanced slowly into the occlusion. It helps to advance the catheter only a few centimetres and then pull it back and repeat the procedure. This is continued until the vessel is clear. Some manufacturers advocate inflating a blood pressure cuff around the limb distal to an occlusion to prevent distal embolization.

Fragmentation baskets are confusingly the reverse in use. The catheter containing the constrained basket is advanced beyond the thrombus then the catheter pulled back to allow the basket to open. The battery-powered impeller is started and the device slowly withdrawn. It's vital that you slowly withdraw the rotating basket – advancing while the basket is rotating is not recommended. If you want a second run at it, collapse the basket by carefully advancing the outer catheter before advancing the device.

# Troubleshooting

**The catheter will not pass down the vessel** If there is stenosis or occlusion blocking the way, treat with angioplasty. If the vessel is tortuous, try directing the catheter with a guide-catheter.

**The Amplatz thrombectomy device stops working** The device will only function for about 15 minutes before it seizes. Use the device intermittently and switch off when not advancing the catheter. Do not forget to turn on the saline 'coolant'.

**The catheter has been kinked and the drive shaft has fractured** Keep the catheter as straight as possible because once kinked it is useless.

**The catheter clears a central core but leaves residual thrombus** This is a limitation of the technique. Ensure that the catheter is correctly sized for the vessel – an 8Fr Amplatz thrombectomy device is necessary for the SFA and most grafts; the 6Fr device is suitable for the popliteal artery. Consider adjunctive thrombolysis to clear any remaining thrombus and distal emboli.

**The device does not clear the thrombus** Unfortunately, this is not rare – check that the device is activated properly. If it is, then the thrombus is probably too organized to break down; consider other techniques.

## Suggestions for further reading

### Thrombolysis

Belli A-M. Thrombolysis in the peripheral vascular system. Cardiovasc Intervent Radiol 1998;21:95–101.
The big picture of thrombolysis, how and when to do it.
Kessel DO, Berridge DC, Robertson I. Infusion techniques for peripheral arterial thrombolysis (Cochrane Review). In: The Cochrane Library, 1. Chichester, UK: John Wiley & Sons, Ltd, 2004, CD000985.
As sexy as new techniques sound there is no evidence that they improve the key outcome measures of amputation rates or mortality.

### Percutaneous aspiration thrombectomy

Wagner HJ, Starck EE. Acute embolic occlusions of the infrainguinal arteries: percutaneous aspiration embolectomy in 102 patients. Radiology 1992;182:403–407.
Excellent results from the men who started it all. NB: Uses a selected group of patients without underlying peripheral vascular disease. Note also the high complication rate.

### Mechanical thrombectomy

Gorich J, Rilinger N, Sokiranski R, et al. Mechanical thrombolysis of acute occlusion of both the superficial and the deep femoral arteries using a thrombectomy device. AJR Am J Roentgenol 1998;170:1177–1180.
Rilinger N, Gorich J, Scharrer-Pamler R, et al. Short-term results with use of the Amplatz thrombectomy device in the treatment of acute lower limb occlusions. J Vasc Intervent Radiol 1997;8:343–348.
Sends a clear message that best results are with emboli.
Rousseau H, Sapoval M, Ballini P, et al. Percutaneous recanalization of acutely thrombosed vessels by hydrodynamic thrombectomy (Hydrolyser). Eur Radiol 1997;7:935–941.
Contains a mixture of dialysis access, peripheral grafts and native vessels and concludes that best results are obtained in dialysis access.

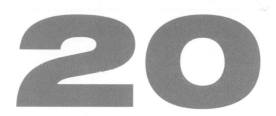

# Venous intervention

Percutaneous placement of IVC filters and treatment of SVCO are the cornerstones of venous intervention. Venous angioplasty, stenting and thrombolysis are sometimes performed but remain controversial techniques except in the management of haemodialysis access. The principles of negotiating and treating venous stenoses and occlusions are exactly the same as in the arterial system. This chapter covers some established indications for venous intervention and details aspects of intervention specific to the venous system.

## IVC filters

IVC filters are placed to prevent pulmonary embolism from sources in the lower limbs, pelvis and IVC. Contemporary devices are readily placed percutaneously via the right IJV or femoral veins. Several permanent and retrievable filters are commercially available. Most retrievable filters can be left permanently in place.

### Indications for IVC filtration

There is little evidence to support the use of IVC filters, but most would consider two unquestionable indications for placement of a permanent IVC filter; several further indications may also be valid and should be considered on a case-by-case basis (Table 20.1). Thrombosis rates vary between devices; overall, about 10% of permanent IVC filters will thrombose within 5 years. Permanent filters should be avoided whenever possible in those patients with a long life-expectancy.

There are a few contraindications to caval filtration when there is a high risk of major pulmonary embolus. Introducer sheaths for IVC filters start at 7Fr; insertion of large catheters into the femoral vein is itself a cause of deep vein thrombosis (DVT), hence the jugular approach has a distinct advantage!

### Equipment

- Ultrasound for right IJV puncture.
- Basic angiography set.
- Cobra catheter.
- 3-mm J guidewire.
- An appropriate IVC filter set (see below).

IVC filters are supplied with different delivery systems designed for use from either the jugular or the femoral approach. These systems are not interchangeable, so make sure that

**Table 20.1** Indications for caval filtration and recommended filter type

| Indication | Filter type |
| --- | --- |
| **Unequivocal** | |
| Recurrent PE despite adequate anticoagulation | P |
| PE with contraindication to anticoagulation | P |
| **Relative** | |
| Free-floating ileofemoral/IVC thrombus with a high risk of embolization | P/R |
| Patients with PE and severely limited cardiorespiratory reserve | P |
| Spinal cord injury with paraplegia | P |
| Severe trauma | P/R |
| Prophylactic – before surgery on patients at high risk of DVT or PE, e.g. before hip surgery in the presence of ipsilateral femoral DVT | R |

*P, permanent; R, retrievable.*

you have the correct device! Check also that you have an appropriately-sized device for the IVC. The bird's nest filter is currently the only filter that can be placed in a megacava.

## Procedure

*Access* The right IJV is the 'universal gateway' and can be used for access even in the presence of ileofemoral DVT. Some filters have inflexible delivery systems and cannot be delivered from the left jugular or the left femoral vein.

Make sure that there is a contemporary ultrasound to document the site and extent of thrombus. Placing a catheter through a thrombosed vein is likely to result in iatrogenic pulmonary embolism (PE)!

*Catheterization* From the jugular route, use a Cobra catheter and 3 mm J guidewire to carefully negotiate through the right atrium to the IVC. From the femoral route, simply place a pigtail catheter at the iliac venous confluence.

*Runs* Angiography is required for three reasons:
* To demonstrate the patency of the IVC, assess its size and any angulation
* To confirm conventional anatomy, i.e. single IVC
* To document the position of the renal veins
* To perform pulmonary thrombectomy.

It is usually sufficient to perform a simple IVC injection through a pigtail catheter placed just above the confluence of the iliac veins. An initial gentle hand injection will ensure that there is no thrombus adjacent to the catheter; perform a more vigorous injection to demonstrate the entire IVC. The position of the renal veins is usually apparent because of streaming of unopacified blood (Fig. 20.1). If the renal veins cannot be identified, use a Cobra catheter to engage them and perform selective hand injections to demonstrate their position.

 **Tip:** Use the patient's spine as a reference for the position of the renal veins and to measure the IVC. If your angiography equipment does not include measurement software, it is helpful to place a radio-opaque ruler to the left of the spine.

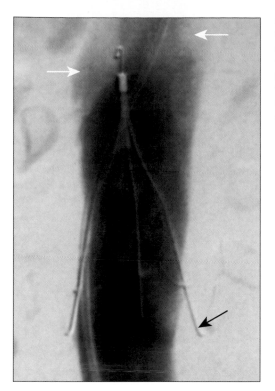

**Fig. 20.1** ■ IVC venogram performed prior to removal of IVC filter. Note the streaming effect of unopacified blood from the renal veins (white arrows). It is not uncommon to see a filter leg protruding through the IVC wall (black arrow); this does not preclude removal but should encourage you to be alert to possible difficulty.

Once the position of the renal veins has been established, do not move the table or the image intensifier. Do not forget to measure the diameter of the infra-renal IVC. Most IVC filters can only be used within a specified range of IVC diameters; if the filter is too small, the first place it will lodge is the tricuspid valve!

*Positioning the filter* There are two sites to place an IVC filter, and the position is determined from the cavogram.

- Infrarenal: this is the optimal site; if the filter causes IVC thrombosis, the renal veins will be spared. Conical filters should be placed with the filter apex at the level of the renal veins; the high flow promotes dissolution of thrombus trapped or formed within the filter.
- Suprarenal: in the presence of infrarenal thrombus, a filter can be sited between the renal and hepatic veins. In this position, filter thrombosis can lead to renal vein thrombosis and renal infarction.

*Deploying the filter* Each type of filter is deployed differently and there may even be differences for a single type of filter depending on whether the jugular or femoral route is used. Read the instructions carefully before use; if you do not understand them, seek help!

 **Alarm:** If there is no contraindication, the patient should be anticoagulated while the filter is in situ to minimize the chance of filter thrombosis.

**Bird's nest filter** The bird's nest filter comes with a long and very comprehensive set of instructions. The filter comprises two V-shaped anchoring struts and a very fine mesh of wire

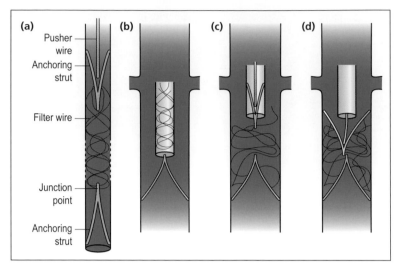

**Fig. 20.2** ■ Key steps in the deployment of the bird's nest filter (jugular deployment): (A) Filter in delivery catheter. (B) Deploy the proximal anchoring struts – the sheath is retracted. (C) Deploy the filter wires – the inner pusher wire is advanced. (D) Deploy the distal anchoring struts – the sheath is retracted.

that sits between the struts rather like an IVC Brillo pad! The deployment device consists of an outer sheath with an inner wire pusher that is attached to the filter. The device is fairly complicated to use but has the advantage of placement in caval diameters up to 45 mm.

The deployment can be thought of in three stages (Fig. 20.2):

1. Deploy the first anchoring strut – the pusher is held in place and the sheath retracted.
2. Deploy the bird's nest wires – the pusher is held stationary and the sheath is retracted by 2–3 cm to give the nest space to form. Holding the sheath stationary, the filter wires are then deployed by advancing the inner pusher until the junction point of the proximal hook wires is seen.
3. Deploy the second anchoring strut – the pusher and sheath are advanced to overlap the struts, then the sheath is retracted to deploy the proximal anchoring strut. The filter is then released from the deployment mechanism using the push button at the end of the mechanism.

The instructions are essential and referred to during the procedure even by experienced operators!

**Gunther tulip filter** This can be used as either a temporary or a permanent filter. It is a simple conical filter that can be placed from either the jugular or the femoral approach. The filter has a small hook at the apex, which allows retrieval using a snare and specialized retrieval kit. Check whether you have a jugular or femoral device.

*Filter removal* There is no absolute consensus on the length of time a filter can be left in place before removal is attempted. However long the filter has been in place be gentle; stripping the IVC would be a fatal error. Perform a cavogram (Fig. 20.3) to see if there is any residual thrombus either in the filter or which would threaten significant PE. If there is less than 1 cm³ of thrombus in the filter, it can be removed. The filter has a hook at its apex, which is snared from the jugular vein. The snare must be placed at the top of the hook; the

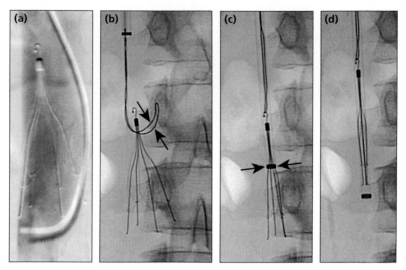

**Fig. 20.3** Removal of a Gunther tulip IVC filter. (A) Initial IVC angiogram demonstrates that the filter is free of thrombus. (B) The snare (arrows) is passed over the filter and the apex of the hook is snared. (C) The filter closes as the sheath (arrows) is advanced over it. (D) When the filter is fully inside the sheath, they are removed together.

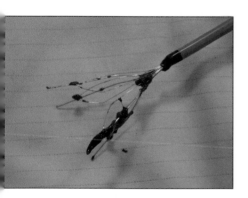

**Fig. 20.4** ■ Thrombus on filter struts despite normal venogram.

snare is held in place and the sheath advanced over it to close the filter (Fig. 20.3). There is almost always thrombus/tissue on the filter struts (Fig. 20.4).

 **Alarm:** If there is difficulty STOP! DO NOT USE FORCE. Accept that it may not be possible to remove the filter. It is better to leave a permanent filter than cause an IVC laceration.

## Complications

Significant procedure-related complications are rare and include:

*Access site thrombosis* Femoral vein thrombosis was particularly common with early devices but is only seen in 2–3% of patients with smaller contemporary devices.

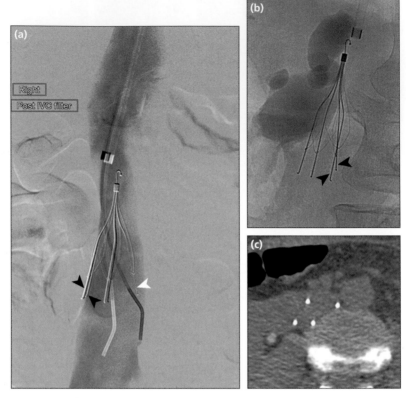

**Fig. 20.5** ▣ Images of IVC filter. (A) The initial frontal projection shows two struts that appear to lie close together (black arrowheads) and a further strut (white arrowhead) that does not seem to reach the vein wall. (B) In the oblique projection the filter struts appear crossed (black arrowheads). (C) The patient was sent for a CT scan, which shows the IVC is flattened, accounting for the proximity of the struts. The legs are all in apposition with the wall.

*IVC perforation* Filter struts may perforate the caval wall; this is rarely clinically significant but may make the filter irretrievable.

*Incorrect deployment* There are four forms of incorrect deployment:
* Malposition in relation to the renal veins
* Incorrect filter sizing. At worst, this will result in fatal embolization of the filter. More commonly, it results in tilting or incorrect opening
* Conical filters can be tilted; this may impair filter function
* The filter may open incorrectly so that the struts are not evenly distributed or appear not to reach the IVC wall. This may impair filter function. If you have any doubt, perform a limited CT to clarify the situation (Fig. 20.5).

If you have placed a permanent filter, you are stuck, whereas a removable filter can be repositioned. If there is severe misalignment, a second filter may have to be placed above the first.

 **Tip:** Try to deploy the filter in a straight portion of the IVC; it is more likely to be effective and much easier to remove.

## Late complications

*IVC thrombosis*
- This is seen in at least 10% of patients with Greenfield and bird's nest filters. Caval thrombosis is serious if suprarenal. Thrombosis of the infrarenal IVC is usually compensated by the development of ascending lumbar collaterals. Remember that surgical ligation of the IVC used to be the treatment for recurrent PE until recently!

*Structural failure of the filter*
- This has led to several filter designs being withdrawn from the market and is another reason to remove filters whenever possible.

The long-term structural integrity and patency of the newer designs of IVC filters remain to be established.

# Superior vena cava obstruction

SVCO causes distressing symptoms, including facial and upper limb oedema, headache and drowsiness. The majority of cases are secondary to intrathoracic malignancy, particularly central bronchogenic carcinoma. Patients with malignant SVCO usually have a poor life expectancy and the aim of therapy is palliation of symptoms. SVCO can also occur in patients with benign conditions, particularly with dialysis catheters. Unless SVCO is treated promptly, extensive venous thrombosis can develop and greatly increases the complexity of intervention.

 **Alarm:** Stenting SVCO is a palliative treatment; there is a procedure-related mortality rate of approximately 2–4% related to pulmonary embolism and the underlying condition.

SVCO is one of the most gratifying conditions for the interventional radiologist to treat. Patients often feel marked improvement immediately the stent is deployed.

## Assessing SVCO

The aim of investigation is to delineate the extent of the venous obstruction and thrombosis and to plan the subsequent intervention. Many patients will have had chest CT with coronal reformats, which will usually serve to delineate the cause and extent of the problem (Fig. 20.6). It will also demonstrate complicating factors such as tumour invasion or thrombosis (Fig. 20.7). Neck ultrasound should be performed to demonstrate patency of the jugular veins; if they are thrombosed, treatment is much harder. Patients may have had bilateral upper limb venography to assess the peripheral and central veins. Remember peripheral injection often fails to opacify the central veins (Fig. 20.8A). If the jugular veins are patent, then simply place a 4Fr dilator in the RIJV to perform venography; otherwise, central catheterization should be performed using 4Fr catheters placed via the basilic veins (Fig. 20.8B).

 **Tip:** You can get a good idea whether there is significant SVCO by looking at the IJV with ultrasound. If the IJV has collaterals, is distended, non-pulsatile or shows spontaneous contrast, there will be a problem.

## Treatment of SVCO

There are two very different clinical scenarios.

*Uncomplicated stenosis or occlusion*
- This is quick and easy to treat. Benign strictures may respond to angioplasty alone but the majority of neoplastic lesions will be treated by primary stenting (Fig. 20.8C).

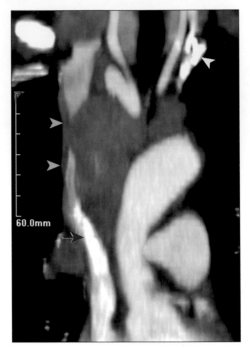

**Fig. 20.6** ■ CT reformat showing SVCO (turquoise arrows) due to a large mediastinal mass. Note collateral veins in the left side of the neck (yellow arrow) and dense contrast in the lower SVC due to filling from the azygous vein.

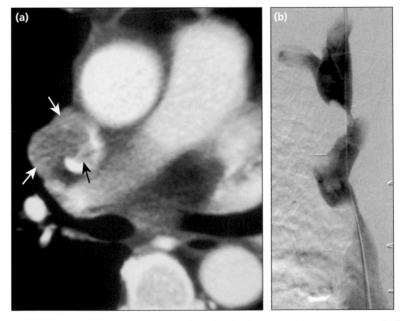

**Fig. 20.7** ■ SVCO. (A) Initial CT shows tumour adjacent to (white arrows) and invading the SVC (black arrow). (B) The venogram performed via a sheath in the right IJV confirms the findings.

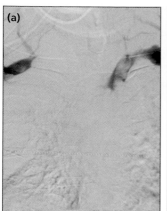
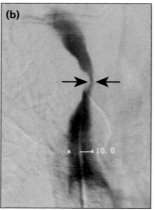
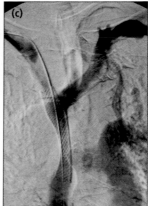

**Fig. 20.8** ▇ SVCO. (A) Peripheral injection does not demonstrate the central veins. (B) Injection through a catheter in the innominate vein demonstrates a simple stenosis (arrows). Note measurement of the SVC diameter. (C) Following deployment of a single Wallstent, excellent bilateral drainage is restored.

*SVCO complicated by thrombosis* The aim of treatment is to re-establish flow without causing pulmonary embolism. There are two distinct strategies: primary stenting or stenting following thrombolysis and thrombectomy. The former is quick but may require additional stents. The thrombus is often organized and difficult to clear, making thrombolysis and thrombectomy a more complicated and time-consuming option.

 **Tip:** Teach your physicians to refer earlier and make life simpler for everyone.

# Equipment

- Basic angiography set.
- Guidewires: curved hydrophilic wire, Amplatz super-stiff wire 180 and 260 cm.
- Catheters: 4Fr straight, Cobra II, Berenstein, 80 cm, 8, 10, 12 and 15-mm angioplasty balloons.
- Sheaths: start with a small sheath to cross the lesion and then escalate to the size needed for the balloon/stent.
- Stents: 8–16+ mm diameter.
- Vascular snares: 10 mm and 25 mm are sometimes required.

# Procedure

*Access* The obstruction is often more readily traversed from the right IJV, which is the shortest, most stable route and can readily accommodate large sheaths.

*Catheterization* Cross stenoses in a standard fashion using a shaped catheter and a hydrophilic wire. Exchange for an Amplatz wire before angioplasty/stenting. If necessary, cross the lesion from the arm and then exchange for a 260-cm guidewire, which can be snared and brought out of a femoral sheath.

*Runs* Perform venography to delineate the obstruction and demonstrate the major collateral channels. Assess the extent and distribution of any thrombus.

*Technique* As a general rule, use angioplasty for benign disease and stents for malignant disease. Thrombus can sometimes be stented over directly. When there is extensive fresh thrombus, an attempt can be made to debulk it by mechanical thrombectomy or thrombolysis using a low-dose infusion. Before starting thrombolysis, it is essential to exclude cerebral metastases and other potential bleeding sites such as the primary tumour. Thrombectomy will not clear all the venous thrombus but rather will create a central channel that will allow it to be stented over.

Choose a stent which will completely cover the lesion and be firmly anchored in the stricture and adjacent vein; in practice, 12–16 mm. Do not leave the end of the stent in the right atrium as it may cause emboli or even perforation.

 **Alarm:** In the presence of thrombosis there is a risk of pulmonary embolus during stent placement, especially if the stent is placed from the femoral approach, as the stent opens from the jugular end towards the SVC. Stents deployed from the jugular vein open from the SVC towards the jugular vein, hence tend to trap the thrombus against the SVC wall as the stent is deployed.

The stent can be dilated with a balloon to an appropriate diameter. Following deployment, perform a venogram to demonstrate patency.

## Troubleshooting

**Poor flow or extensive collateral filling** Perform further angioplasty/stent deployment.

**Both brachiocephalic veins are involved** When there is bilateral obstruction, it is usually only necessary to treat one side.

**There is a large discrepancy in size between the venous segments to be stented** This is an indication to use a Wallstent, which will taper to fit the narrower vessel. This will significantly increase its final length; make sure that you allow for this.

**The patient becomes hypoxic or hypotensive** Resuscitate them promptly and consider the possibility of pulmonary embolism or SVC perforation. Perform a venogram; if there is evidence of a leak, then a covered stent should be deployed. SVC perforation can lead to rapid cardiac tamponade and death. If the venogram is negative, then perform a pulmonary angiogram, and if there is a large embolism, try to macerate it with a catheter.

## Inferior vena cava obstruction (IVCO)

ICVO is considerably less common than SVCO but again mainly secondary to advanced tumour. Affected patients often have gross leg and lower body oedema. The basic principles are identical to SVCO, but particular care should be taken to avoid stenting over the renal or hepatic veins. The IVC has a large calibre and there is a significant potential for stent migration, so choose a suitable stent diameter carefully.

## Iliac vein obstruction

This often presents with iliofemoral deep vein thrombosis and massive leg oedema. The left side is more often affected due to compression by the overlying right CIA (May Thurner syndrome). Treatment is by thrombolysis followed by placement of a large stent.

# Transjugular intrahepatic porto-systemic shunt

The TIPS procedure involves forming a tract between the hepatic vein and the portal vein, thus shunting blood away from liver sinusoids and reducing portal venous pressure. The principal indications for TIPS are variceal haemorrhage not controlled by endoscopic therapy, refractory ascites and Budd–Chiari syndrome. TIPS is a complex procedure with a limited durability that requires follow-up and reintervention in a significant number of patients. There is a 1% procedure-related mortality and a risk of new or worsening hepatic encephalopathy.

 **Alarm:** Patients with poor synthetic liver function are at greatest risk of encephalopathy. When associated with variceal haemorrhage and high APACHE scores, almost all will die within 30 days.

## Anatomy for TIPS

Conventional TIPS tracts are formed between a hepatic vein and either the left or right branch of the portal vein. Although any of the hepatic veins can be used, it is easiest and safest to pass from the right hepatic vein (RHV) into the right portal vein (Fig. 20.9). The RHV bears a reasonably constant position posterior and superior to the right portal vein (RPV). Bile ducts and hepatic artery branches frequently lie in between the RHV and the RPV and are often opacified during the procedure.

The middle hepatic vein may lie anterior to the RPV and therefore punctures may need to be angled posteriorly. Anterior punctures from the middle hepatic vein risk capsular perforation. It can be difficult to differentiate the RHV from the middle hepatic vein in the AP projection but this is easily done from a lateral projection.

## Guidance for TIPS procedure

The principal difficulty with the procedure is targeting the portal vein puncture. It is common for patients to have had MR or CT. Use these to assess patency and position of the portal vein. During the procedure, the portal vein can be imaged by wedged hepatic venography using conventional contrast or $CO_2$ can be used to fill the portal vein retrogradely (Fig. 20.10). Ultrasound allows real-time targeting, but relying on a colleague to direct the

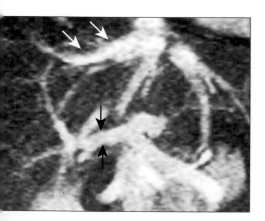

**Fig. 20.9** ■ MRI showing the relationship of the hepatic veins to the portal bifurcation. The right hepatic vein (white arrows), which lies posterior and superior to the right portal vein (black arrows), is the optimal approach.

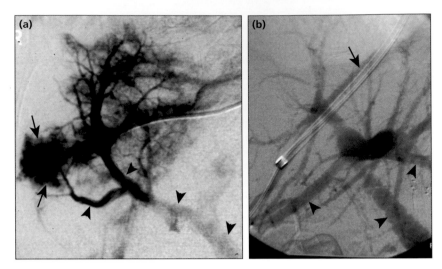

**Fig. 20.10** ■ Wedged hepatic venography. (A) Conventional contrast is forced into the sinusoids causing a dense parenchymal blush (arrows) and then flows retrogradely into the portal vein (arrowheads). The portal bifurcation is clearly seen. (B) $CO_2$ wedged venogram showing the portal vein (arrowheads). Contrast can be seen adjacent to the sheath in the hepatic vein (arrow).

puncture with ultrasound will strain all but the best relationships. Ultrasound is essential if performing portal vein puncture for targeting or as a component of percutaneous TIPS.

 **Tip:** If you don't have $CO_2$ angiography and want to show the relative positions of the RHV and RPV, perform a hepatic venogram during the portal vein phase of an arterioportogram.

## Equipment

- Basic angiography set.
- Guidewires: 3-mm J, curved hydrophilic wire (regular and stiff), Amplatz wire (regular and short tip).
- Cobra catheter, angioplasty balloons 8, 10 and 12-mm by 4-cm.
- 5Fr sheath.
- TIPS set (e.g. Cook UK):
    - 40-cm 10Fr sheath with end marker
    - 51-cm curved guide-catheter with metal stiffener
    - 60-cm long sheathed needle.
- TIPS stents and stent grafts 8, 10 and 12-mm.
- Vascular pressure transducer (to measure portosystemic pressure gradient).
- Ultrasound for right IJV puncture.

## Procedure

TIPS is a painful procedure, sometimes for the operator as well as the patient, which will probably take you a long time to master. Leave yourself 3–4 hours for the case. Think of the patient and consider general anaesthesia; if you do not do this, the patient will require heavy sedation. Anaesthetic assistance is mandatory in variceal bleeders with hepatic encephalopathy.

Before starting, review the pre-procedure imaging to establish that the portal vein is patent; if not available, perform Doppler ultrasound. If there is portal vein thrombosis, stop and seek expert advice.

*Access*  Ultrasound-guided right IJV puncture.

*Catheterization*  Introduce the TIPS sheath into the SVC. Pass the J wire and Cobra catheter into the IVC, taking particular care steering through the right atrium. The RHV is the target vein. Rotate the catheter so that its tip points towards the patient's right, and slowly withdraw it until the tip engages the vein. Advance the hydrophilic wire and Cobra catheter into the vein.

*Runs*  To perform a wedged hepatic venogram advance a 4Fr catheter into a distal and peripheral tributary of the hepatic vein (Fig. 20.10). If the catheter is wedged there will usually be a satisfying sucking sound when the wire is removed. A gentle injection of contrast or $CO_2$ will demonstrate enhancement of the hepatic parenchyma and may even show the portal vein. If the catheter is not wedged, try a different position; if it is wedged, perform a run centred over the portal bifurcation (about 4 cm lateral to the spine, on the right!), including from the bottom of the right atrium down. This will show the relative positions of the portal vein confluence and the hepatic vein origin. If wedged venography fails, consider arterioportography with simultaneous hepatic venography. When you have obtained a good image, mark the positions of the portal veins and the hepatic vein on the screen with a chinagraph pencil and lock the tabletop in position.

*Further catheterization*  Place an Amplatz wire into the RHV and advance the TIPS sheath 4–5 cm into the vein. Exchange the Cobra catheter for the curved guide-catheter and advance this just beyond the tip of the sheath. The angled stiffener within the sheath gives excellent torque control but poor cornering ability, and will only negotiate suitably angled veins.

*Puncturing the portal vein*  This is easy to describe but is one of those practical procedures that takes quite a lot of experience to really get the hang of. Remove the guidewire; remember that the RPV lies anterior to the RHV; and turn the guide-catheter so that the metal arrow points anteriorly and slightly to the right. Slowly pull the guide-catheter back until its tip is 2–3 cm into the RHV. Now advance the sheathed needle through the guide-catheter; aim to hit the RPV 1–3 cm from the portal bifurcation. Resistance is felt as the needle passes into the liver parenchyma; cirrhotic liver is particularly tough. Do not go beyond the projected portal vein position. It is common to feel increased resistance as the portal tract is reached and a 'give' as the portal vein is entered. Withdraw the needle and attach a 5-mL syringe containing 2 mL of contrast to the catheter. Slowly pull the catheter back, aspirating as you go. Stop as soon as it bubbles or you aspirate blood; perform a short contrast run. There are three possibilities:

- Contrast flows towards the right atrium – you are still in the hepatic vein.
- Contrast flows towards the periphery of the liver – you are either in the portal vein or the hepatic artery. Portal vein branches are larger and are often visible to the periphery of the liver.
- Contrast flows towards the portal bifurcation if there is reversed flow in the portal vein. If it does not clear – you are in the bile duct.

If you are in the portal vein, congratulations! If not, continue pulling back until the catheter is in the guide-catheter. Put the needle back, redirect the guide-catheter and try again. Remember Robert the Bruce and his spider and, try, try and try again until the portal vein is entered.

*Catheterizing the portal vein* Once the vein has been punctured, introduce a hydrophilic wire well down into the main portal vein. Advance the catheter from the sheathed needle until it is in up to its hub. If there is any doubt about whether you are in the portal vein, check now with an injection of contrast. Gird your loins and advance the entire guide-catheter and sheath through into the portal vein; this is the defining moment of the procedure. Exchange the hydrophilic wire for the Amplatz wire and remove the catheter and guide-catheter over the wire. Put the Cobra catheter into the portal vein and pull the sheath back into the right atrium. Measure the portosystemic pressure gradient between the portal vein and right atrium.

*Forming the TIPS tract* Once you are in the portal vein, make sure that you do not lose access! Keep the tip of the Amplatz wire under control; it will readily perforate the liver or the mesentery! Dilate the tract with an 8-mm angioplasty balloon. If the patient is awake, now is the time for some heavy sedation and analgesia, as dilating the tract is very painful. The balloon will usually waist at the hepatic vein and portal vein.

*Stenting the TIPS tract* The tract must be stented if it is to stay open. Most operators use either the Viatorr stent graft or the Wallstent. Obtain a venogram by simultaneously injecting into the portal and hepatic veins (Fig. 20.11A) and measure the length of stent needed: either use a calibrated catheter (Fig. 20.11) or the measurement software on your angiography unit. The stent should be long enough to cover from the origin of the hepatic vein, through the parenchymal tract (≈4 cm) and project about 2 cm into the portal vein. Do not leave stent protruding into the right atrium or dangling down the main portal vein as these can interfere if the patient has a liver transplant!

There is evidence to suggest improved patency using PTFE covered stent grafts. The Viatorr (Gore) has been designed specifically for TIPS and comprises bare stent that extends into the portal vein and a PTFE-covered portion intended to cover the intrahepatic tract and hepatic

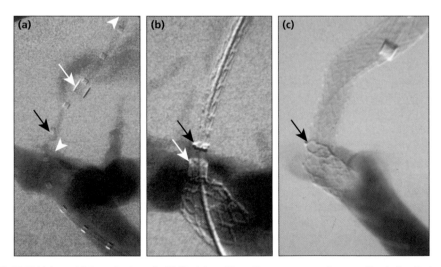

**Fig. 20.11** ▪ Using a Viatorr stent-graft. (A) Portal and hepatic venogram using a calibrated catheter (black arrow); the end of the TIPS sheath is in the hepatic vein (white arrow). Chevrons indicate the end of the hepatic vein and the portal end of the TIPS tract. (B) The sheath is placed in the portal vein, the stent is positioned so that the marker indicating the transition between the bare stent and covered stent is at the distal end of the TIPS tract (black arrow); the sheath (white arrow) is then pulled back to deploy the bare stent. (C) Completion venogram showing correctly positioned stent-graft.

vein (Fig. 16.9 in Chapter 16, Stents and Stent-Grafts). The length of the covered part of the stent graft is the distance from the portal vein end of the TIPS tract to the end of the hepatic vein, the diameter is that of the desired shunt. The tract is dilated according to the pressure gradient. As neo-intimal hyperplasia does not narrow the stent-graft, there is a tendency to use smaller grafts. Most operators would use a 10-mm stent-graft for bleeding and an 8-mm stent graft for ascites.

*Finishing off* Dilate the tract to 8 mm and then measure the portosystemic gradient. If the gradient is greater than 12 mmHg, dilate the tract to 10 mm and then 12 mm until the gradient is abolished.

   If the gradient is less than 12 mmHg, perform a completion venogram. A satisfactory venogram shows almost all portal vein flow passing through the stent into the hepatic vein (Fig. 20.11C).

## Troubleshooting

This section could potentially be as long as the procedure section.

**Unable to catheterize the hepatic vein** This is either due to an obstruction or unfavourable angulation. Review the previous imaging to ensure vein patency and perform a venogram to look for obstruction (Fig. 20.12). If there is a hepatic vein web, consider angioplasty rather than TIPS. If there is modest cranial angulation, consider shaping the introducer accordingly.

**Unable to hit the portal vein** Only practice helps here. Check that you are in the RHV and not the MHV. Try different points along the RHV and different degrees of torque on the metal stiffener. Consider bending the sheathed needle to alter the approach.

**Hit an intrahepatic bile duct** This is of little consequence in its own right. The cholangiogram will help indicate the position of the portal bifurcation. The main importance is that TIPS tracts contaminated by bile have an increased incidence of pseudointimal hyperplasia and thrombosis.

**Hit the hepatic artery** This is less common than biliary puncture but more likely to cause problems. If intrahepatic, you are likely not to be in too much trouble – simply carefully observe the patient during the remainder of the procedure. If extrahepatic, the potential to

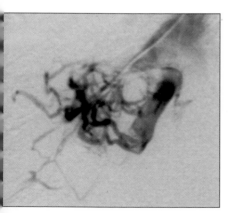

**Fig. 20.12** ▪ Budd–Chiari syndrome. The hepatic veins could not be catheterized. Injection into the stump of the right hepatic vein reveals the network of spidery veins typical of Budd–Chiari syndrome.

bleed is higher. Wait a few minutes and perform an angiogram. If necessary, embolize to stop the bleeding.

**Hit peripheral portal vein** You are unlikely to succeed unless the tract has a favourable course. If you are not too far peripheral and too angulated, proceed as normal. If not, start again.

**Hit the main portal vein** This is a dangerous thing to do, as there is a risk of massive bleeding if the vein tears, e.g. during angioplasty/stenting. Consider leaving a guidewire in situ to mark the position of the vein while you try again.

**Unable to advance the TIPS catheter/sheath into portal vein** Not uncommon in cirrhotic livers. Exchange the sheathed needle catheter for an 80–100-cm 4Fr catheter and advance the 4Fr catheter into the portal vein, then exchange for the Amplatz wire. If it is still impossible, then carefully remove the curved guide-catheter, keeping the Amplatz wire in situ and dilate the tract with a 4-mm angioplasty balloon. If this fails, exchange for a supportive 0.018-inch wire (e.g. platinum plus) and use a low-profile angioplasty balloon to dilate the tract.

**The portal vein tears** This is an emergency. Call for help and resuscitate the patient. The best advice is to stent or stent-graft the tract immediately. The drop in portal pressure will usually stop the bleeding. If this fails, gain control by placing an occlusion balloon in the portal vein, and breathe deeply. Surgery is the only solution.

**Residual pressure gradient post TIPS** If a >12 mmHg gradient persists following stenting and angioplasty, perform a venogram and measure pressures to identify the point of obstruction. Use further stents as necessary. If a gradient persists, a parallel TIPS may be necessary.

**The patient is still bleeding** Embolize the dominant varices through the TIPS tract. There is no need to routinely embolize varices.

**Encephalopathy** Severe encephalopathy is usually associated with a very low portosystemic pressure gradient and will require either reduction of the diameter of the TIPS tract or occlusion. There are a variety of different ways to reduce the flow through the graft. The simplest method TIPS is performed by placing a Prolene suture around the centre of an angioplasty balloon and then using this to deploy a balloon-mounted stent-graft (e.g. Jomed). This will leave a waist in the stent. Measure the pressure gradient and progressively dilate the waist until a suitable pressure drop is obtained, usually about 12–14 mmHg.

## TIPS follow-up

Make sure that the patient is followed-up with Duplex ultrasound to confirm shunt patency and exclude stenosis. Intervention is frequently necessary; bare stents have only 50% primary patency at 1 year. Without intervention, virtually all TIPS have thrombosed by 2 years. At any sign of trouble, perform a venogram and measure pressures. If the gradient is >12 mmHg, then intervention is indicated. Stenoses tend to occur in the hepatic vein and within the TIPS tract. These are normally treated by stenting. These procedures can usually be performed as a day case via a 7Fr jugular puncture.

## Transjugular liver biopsy

See Chapter 25, Biopsy and Drainage.

# Tunnelled central lines

Tunnelled central lines are used when long-term central venous access is required for dialysis, chemotherapy and total parental nutrition. All tunnelled lines are anchored by a subcutaneous cuff that induces fibrosis and prevents inadvertent removal.

The advantages of radiological placement are reliable venous access, accurate positioning and minimal procedural complications. Interventional techniques can also be used to gain vascular access in difficult cases and also to salvage failing lines.

## Learn your lines!

It is essential you understand what type of line you are dealing with, as this affects the sequence of tunnelling and line positioning. All tunnelled lines are variations on two designs:

- Lines that are cut to length, e.g. Hickman line. With this type of line, tunnelling is performed before positioning. Infiltrate local anaesthetic at the desired exit site on the anterior chest wall and make a small incision the width of a size 11 scalpel blade (~ 5 mm). The tunnel is fashioned back to the point of venous access; go slowly and take care not to make a carotid jugular kebab! The catheter is attached to the tunnelling device and pulled through the tunnel until the cuff is 2 cm into the tunnel. The line is placed on the skin to mimic the curve of the guidewire and is then cut to the appropriate length to leave the tip in the right atrium.
- Lines that are fixed length, e.g. some dialysis catheters and Groshong lines. Tunnelling is performed before or after positioning, depending on whether the hub is an integral part of the catheter. The line is inserted to optimum position and then laid on the skin to define the exit point roughly 3 cm beyond the cuff. The tunnel is then made from the venous access site to the exit site using the sharp steel tunneller provided. Altenative dialysis catheter designs are fixed length with tunnelling occurring before final catheter placement.

## Equipment

- Most proprietary devices come complete with the basic equipment necessary for placement. It is helpful to have some catheters and wires in reserve for difficult cases.
- Guidewires: angled hydrophilic, Amplatz super-stiff.
- Catheters: Cobra II.
- Ultrasound machine: this is essential; a 5 MHz or 7 MHz probe with a biopsy guide is ideal.

## Procedure

There are three stages to the insertion of all tunnelled lines:

- Venous access – always the first stage
- Tunnelling
- Line positioning.

*Access* The right IJV provides the straightest route for central venous catheterization. The jugular vein seems less prone to thrombosis than other routes. Alternatives are the left IJV and the subclavian veins. Access may be limited by the presence of local disease, radiotherapy or stenosis/occlusion of the target vein. A 1 cm transverse skin incision is necessary to allow side-by-side placement of the line and the tunnelling device. Forceps can be used to perform subcutaneous blunt dissection, which will ease introduction of the catheter.

Use ultrasound to guide the venous puncture. Advance the guidewire into the right atrium/ IVC under fluoroscopic guidance.

*Tunnelling* The aim is to tunnel in the subcutaneous plane; this is painless for you and the patient. Introduce the tunneller and apply gentle forward pressure while rocking it from side to side. The exit site is usually on the anterior chest wall. Tunnelling over the clavicle from an internal jugular entry can be difficult; if using a metal tunneller, bending the shaft makes it considerably easier. Many tunnellers have a sleeve which is pulled over the line end to prevent detachment during passage through the subcutaneous tunnel. If the line does detach, pass a long sheathed needle through the tract, exchange the needle for a stiff guidewire and:

- Either – pass a suitably sized peel-away sheath (e.g. 16Fr) through the track. Once the sheath is in position this guarantees success and you will wonder what the fuss was all about
- Or – dilate the tract with serial dilators or an angioplasty balloon. Save this for cases where you don't have a peel-away sheath of the appropriate size.

**Tip:** Think about the exit site, as a carelessly positioned line will cause discomfort by rubbing on clothing. The cuff should be 1–2 cm from the exit site. If it is further than this, line removal will be difficult and can require significant dissection!

*Line insertion* The line is always introduced through a peel-away sheath (Fig. 24.2, Chapter 24, Equipment for Non-vascular Intervention). This is inserted just like a standard sheath. Remember the basic rules of vascular access; keep the guidewire under tension to avoid kinking. Tell the patient to stop breathing and take out the dilator and guidewire. Put your thumb over the end of the peel-away sheath and allow the patient to breathe normally.

**Alarm:** Air embolism can be fatal but is readily prevented. Instruct your patient to stop breathing while you remove the dilator. Keep your thumb securely over the end of the sheath after the dilator has been removed. Everyone can now breathe normally. Tell the patient to stop breathing again when you insert the catheter.

Ask the patient to stop breathing again and advance the catheter into the peel-away sheath until correctly sited.

*Line positioning* The tip should be advanced just into the right atrium. The line invariably ends in the SVC when the patient is erect and takes a full inspiration for the check chest X-ray. The sheath is then removed by splitting and peeling the sheath. Remember to keep your index finger on the catheter to hold it in position.

*Final assembly* Close the venous access site with a Steri-Strip. If your boss insists on a suture, try not to puncture the line as you insert it! Using a suture set with toothed forceps to hold the skin edge up will minimize the risk of a sharp stick injury to you and the line.

Lines that are tunnelled towards the exit site need to have Luer lock fittings attached after tunnelling. The mechanism of attachment varies from system to system and is clearly described in the instructions. Test that blood can be aspirated and flush the line thoroughly. The line needs to be anchored by a suture for the first week until there is tissue ingrowth into the cuff. Cover both sites with a clear occlusive dressing to minimize the risk of infection.

*An additional note on dialysis lines* Successful dialysis depends on removing blood from one site (arterial line) and returning it to a separate site (venous line), typically more centrally in the venous circulation. If the lines are too close together or the venous line is proximal to the arterial line, dialysis will not be effective as the blood will simply recirculate. The separation is ensured in two ways:

- Use of 2 separate lines, e.g. Tessio lines. This requires two separate venous punctures and tunnels. The venous line is longer than the arterial line. Two lines are fine when there is good venous access but increases the problem when there is limited access.
- Use of a dual lumen line, e.g. Ash split catheter. These involve a single puncture and tunnel. The line is typically large, e.g. 14.5Fr.

All dialysis catheters are intended to have high flow rates. This can only be achieved if the line is not kinked. The dual lumen lines are more prone to kinking and some come precurved with reinforcement intended to prevent this.

## Troubleshooting

**Arterial puncture** Take the needle/dilator out and get the ultrasound machine while you obtain haemostasis!

**Doubt about position** Use fluoroscopy at the first sign of trouble. Put in a 4Fr dilator and inject contrast to confirm the anatomy.

**Unable to advance the sheath** Put in a 4Fr dilator to secure vascular access. If this fails, use serial dilators.

- Use the hydrophilic wire and Cobra catheter to access the IVC.
- Exchange for an Amplatz wire and use this to introduce the sheath.

**Unable to introduce the line through the sheath** This can be tricky; the sheath is thin-walled and tends to kink at bends.

- Try to pull the sheath back while maintaining forward pressure on the catheter. Do not split the sheath yet.

If this fails:
1. Replace the dilator and use a hydrophilic guidewire to try to negotiate the kink. Then reinsert the sheath fully and this may straighten the sheath sufficiently to use.

If this fails:
2. Insert the catheter as far as it will go and peel away the sheath. Remember to apply forward pressure to keep the catheter in position. The catheter can usually be advanced once it is within the vein.

**Unable to aspirate blood from the line** Check the line position on fluoroscopy; check for kinking at the venous puncture site.

- Sit the patient up and try other postural manoeuvres to alter line position.
- If all else fails, inject contrast through the line to delineate the problem.

**Kinking** This occurs most commonly deep to the puncture site at the point the line enters the vein. It can be difficult to rectify; try passing a stiff hydrophilic guidewire through the line to open out the bend (this seldom works in isolation). If using a dual lumen catheter, try gently rotating the shaft of the catheter during fluoroscopy:

- Blunt dissection around the line to increase the space
- Exchanging for another catheter over a stiff hydrophilic wire
- Swapping for a precurved line.

**Tip:** Try to prevent kinking. Use a more lateral puncture into the vein and make a two-stage tunnel come out 2–3 cm lateral to the puncture site and then tunnel across to the puncture site.

# Awkward venous access

Last ditch venous access can literally be a lifeline for some patients; this is particularly true of haemodialysis patients. By the time a patient has had multiple tunnelled lines, all of the central veins may be stenosed or occluded. At this stage, the renal team usually resorts to temporary femoral access, but this is uncomfortable and usually results in infection. It is essential to re-establish long-term central venous access. There are descriptions of using the hepatic veins and the IVC but this is rarely necessary. The vast majority of patients can have access established via collateral veins using the same techniques to cross stenoses and occlusions that are described in the section on angioplasty and stenting. Remember that the aim is to establish venous access not venous patency: if necessary, dilate stenoses or occlusions to allow introduction of the line. Only place a stent if there is symptomatic venous obstruction.

The first stage in the procedure is to perform an ultrasound scan of the neck veins. If an internal jugular vein is patent, this is the optimal approach. There are always plenty of tortuous veins which cross the midline of the neck; these are seldom useful. Look for the patent anterior and external jugular veins or veins that lie more laterally in the neck.

Puncture the chosen vein under ultrasound guidance and insert a 4Fr dilator to perform venography. If there is a direct route to the central veins, then go for it. Dilate underlying stenoses as necessary in order to introduce the catheters. More often there is no direct route, but with knowledge of the likely course of the vein it is often possible to find a way through. Perseverance is the key – if the vein you have punctured is not 'the one', the venogram will often suggest an alternative (Fig. 20.13).

**Fig. 20.13** ■ Awkward access. (A) Injection into a vein in the left side of the neck shows collaterals communicating with the azygous vein (arrowheads) and into the SVC (arrows). (B) The Groshong line follows this tortuous path.

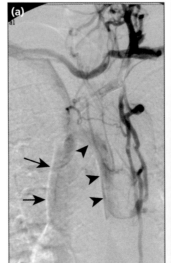

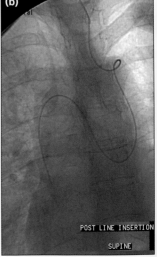

**Impossible access – keys to success**

- Good ultrasound.
- Plenty of time and determination.
- Use low-profile wires and balloons to cross tight strictures and occlusions.
- Once you have access into a central vein, don't lose it! Get a supportive wire (e.g. an Amplatz wire) in place, preferably through to the IVC.
- If dual catheters are required, e.g. for haemodialysis, resist the temptation to use the same puncture site for two wires. This only results in a venous tear and excessive bleeding. Instead, use ultrasound or fluoroscopy to perform a second puncture into the same vein about 1 cm from the first puncture. Better still, use a dual lumen line!
- Use a long peel-away sheath – the sheath supplied with the catheter will not be long enough to support the catheter all the way through to the SVC/right atrium.
- Leave a stiff hydrophilic wire through the sheath to minimize kinking when the dilator is removed.
- Use a snare to grasp the catheter and pull it through very tortuous veins if the peel-away sheath kinks.

# Maintenance of tunnelled central lines

All long-term central venous access is prone to four problems: **infection, venous thrombosis, fibrin sheath** and **mechanical failure**.

Infection limited to the exit site can be successfully treated with antibiotic treatment; however, for tunnel infections and infected lines, removal is usually required. Don't be tempted to place a new line until the patient has been clear of infection for several days or you will be removing that line as well. If access is needed in the interim, then use in and out catheters.

Line-related venous thrombosis is usually associated with symptomatic limb oedema, in which case the line is removed and the patient treated as for a DVT. IF the thrombosis is asymptomatic, then anticoagulation alone is adequate.

Mechanical failure usually results in line fractures; extravasation then causes pain during injection and sometimes leak of fluid from the skin entry site. Occasionally, a line fractures or a totally implanted device such as a vascular port separates from its hub, leading to migration of the line and retrieval by snare (Chapter 22, Rendezvous and Retrieval Procedures).

Fibrin sheath formation is a common occurrence. Fibrin deposits envelop the line to form a condom-like cover. This obstructs the line tips, prevents aspiration of blood and may lead to extravasation. In dialysis lines, it results in markedly reduced flow, which compromises dialysis.

When there is a problem with a line, the first step is to establish the diagnosis with a linogram. This is simply an injection of contrast down the line under fluoroscopic control. Check the entire line from the skin to its tip. Look for:

- Extravasation. This most commonly occurs at points of flexion or compression.
- Free flow of contrast from the line lumen via the end- and side-holes. Sometimes it is necessary to perform a run to establish what is happening. Due to cardiac motion, unsubtracted images may be clearer.
- Reflux of contrast back around the line, often with a thin radiolucent 'membrane'; this indicates a fibrin sheath (Fig. 20.12).
- Line migration, typically into the pulmonary artery (see Chapter 22, Rendezvous and Retrieval Procedures).

If there is a fibrin sheath, the first-line treatment is to flush the line vigorously. This may disrupt the sheath sufficiently to restore flow. The next step will usually be to try a low dose of thrombolysis; this is best given by infusion rather than as a bolus. The ward team can do this without your help. If this fails, then mechanically stripping the fibrin sheath with a

Gooseneck snare is usually the answer. Warn the patient that even if this is successful the fibrin sheath is likely to recur and require further treatment.

## How to strip

The lines often abut the wall of the SVC, which makes them difficult to snare. In this case simply pass a guidewire through the line and into the IVC if it will go. If you are dealing with a Groshong line, only a hydrophilic wire will pass through it. It may take a little pushing to get it through the valve but don't be deterred, it will go. Pass a Gooseneck snare from the femoral vein to catch the wire and then advance it over the line. If there are two lines, e.g. dialysis catheters, both can be snared at once. Take the snare as far up the line as it will go. Tighten it so that it grips the line fairly firmly (Fig. 20.14).

Pull the snare back; if it is gripped tightly enough it will tug the line down when you pull. It is best to warn the patient that they will feel as though someone is pulling on the line, because they are. You are aiming to get enough grip to remove the sheath but leave the line in-situ. Repeat this once or twice, then repeat the linogram. If flow is restored and the lines aspirate freely, then stop. If not, try again.

Sometimes when there are two lines that are stuck together, success is indicated by the line tips separating.

 **Tip:** Leave the wire through the catheter while stripping, as this allows the snare to be passed straight back up again. When performing the linogram, you need to remove the wire, so park the snare high up the line so that you don't have to catch it again.

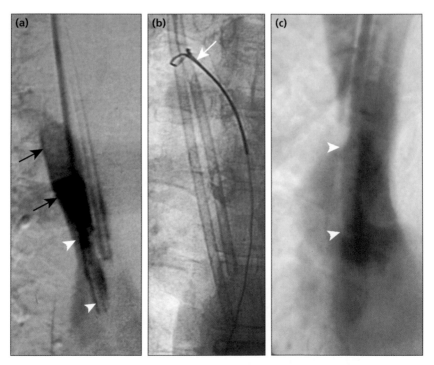

**Fig. 20.14** ▧ Stripping a poorly functioning Tessio line. (A) Injection through the venous line. The line tip is occluded (arrowheads) and contrast outlines a fibrin sheath (arrows). (B) A Gooseneck snare (white arrow) has been placed around both lines. (C) Following stripping, the line fills to the tip (arrowheads) and contrast flows normally into the SVC. Normal function was restored.

# Suggestions for further reading

## Venous intervention

Becker DM, Philbrick JT, Selby JB. Inferior vena cava filters: Indications, safety, effectiveness. Arch Intern Med 1992;152:1985–1994.

Linsenmaier U, Rieger J, Schenk F, et al. Indications, management and complications of temporary inferior vena cava filters. Cardiovasc Intervent Radiol 1998;21:464–469.
A useful overview.

McFarland DR (ed) Interventional radiology in the venous system. Semin Intervent Radiol 1994;11.

Vesely TM. Technical problems and complications associated with inferior vena cava filters. Semin Intervent Radiol 1994;11:121–133.

## SVCO

Nicholson AA, Ettles DF, Arnold A, et al. Treatment of malignant superior vena caval obstruction: metal stents or radiation therapy. J Vasc Intervent Radiol 1997;8:563–567.
What can be achieved in good hands, the biggest series to date.

## TIPS

LaBerge JM. Anatomy relevant to the transjugular intrahepatic portosystemic shunt procedure. Semin Intervent Radiol 1995;12:337–346.
Why we try to use the right hepatic vein to approach the portal vein.

Saxon RR, Keller FS. Technical aspects of accessing the portal vein during the TIPS procedure. J Vasc Intervent Radiol 1997;8:733–744.
Guidance and practical TIPS tips.

## Central lines

Hall K, Farr B. Diagnosis and management of long term central venous catheter infection. J Vasc Intervent Radiol 2004;15:327–334.

Mauro MA, Jaques PF. Radiologic placement of long-term central venous catheters: A review. J Vasc Intervent Radiol 1993;5:127–137.

Ramsden WH, Cohen AT, Blanshard KS. Central venous catheter fracture due to compression between the clavicle and first rib. Clin Radiol 1995;50:59–60.
A potential pitfall of the subclavian approach to central lines, which applies equally to stents and stent-grafts.

Trerotola SO, Johnson MS, Harris VJ, et al. Outcome of tunneled hemodialysis catheters placed via the right internal jugular vein by interventional radiologists. Radiology 1997;203:489–495.
The RIJV is the approach to use with excellent patency and few complications.

# 21

# Haemodialysis access – imaging and intervention

Referrals for management of vascular access problems will be among the most common requests for vascular intervention in centres where haemodialysis is performed. The dialysis patient is currently one of the most important learning and training grounds for vascular access, catheter and wire manipulation, thrombolysis and angiography!

For patients on haemodialysis, their fistula, graft or dialysis catheter is a lifeline. Unfortunately, problems are not rare and anyone working on a site with a dialysis unit will frequently see patients with problematic access. Stenoses lead to inadequate dialysis, prolonged bleeding, arm oedema and thrombosis. Large shunts may cause steal phenomena. The key to these procedures is to understand the anatomy and the physical examination.

*Fistula examination* Feel the fistula for the 'thrill' at the anastomosis and in the draining vein. The vein adjacent to the anastomosis usually has a spongy feeling. If the fistula is underfilled, there is a problem with the inflow. A tense, distended vein indicates venous outflow obstruction. A swollen arm indicates central venous obstruction (Fig. 21.1). Venous stenoses are often palpable as 'defects' in the draining vein associated with a change in the degree of venous filling and thrill.

*Graft examination* There is usually a thrill at the venous anastomosis and examination is in essence the same as that for a fistula.

*Diagnostic imaging* Ultrasound is invariably the first test, as it can show the inflow, anastomosis, stenoses and also flow; if ultrasound is abnormal, invasive imaging is usually, required. Imaging is required if the fistula shows problems related to dialysis:

- **Before**: reduced thrill, aneurysm development, difficulty needling, arm swelling
- **During**: poor flow rates, recycling
- **After**: prolonged time to stop bleeding.

*Arteriovenous fistulae* The commonest fistula is the radio-cephalic (Brescia–Cimino) fistula fashioned at the wrist of the non-dominant arm (Fig. 21.2). If this fails, it may be revised or a more proximal fistula formed, usually between the brachial artery and the cephalic or basilic vein. Sometimes the basilic vein is 'transposed' onto the brachial artery to increase the options. Once the non-dominant arm sites are exhausted, the dominant arm is used; if this fails, a fistula may be formed at the groin.

*Haemodialysis grafts* These are an alternative to fistula formation and have the advantages of being ready to use immediately and allowing higher flow rates. The price for this is the frequency with which they develop stenoses and thrombose. Grafts often have a loop

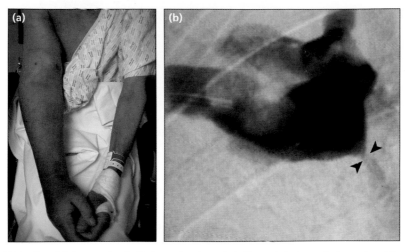

**Fig. 21.1** ■ Swollen fistula arm due to high-grade stenosis in the subclavian vein (arrowheads).

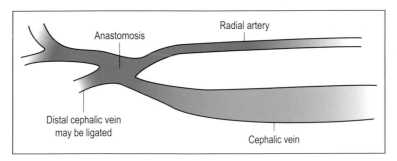

**Fig. 21.2** ■ Brescia–Cimino fistula (distal radial artery to cephalic vein).

configuration. Typical sites are between the brachial artery and the cephalic or basilic vein or between the femoral artery and vein.

## Equipment

- Basic angiography set with a 3Fr straight catheter.
- Ultrasound.

## Procedure

The same questions need to be answered for both fistulae and grafts, namely, the state of the inflow, the condition of any anastomoses and the condition of the draining veins from the periphery to the central veins.

*Access* Retrograde arterial puncture of the ipsilateral brachial artery or the inflow limb of the loop graft is the ideal method. Performing the study via a 3Fr arterial puncture optimizes visualization of the inflow and allows complete assessment. The alternative, which seldom produces as satisfactory images, is to place a needle in the draining veins of the fistula and use a supra-systolic tourniquet to achieve retrograde flow through the arterial anastomosis.

Remember that the patient will be heparinized during dialysis so do not perform the study straight afterwards.

*Catheterization* Selective catheterization is only required for intervention.

*Runs* The principle is the same as in graft angiography: show the anastomosis in profile. Because of the high flow rates through fistulae, a high frame rate (4–6 FPS) may be needed to study the anastomosis and the peripheral draining veins. As flow slows in the more central veins, the flow rate is decreased to 1–2 FPS. For arm haemodialysis access sites, the venous return should be studied as far as the right atrium.

As always for arm angiography, it is necessary to rotate the angiography table to obtain views down to the hand. Start with the patient's arm in the anatomical position (palm up). Multiple oblique views are often necessary to sort out the anatomy.

 **Tip:** To obtain oblique views, consider turning the patient's arm rather than rotating the C-arm.

## Interpretation

- Significant stenoses are those causing greater than 50% diameter narrowing.
- There are often occluded venous segments with collaterals and retrograde flow. This may only be appreciated when the runs are reviewed frame by frame at the console.
- Filling of collateral veins around the central veins is always abnormal. If you cannot see a lesion, try another view.

## Troubleshooting

**Unable to puncture the fistula** Use ultrasound to target the puncture.

**The arteries distal to the fistula do not fill** This is usually secondary to a steal phenomenon through the fistula. Apply a tourniquet to occlude the venous drainage. The arteries will normally now fill.

## Angioplasty and stenting

There is controversy about whether to intervene on asymptomatic dialysis access stenoses but symptomatic stenoses must be treated to improve dialysis, relieve swelling and prevent thrombosis. The commonest sites for stenoses are at the venous anastomosis and dialysis puncture sites. Central venous catheterization also predisposes to stenosis.

 **Tip:** You can learn all the essentials of angiography, catheterization and angioplasty on the humble fistula. Do lots!

Before treating any stenosis or occlusion, make sure that everyone is aware of the objectives of the procedure, i.e. to preserve the function of the dialysis access site. Restenosis is frequent and repeat intervention is often necessary. Explain to the patient that treatment is a temporizing measure and not a miracle cure.

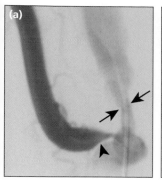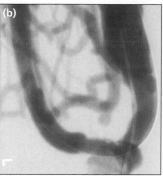

**Fig. 21.3** ■ (A) Brescia–Cimino fistula with stenoses at the anastomosis (arrowhead) and in the draining vein (arrows). (B) Following angioplasty, excellent flow is restored.

*Access* Choose the approach according to the location of the lesion and the condition of the adjacent vessels. For direct arteriovenous fistulae, the dominant draining vein is usually catheterized; this is almost always the vein that is used during dialysis. It is sometimes necessary to approach Brescia–Cimino fistulae via an antegrade brachial artery puncture. Haemodialysis grafts are directly punctured at a point that allows space to manoeuvre under the C-arm with respect to the lesion. Think about where to position the ultrasound, trolley, C-arm, etc. It is often useful to stand towards the patient's head and sometimes helps to work from the contralateral side across the patient's chest when working on the basilic vein.

 **Tip:** The apex of some loop grafts is reinforced to prevent kinking. Check with the surgeon or puncture away from the apex.

   **Angioplasty** is performed in the conventional fashion (Fig. 21.3). Consider sending the patient for dialysis immediately after treatment. The sheath can be exchanged for a dialysis catheter which is left in situ; discuss the best arrangement with the dialysis unit.
   **Stenting** is reserved for those cases in which angioplasty alone is unsuccessful. Only stent if it will achieve good outflow; if not, the patient is better off with surgery. Take care when stenting the central veins as stent compression is common between the clavicle and the first rib. Try not to stent across other vessels that may be needed for central access in the future, especially the jugular veins. Make sure that the patient and clinician are aware of the position of the stent so that it is not inadvertently punctured. Long-term stent patency, particularly in peripheral veins, is poor.

## Troubleshooting

**Unable to puncture the draining vein** Use ultrasound guidance; colour flow is invaluable for this.

**Unable to dilate a stenosis** It is often necessary to consider using a cutting balloon or use prolonged high-pressure inflation to overcome fibrotic strictures (Fig. 21.4). Make sure that you have suitable angioplasty balloons before starting! Never use a stent when you cannot eliminate the waist on the angioplasty balloon – you are simply lining a stenosis with metal.

**Rupture** Rupture is more common during venous intervention than during arterial angioplasty. It is probably more common when using cutting balloons (Fig. 21.5). Extravasation is managed in a similar fashion to arterial injury; remember that occlusion is often an acceptable outcome if the fistula was not functioning adequately.

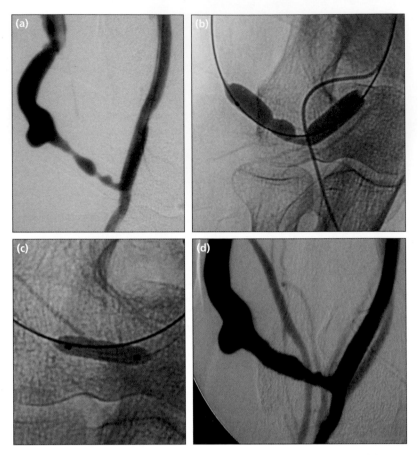

**Fig. 21.4** ■ Brachiocephalic fistula stricture. (A) Complex stricture in the cephalic vein. (B) Persistent waisting in a conventional angioplasty balloon. (C) Elimination of the waist with a cutting balloon. (D) Completion angiogram.

**Spasm**   Spasm is common in the radial artery and in veins. Use vasodilators prophylactically and to treat spasm. Consider gentle dilation of areas of resistant spasm.

# Thrombosis

Unfortunately, thrombosis is often the first sign of a problem. Radiological treatment options are thrombolysis and mechanical thrombectomy; the alternative is surgical embolectomy. Remember that there is almost always an underlying stenosis that must be treated when flow is restored. Ideally, treatment should be performed before the patient requires temporary venous access for dialysis as this preserves central veins.

Remember the contraindications for thrombolysis. CVA during thrombolysis is probably less common in a young dialysis patient than in an elderly patient with peripheral vascular disease. If the patient has a central line, check that there were no complications during placement that might compromise thrombolysis.

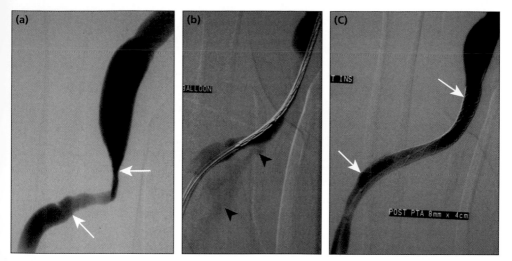

**Fig. 21.5** ■ Extravasation post cutting balloon. (A) Pre-angioplasty flow-limiting basilic vein stenosis (arrows). (B) Brisk extravasation following cutting balloon angioplasty (arrowheads). (C) Completion angiogram following deployment of a covered stent.

*Direct AV fistulae* Puncture the main draining vein about 10 cm away from and aiming towards the anastomosis. Perform gentle venography to confirm the anatomy. Position a 4Fr straight multi-sidehole catheter with its tip as close to the anastomosis as possible. Give a bolus dose of the thrombolytic agent (e.g. 5 mg rt-PA) and then start an infusion (see Chapter 19, Thrombolysis and thrombectomy, p. 228). Perform periodic check angiography to evaluate progress. When flow is re-established, perform check venography and treat any underlying stenoses.

*Haemodialysis grafts* The thrombus is usually confined to the graft but may extend beyond it if there is a stenosis in the draining vein (Fig. 21.6). Occluded grafts can be treated by thrombolysis or thrombectomy using a crossed catheter technique (Fig. 21.7).

1. Punctures are made into the arterial and venous limbs and catheters manipulated round the graft. Puncture of the graft is usually straightforward but if it is difficult to palpate, use ultrasound.
2. Using a hydrophilic guidewire and a Cobra catheter, negotiate into the draining vein beyond the venous anastomosis and perform a venogram to demonstrate the venous anatomy. If there is no direct venous drainage, stop now as the graft needs to be surgically revised.
3. Either perform thrombolysis, usually with boluses of rt-PA, or thrombectomy using a mechanical thrombectomy device. Aim to treat the venous outflow first, then deal with the arterial limb. It is not essential to clear all the thrombus at this stage but just enough to allow flow to occur.
4. There is usually a platelet-rich plug of thrombus at the arterial end of the graft, which is resistant to thrombolysis. Use a hydrophilic guidewire to manipulate into the native artery and pass a small balloon catheter above the arterial anastomosis. Gently inflate it and pull it back into the graft (an over-the-wire Fogarty embolectomy catheter is ideal although conventional angioplasty balloons will work). The platelet plug disimpacts and flow is restored.
5. Now is the time to tidy up the residual thrombus; often simple balloon angioplasty will macerate it.
6. Remember to look for the underlying lesion and treat it with angioplasty or stenting.

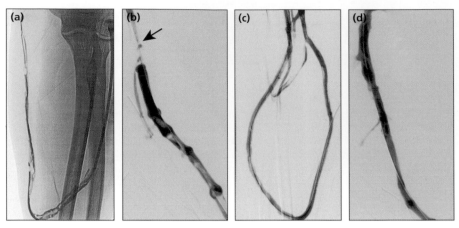

**Fig. 21.6** ■ (A) Thrombosed forearm loop graft. (B) Stenosis in the draining vein (arrow). (C) Following mechanical thrombectomy, the graft is clear. (D) The cephalic vein is widely patent following angioplasty.

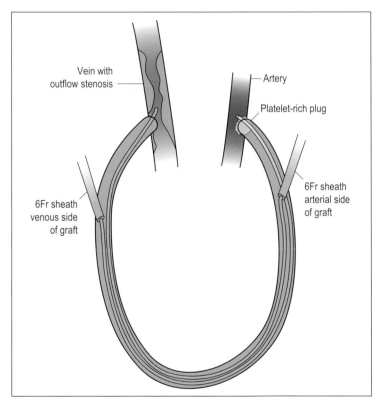

**Fig. 21.7** ■ Crossed catheter technique for loop graft thrombolysis.

# Troubleshooting

**Uncertain anatomy** Try hard to establish the type of fistula or graft before starting. Look for operation notes and speak to the surgical team in charge. Ultrasound will often clarify the anatomy. If not, adopt a 'suck it and see' approach.

**Extravasation occurs during thrombolysis** This is almost inevitable when treating dialysis access grafts that have had frequent punctures. Warn the patient about this in advance. It is usually possible to complete treatment unless there is marked extravasation.

**Intra-procedural thrombosis** Particularly with thrombectomy, it can be difficult to stop re-thrombosis during the procedure. The key is avoiding delay between steps 4 and 5; it is essential to get flow through the fistula. Minor amounts of residual thrombus are easily resolved after flow has been established.

## Suggestions for further reading

Beathard GA. Percutaneous transvenous angioplasty in the treatment of vascular access stenosis. Kidney Int 1992;42:1390–1397.

Beathard GA, Welch BR, Maidment HJ. Mechanical thrombectomy for the treatment of thrombosed hemodialysis access grafts. Radiology 1996;200:711–716.

An interesting paper on pulse-spray technique with saline replacing the thrombolytic agent.

Lammer J, Vorwerk D. Hemodialyis fistulas and grafts. Semin Intervent Radiol 1997;14:1–110.

Everything you wanted to know … well almost. The authors have not included thrombolytic therapy, but still a very good read.

Schuman E, Quinn S, Standage B, et al. Thrombolysis versus thrombectomy for occluded hemodialysis grafts. Am J Surg 1994;167:473–476.

A thoughtful paper that reminds us of the established primary role of surgical thrombectomy and that the principal advantage of radiology is to treat the underlying lesion.

Valji K. Transcatheter treatment of thrombosed hemodialysis access grafts. AJR Am J Roentgenol 1995;164:823–829.

An excellent overview with an extensive reference list.

Valji K, Bookstein JJ, Roberts AC, Davis GB. Pharmacomechanical thrombolysis and angioplasty in the management of clotted hemodialyisis grafts: early and late clinical results. Radiology 1991;178:243–247.

The strongest advocates of pulse-spray thrombolysis.

# 22

# Rendezvous and retrieval procedures

Foreign body retrieval is usually for iatrogenic problems, most of which will have been of your own making. The techniques and equipment described can also be used for snaring guidewires for pull-through procedures or to reposition misplaced central lines. The majority of foreign body retrieval is within the vascular system, although occasionally these techniques are required in the biliary or urinary system. There are not many tools at your disposal so a thorough knowledge of how they work and an inventive mind are the keys to success.

## The toolkit

### Amplatz Gooseneck snare (Figs 22.1, 22.2, see also Chapter 9, Equipment for Angiography, Fig. 9.13)

This is the best-known and most popular snare. The snare loop comes in a range of sizes from 2 mm to 25 mm and the chosen diameter should correspond to the target vessel. The snare is supplied with its own guide-catheter; this varies in size from 4Fr to 6F according to the snare chosen. The guide-catheter has a radio-opaque tip marker and can be shaped if necessary to increase manoeuvrability.

### The EnSnare (MD Tech) (Fig. 22.2)

This snare is constructed with three snare loops and comes in different sizes. Each is designed to function in a range of vessel diameters, e.g. the mini snare will function from 4 mm to 8 mm and the large snare from 12 to 20 mm. This is a distinct advantage when working in a confined space or when it is difficult to turn the snare.

Snares are simple to use; rather harder is deciding when a 'foreign body' will be relatively innocuous if left in situ and when removing it is likely to cause more harm than good. A 'foreign body' that is free in the right atrium has the potential to be injurious while an unexpanded stent in a minor branch vessel is not a big problem.

**Using a snare in eight easy steps**

1. First position a guidewire adjacent to the object to be removed; if you cannot manage this, then you will not be able to remove it!
2. The guide-catheter is passed along the guidewire in the normal fashion and the guidewire removed.
3. The snare is compressed within an introducer and then advanced into the catheter.
4. As the snare loop emerges from the catheter, it opens like a lasso (Fig. 22.1).

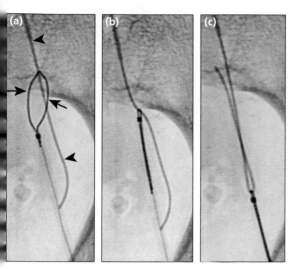

**Fig. 22.1** ■ Snaring a guidewire. (A) The open snare (arrows) is positioned over the guidewire (arrowheads). (B) The snare is tightened to grip the wire. (C) The snare is pulled back into the sheath bringing the guidewire with it.

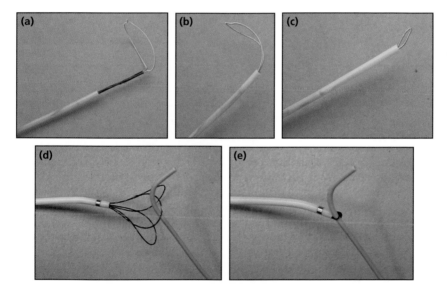

**Fig. 22.2** ■ Upper panel: Amplatz Gooseneck snare fully open, partially open and closed. Lower panel: EnSnare with catheter open and closed.

5. Allow the snare loop to open so that occupies the entire vessel lumen. The snare loop can be rotated, advanced or withdrawn to position it over the target.
6. Once the target is in the loop, it is kept still and the guide-catheter is advanced. This tightens the snare and grips the target (Fig. 22.1).
7. The snare and its prey can now be pulled back to the access site.
8. The prey is either removed (Fig. 22.1), parked somewhere safe or, in the case of a large object, held onto until the vascular surgeon can remove it safely.

**Tip:** Remember, many objects can be snared and retrieved, but not all can be removed; frequently, a large sheath will be necessary, e.g. to remove a kinked catheter.

# Clinical scenarios

It is essential to decide whether the foreign body needs to be removed. Stents, embolization coils, and fragments of catheter and guidewire will probably cause vessel thrombosis. Only if thrombosis is likely to be clinically relevant should retrieval be attempted; if not, leave the foreign body where it is. If something does need to be removed, it is a good idea to heparinize the patient to prevent thrombosis during the procedure.

*Catheter and guidewire fragments* Guidewire fragments are fairly straightforward. Find a free end and snare the wire fragment. Fortunately, wire fragments are small enough to be withdrawn through a 6Fr sheath even when doubled back. Catheter fragments and bits of central venous catheters are usually easy to capture but will not come through a standard sheath. The first option is to increase the sheath size to a size approximately twice the size of the target – this is often fairly large. Alternatively, bring the snared object back to the sheath and pull it snugly into the end of the sheath and withdraw the fragment, snare and sheath simultaneously. In practice, this is the most frequently used option.

*Embolization coils* The ease of retrieval for coils is critically dependent on the size of the target vessel. If the coil has migrated into a small-calibre vessel, retrieval may require a micro-snare. In many situations, vessels of this calibre are not vital and the safest option is to leave the coil alone. Particular care should be taken if the target coil is adjacent to a nest of coils, e.g. when the last coil of an embolization has extruded back into the main trunk. It is very easy to drag entangled coils back during the retrieval and make the situation much worse.

*Stents* Partially and even completely deployed stents have been successfully retrieved using snares. It is possible to progressively crimp down stainless steel stents with a lot of patience but this is not a technique for stents that have undergone minor mispositioning. The stent must be in a site that poses a significant threat to the patient, e.g. embolization to the heart or pulmonary circulation. Unfortunately, the majority of stents will not line up neatly and require a large sheath or an arteriotomy or venotomy for removal. Consider deploying the stent in a less harmful position, e.g. an iliac vessel. Remember that any of these options is a lot better than a thoracotomy. Self-expanding stents are even more difficult, as only a portion can be compressed and many have 'sharp edges'. They almost always need to be 'parked' safely (Fig. 22.3). This is definitely an area for expert hands only.

*Bullets and exciting projectiles* Intravascular bullets, shot or fragments are occasionally seen in arteries and veins. They are usually brought to a safer place for surgical removal, but a small lead shot can sometimes be safely extracted.

## Repositioning central venous lines

The majority of these are subclavian central venous lines that have passed from the subclavian vein into the IJV or from the right subclavian into the left brachiocephalic vein. Either way, non-tunnelled lines can often be readily exchanged by simply directing a guidewire through the original line into the SVC, then exchanging for a new line. Only in exceptional circumstances is it worth performing more elaborate manoeuvres for a non-tunnelled line. In addition, these lines are relatively stiff, making hooking the line down more difficult.

Tunnelled central lines deserve more effort. The tunnel means that it is less easy to simply exchange the catheter and therefore more ingenious solutions are required.

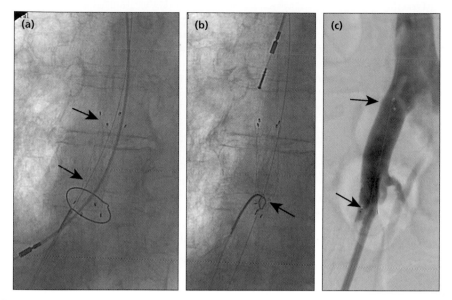

**Fig. 22.3** ▦ Retrieving a self-expanding stent from the right atrium. (A) An innominate vein stent (arrows) has been displaced during placement of a pacing wire. A 0.018-inch wire has been passed through the stent and a gooseneck snare advanced over this. (B) The lower end of the stent is grasped and compressed (arrow); the upper end remains expanded. (C) The stent (arrows) has been pulled back and parked in the common iliac vein.

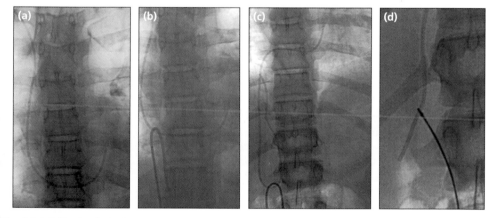

**Fig. 22.4** ▦ Retrieval of a broken catheter fragment. (A) The catheter tip has migrated into the right ventricle. (B, C) The catheter is hooked with a Sidewinder catheter and pulled down into the inferior vena cava. (D) The catheter is snared prior to being pulled out through the femoral vein sheath.

1. The first step is to pass a stiff Terumo wire through the line. This simple manoeuvre can deflect it into the correct position.
2. Next, attempt to hook the line down into the target vessel. Perform a femoral puncture and negotiate a pigtail catheter to the target line. Try to hook the line down using the pigtail; occasionally, it can be helpful to stiffen the pigtail by passing a guidewire partially round the loop. If this fails, it may be worth trying the same manoeuvre with a Sos Omni catheter (Fig. 22.4).

If neither of these options is successful, then try using a gooseneck snare. The difficulty with snaring is that the target object has to present a free end to capture. If the end of the misplaced line is in a decent sized vessel, it is possible to manipulate the snare and the guide-catheter into an appropriate position. If the line is in a small vessel, access with a snare can be difficult. It is sometimes possible to move the end of the misplaced line into a more favourable position by simply performing a rapid hand injection of saline down the line.

## Rendezvous, pull-through technique or 'bodyflossing'

This is a special form of guidewire retrieval and refers to putting a guidewire in at one site and bringing it out at another. This gives enormous strength and stability as the wire can be held under tension and catheters can be placed end to end. It is typically used when it is simpler to traverse a lesion from one site while the other is the optimal route for intervention, e.g. large stents are best placed via femoral access rather than from the arm.

In the first instance, an attempt should be made to steer a hydrophilic guidewire into the target sheath using a shaped catheter. Opacification of the target sheath with contrast will make it much easier to see. This will usually succeed but may be quite fiddly. You will find that the wire will not pass through the haemostatic valve. In this case, pass a smaller sheath inside the larger one; the wire will pass into this. Advance the wire as you retract this sheath (Fig. 22.5). The wire will come out of the valve. If you cannot make this work, use a gooseneck snare to grasp the wire in the iliac artery or the aorta. This is quick but much more expensive. The wire will usually get damaged during snaring, so do not use it again.

**Tip:** It is surprisingly easy to steer a guidewire into a vascular sheath but it is much harder to get it out through the haemostatic valve. The simplest way to solve this problem is by placing a smaller sheath halfway into the larger one and pushing the wire into this up to the valve. Pull the sheath back out, and hey presto! there is the wire (Fig. 22.5).

There are three scenarios where rendezvous is likely to be needed:

- When the iliac artery has been recanalized from the contralateral approach.
- When there is difficulty catheterizing the contralateral limb during aortic stent grafting. In these circumstances simply use a small Sidewinder-shaped catheter from the ipsilateral side. This will always pull back into the contralateral limb stump. This allows a guidewire to be passed into the aneurysm sac; don't hesitate to grab a large snare and capture it!
- When there is difficulty advancing a stent-graft through tortuous iliac vessels, despite a Lunderquist wire.

In the first two scenarios the wire will be passed over a bifurcation. This has two ramifications. Firstly, when applying tension to the wire to deliver devices, always place a catheter over the bifurcation to prevent a cheesewire effect. Secondly, the catheter can actually be brought out at the contralateral groin. If you then need to pass a catheter up into the aorta in order to deploy a stent or stent-graft, it is often possible to push a loop of catheter up into the aorta by simultaneously advancing the catheter from both sides. When the apex of the loop is well above the bifurcation, simply insert a short-tip Amplatz wire from the contralateral side up to the apex then pull back the catheter to leave the wire in the aorta.

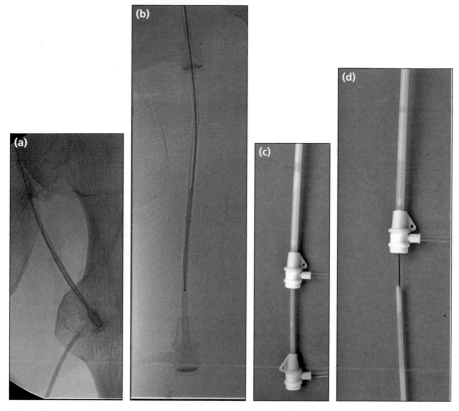

**Fig. 22.5** ■ Bringing a wire out through a sheath. (A) The hydrophilic wire will not pass through the haemostatic valve. (B, C) Sheath in sheath. A smaller sheath has been inserted into the original sheath and the wire has been advanced into it. (D) The smaller sheath is pulled back to reveal the wire.

## Suggestions for further reading

Brown PG, McBride KD, Gaines P. Technical report: Hickman catheter rescue. Clin Radiol 1994;49:891–894.

Egglin TPK, Dickey KW, Rosenblatt M, et al. Retrieval of intravascular foreign bodies: experience in 32 cases. AJR Am J Roentgenol 1995;164:1259–1264.
This is a large series of a variety of devices with a good reference section.

Hartnell GG. Techniques for intact removal of vascular foreign bodies. J Intervent Radiol 1996;11:29–37.
A how I do it approach with references.

Hartnell GG, Gates J, Soujanen JN, et al. Transfemoral repositioning of malpositioned central venous catheters. Cardiovasc Intervent Radiol 1996;19:329–331.

# Section Three

# Non-vascular intervention

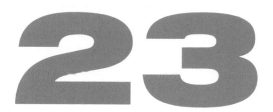

# Imaging guidance for intervention

A wide range of interventional procedures can only be safely performed with accurate imaging guidance. The aim of this chapter is to outline the basic principles of imaging-directed intervention. Ultrasound, CT and fluoroscopy have complementary roles; individual circumstances dictate the optimal modality.

## Ultrasound guidance

Ultrasound is ideal for many biopsy and drainage procedures and allows the procedure to be visualized in real time. Use ultrasound if it clearly demonstrates the target and a suitable approach. Usually this is achieved in solid organs or for larger abdominal collections. As a basic principle, use the highest frequency probe that gives a good image from the skin to the target site. Use a 7.5 MHz probe for superficial structures and a 3.5–5 MHz probe for deeper structures. It is exceedingly helpful to have a probe with a small footprint, as this improves access.

*Sterility* All invasive procedures should be performed with aseptic technique. Sterile ultrasound probe covers and ultrasound gel are readily available. Sterile ultrasound gel is used outside the ultrasound probe cover, but ordinary ultrasound gel can be used inside the probe cover. A clean drape should be used to cover the probe cable. Attach the cable to the drapes with a towel clip to save dropping an expensive probe.

 **Tip:** If you do not possess a suitably sized probe cover, improvise with a sterile surgical glove. Cut the cuff off the second glove and use this as a 'rubber band' to attach the glove/drape to the probe.

*Directing punctures* The ultrasound image represents a slice of tissue only 1 mm thick; much less than the width of the probe! For effective guidance, the needle must pass along the scan plane, which runs directly along the midline of the probe; even a small degree of misalignment will mean that the needle is not in the scan plane (Fig. 23.1). The importance of this relationship cannot be overemphasized; this is the single most important factor in successful ultrasound guidance.

 **Tip:** If you cannot see the needle, look to check that the needle and probe are aligned correctly.
Many probes come with a needle guide that can be used for the majority of ultrasound-guided interventions; the alternative is to use the freehand technique.

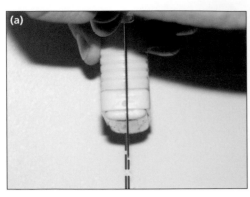
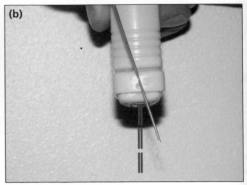

**Fig. 23.1** ■ The importance of keeping the needle in the plane of the ultrasound beam: (A) the needle path will be in the focused ultrasound beam; (B) despite starting in the middle of the probe, the needle is angled out of beam and will not be visualized.

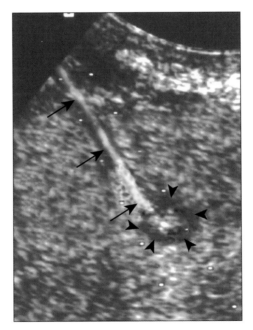

**Fig. 23.2** ■ Biopsy of a small hepatic metastasis using a needle guide (arrowheads). The white dots showing the projected needle path are clearly visible and the needle (arrows) can be seen entering the lesion.

A needle guide is so simple to use that no experience is needed to manage it. The guide attaches to the probe and constrains the needle to a predetermined path. The needle trajectory is displayed as two broken parallel lines superimposed on the image. This usually has to be selected on the ultrasound machine itself. The probe is positioned so that the projected needle path crosses the target. The needle is then advanced to the target (Fig. 23.2).

The freehand technique is required when there is no suitable path within the constraints of the needle guide. As the name suggests, the needle is advanced along the scan plane with one hand, while the probe is fixed with the other. The most common problems are due to angulation or rotation of the probe relative to the path of the needle.

**Tip:** When the needle tip is not clearly seen, gently oscillating the needle backwards and forwards greatly enhances its visibility.

# CT guidance

CT is used to guide biopsies and drainage of areas that cannot be seen on ultrasound, e.g. the lung, mediastinum, bone and areas of the abdomen obscured by bowel gas. There are several disadvantages to using CT compared with ultrasound:

- Needle passage cannot be viewed in real time
- The patient must be brought in and out of the scanner for each needle pass
- It is time consuming and exposes both patient and operator to radiation.

The principles of CT guidance are simple, although the procedure can be technically challenging. When performing procedures in the chest and abdomen, it is important to explain to the patient the necessity to try to take the same size breath during each scan and needle pass.

**Patient positioning** The diagnostic scans are reviewed and a suitable needle path is chosen. The patient is positioned either supine or prone, depending on the position of the target. Remember that, although angled needle trajectories can be used, it is simplest to judge a vertical needle pass.

 **Tip:** Sometimes it can be helpful to tilt the CT gantry as this allows the needle to be angulated cranially or caudally while remaining in the scan plane.

The simplest way to mark the puncture site is to use a reference grid placed over the region of interest. Grids can be purchased or can be readily made from some thin plastic tubing (Fig. 23.3).

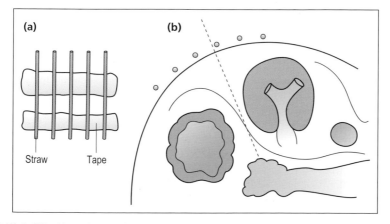

**Fig. 23.3** ■ (A) A CT grid can be readily made using plastic tubing and adhesive tape. (B) The optimal approach is determined by the markers.

## CT guidance: a step-by-step approach

1. The grid is positioned with the markers oriented perpendicular to the scan plane.
2. The patient is rescanned with the grid in place.
3. Select the slice that shows the optimal approach to the target and return the patient to this position.
4. Identify which of the grid lines corresponds to the best approach.
5. Turn on the light beam and simply mark where it intersects the chosen grid line.
6. Move the table to bring the patient out of the scanner gantry.
7. Clean, drape and anaesthetize the skin.
8. Advance the needle along the anticipated trajectory.
9. Rescan the patient.
10. Repeat steps 8 and 9 as necessary.

If you are lucky, your unit will have a CT fluoroscopy module. Don't get too excited as it's not quite as dynamic as real fluoroscopy, but it does speed the procedure up significantly. Exact designs vary, but essentially this system allows the operator to control the X-ray exposure at the table side, doing a very small number of cuts at your chosen level. Some systems have motor-driven movement to the chosen position.

**Tip:** If you are uncertain about judging the approach, then use a 22G needle to verify the approach. A second needle is positioned alongside the first and its position checked again.

A common pitfall is for the needle to pass obliquely through the scan plane. This can be demonstrated by performing one or two cuts above and below the target plane. If the needle tip is still in a satisfactory position, proceed as normal; if not, reposition the needle, compensating for the incorrect angle.

# Fluoroscopic guidance

Fluoroscopic guidance is used principally to guide percutaneous nephrolithotomy and biliary drainage and more rarely to biopsy pulmonary masses and bones. Whenever possible, use an X-ray machine with a C-arm, and avoid machines with overcouch explorers. Remember the basic principle of radiology: two views are necessary for localization.

Position the patient for the procedure and fluoroscope to identify the target lesion. Centre the field on the lesion and mark the position with a pair of sponge forceps. It is nearly always possible to choose an approach that allows the needle to be advanced perpendicular to the skin. For pulmonary biopsy, ask the patient to suspend respiration. Advance the needle part-way to the target and then fluoroscope to confirm that the tract is passing in the correct direction. Rotate the C-arm through 90° and fluoroscope again to determine the position of the needle tip relative to the target. Advance the needle until it reaches the target and reconfirm the position on the original projection.

The situation is slightly different during biliary drainage and nephrostomy, as an oblique approach is required for catheter and guidewire manipulation. When aiming at a specific duct or calyx, it is essential to know whether the needle is passing anterior or posterior to the target duct. This is resolved by rotating the C-arm (the patient can be rotated but remember there is a long needle sticking in them) and observing the movement of the needle relative to the target. If the needle is posterior, when the C-arm is rotated, the needle moves in the same direction as the C-arm rotation; if it moves in the opposite direction, it is anterior to the target. Remember that the reverse is true if you are turning the patient. When you think that you have grasped this concept, just wait until you try it in practice.

# Suggestions for further reading

Matalon TAS, Silver B. US guidance of interventional procedures. Radiology 1990;174:43–47.
Essential ultrasound techniques; well illustrated.
Yeuh N, Halvorsen RA, Letourneau JG, et al. Gantry tilt technique for CT guided biopsy and drainage. J Comput Assist Tomogr 1989;13:182–184.
An invaluable technique for many lesions.

# 24

# Equipment for non-vascular intervention

The majority of catheters and guidewires used within the vascular system are also appropriate for non-vascular intervention. There are, however, several devices that are used mainly for non-vascular applications.

## Co-axial access set (Neff/Accustick)

A co-axial access set converts a 22G puncture to 0.035 inch guidewire access (Fig. 24.1). The set is used mainly for PTC and more difficult nephrostomy insertion, e.g. in an undilated system. The set comes with a 22G needle for the initial puncture, and a short 0.018 inch guidewire, which is inserted through the needle after successful puncture. An interlocked dilator system can then be inserted over the guidewire; essentially this consists of an inner 3Fr dilator with an outer 6Fr dilator. The inner dilator and guidewire are then removed, leaving the 6Fr dilator, which will accept a standard 0.035-inch guidewire.

 **Alarm:** The tip of the 0.018 guidewire is very easily kinked, and once kinked it can be difficult to withdraw through the needle again. Be careful – it is possible to shear the wire off!

## Torcon blue biliary manipulation catheter (Cook)

This is a short, single-endhole braided steel polyethylene catheter, which has excellent torque control and is invaluable for urinary and biliary work. Conventional angiographic catheters can be used but tend to have poorer torque control.

## Peel-away sheath

This is a non-haemostatic plastic sheath that has been bonded along its midline (Fig. 24.2). The peel-away sheath is inserted over a supplied inner dilator which is then removed. Catheters and stents will readily pass down the sheath because of the reduction in friction and improvement in angles. The sheath is peeled apart by grasping the two proximal toggles. It is important to maintain some forward pressure on the device within the sheath to avoid inadvertently pulling it back while removing the sheath. Peel-away sheaths often do not have a haemostatic valve; this generally isn't a problem for non-vascular intervention but recently several sheath types now have a valve designed to slide over the opening; the valve must be slid back to allow the sheath to split.

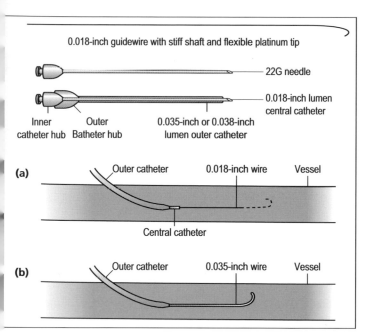

**Fig. 24.1** ■ Mini-access set. (A) Inner and outer catheters are inserted over 0.018-inch wire. (B) Inner catheter and 0.018-inch wire are removed and an 0.035-inch wire can be passed down the outer catheter.

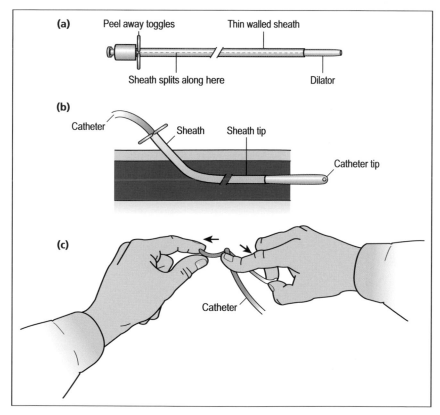

**Fig. 24.2** ■ Peel-away sheath. (A) Sheath and dilator assembled. (B) Dilator and wire are removed to allow passage of the device. (C) Hold the catheter in place with a finger, then pull the hub to split and remove the sheath.

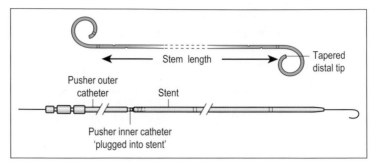

**Fig. 24.3** ■ Double-J ureteric stent system.

## Ureteric stent systems

A variety of ureteric stent systems are available, but, as always, they essentially operate on similar principles (Fig. 24.3). The ureteric stent is usually a double J configuration and straightened on the wire. A pusher is used to deliver the stent into position across a suitably stiff guidewire. The most common variation of design is the mechanism to pull back the stent if it is pushed in too far. In some systems, an inner catheter is 'plugged' into the proximal end of the stent, which allows retraction of the stent. Alternatively, a suture loop may have been passed through the last two stent sideholes. After optimal stent positioning, the inner catheter is withdrawn while maintaining the pusher in position to release the stent. In systems with a suture loop, remember to cut the suture loop and remove it before withdrawing the pusher. There isn't a standard way of describing the length of the stent. Some manufacturers use the total length and others only the straight section between the pigtail loops. As always, get familiar with the kit you are using.

# 25

# Biopsy and drainage

This chapter is divided into three main sections:

- Fine needle aspiration cytology and biopsy
- Draining fluid collections and abscesses
- Biopsy and drainage of specific areas.

Complications of biopsy and drainage are discussed at the end of the chapter. Biopsy and drainage procedures involve traversing normal tissue to reach an abnormal area. To do this requires a safe access route and accurate targeting. The principles of image guidance for intervention were discussed in the preceding chapter. The shortest, straightest route is usually the best approach but there are important exceptions to this rule, e.g. peripheral liver lesion. Take time to plan an approach that avoids important structures, e.g. bowel, lung, major vessels and the gallbladder.

To minimize complications, the patient should be fasted for abdominal biopsy and coagulopathy should be excluded. Make sure that the patient has given consent and that all parties are aware of the potential risks (and their consequences) of the procedure.

**Consent issue:** Explain the benefits of obtaining material for diagnosis/drainage. Problems tend to come from bleeding and traversing other structures, but serious complications are rare.

# Fine needle aspiration cytology and biopsy

The aim of aspiration or biopsy is to obtain a satisfactory tissue specimen for cytology or histology. Ultrasound is used whenever possible as it allows real-time guidance without exposing you or the patient to ionizing radiation.

## The patient

The vast majority of biopsies are performed under local anaesthesia and patient cooperation is essential. Explain what the procedure entails; in particular, stress the importance of breath-holding during the needle pass. If the patient does not understand or cannot cooperate, then stop now! Most biopsies are not painful; emphasize that analgesia is available if needed. Make sure that the patient is aware that regular post-biopsy observations are normal and do not indicate a problem.

# Contraindications

## Abnormal clotting or platelets

- It is mandatory to know the platelet count and clotting status.
- No additional precautions are necessary when the INR is ≤1.5 and the platelet count ≥50000.

  When the clotting is more deranged, consider transfusion of FFP ± platelets.

## Vascular lesion

- Some tumours are highly vascular, e.g. renal cell tumour metastases. Switch on the colour Doppler if there is any doubt. If you need to biopsy a vascular lesion, make sure that the patient is adequately prepared. This may require large bore IV access and cross-matched blood. Try to avoid the main tumoral vessels and be prepared to embolize the lesion if necessary.

## Obstructed system

- The target for biopsy is likely to be the point of obstruction and fistula or intra-abdominal leakage can occur. It is best to drain the system before biopsy. Attempting drainage after a complication can be very difficult.

## Uncooperative patient

- Consider sedation or general anaesthesia.
- Remember that a sedated patient will not be able to breath-hold.

## Diagnosis irrelevant to management

- Do not be persuaded to do the biopsy just because it would 'be nice to know'.

# Which specimen – cytology or histology

There are two sampling techniques: aspiration cytology and cutting needle biopsy. The local pathology service will guide you on the type of specimen they require. Usually only a few cells are needed to diagnose malignancy but a core of tissue is needed to subtype tumours or assess diffuse liver/renal pathology.

# Fine needle aspiration cytology

**Aspiration cytology**, sometimes referred to as fine needle aspiration cytology (FNAC), is performed with a 21G or 22G (Chiba needle). The specimen only contains a few cells, but for many conditions this will establish the diagnosis. The risks involved are very small; FNAC is frequently possible even in hazardous areas.

The needle is placed into the lesion under imaging guidance and then attached to a 20-mL syringe. Draw a full vacuum on the syringe while the needle is passed back and forward through the lesion (Fig. 25.1). If you have an assistant, use a connecting tube or a 21G butterfly needle and get the assistant to aspirate the syringe while you manipulate the needle under guidance.

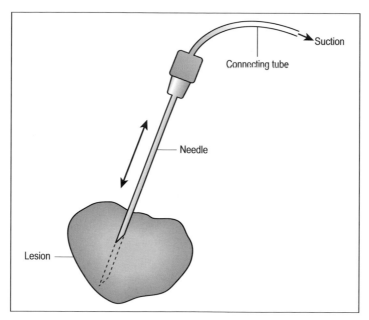

**Fig. 25.1** ■ Aspiration technique. The needle is passed into the lesion under ultrasound control. A connecting tube and 20-mL syringe are attached to the needle. Draw a full vacuum on the syringe and then pass the needle back and forward through the lesion. Slowly release the vacuum as the needle is withdrawn or the tiny sample will disappear into the syringe.

 **Tip:** Withdraw the needle under gentle suction, then remove the syringe. Vigorous suction results in the tiny sample being lost in the syringe; without suction, the sample stays in the patient.

Place the sampling needle onto a slide and gently eject the needle contents onto the slide with an air-filled syringe. Also put any fluid in the sampling syringe onto a slide. Specimens may be simply air-dried but specimen preparation varies from centre to centre; check the preference of your cytologist. Specimens only contain a few cells and therefore it is best to make at least two passes.

 **Tip:** It is helpful to have a cytologist to prepare the slide. The cytologist will make a better film and also be able to make a preliminary inspection of the material to ensure that it is adequate.

# Cutting needle biopsy

Cutting needle biopsy obtains a larger specimen, typically a 1-mm core of 20-mm length. The cutting needle consists of two parts: an outer cutting shaft and an inner stylet (Fig. 25.2). Most centres use automated devices but if using cutting needles manually, it is essential to realize that the specimen is 'cut' when the outer shaft is advanced.

**Manual biopsy needles** Fully manual devices are relatively rarely used now as single-use spring-loaded devices are more reliable and rapid at taking a specimen than most humans. Most are versions of the traditional Tru-cut needle (Fig. 25.3). The needle comes in various

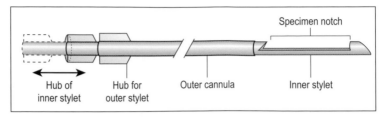

**Fig. 25.2** ■ Construction of a cutting biopsy needle. Tissue prolapses into the specimen notch and is cut by advancement of the outer cutting needle shaft.

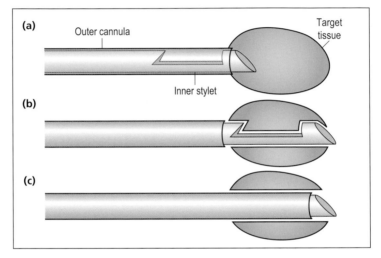

**Fig. 25.3** ■ Mechanism of action of a cutting needle. (A) Needle is advanced to the edge of the target tissue. (B) Inner stylet is advanced into the target tissue. (C) Outer cutting shaft is advanced to resheath inner stylet and cut the specimen core.

sizes from 14G to 18G and with two different specimen lengths, 1 cm and 2 cm. In practice, the 18G 2-cm needle is suitable for the majority of biopsies.

**Tip:** Choose the shortest length of biopsy needle that will reach the target. Particularly in CT, needles that are too long flop about during repeat scanning and are more likely to get accidentally pushed in too far.

**Automated biopsy devices** The needles are always single use but the mechanism may be disposable or reusable. There are two principal mechanisms, which differ in the way in which the central stylet is advanced.

The first mechanism is typified by the Temno needle. In this device, the inner stylet is manually advanced into the target. At this stage, resistance is felt and further pressure on the trigger mechanism fires the outer sleeve to cut the core. Important points to note are:

• The precise position of the core is ascertained before the biopsy is taken; this is particularly important in proximity to hazardous areas

- It is an integral system. There is no handle to attach and detach, but it remains relatively small and light. This is an important consideration for CT biopsy, where the patient must be rescanned to confirm needle position.

The alternative system is fully automatic. At the push of the button both the inner stylet and then, almost instantaneously, the outer cutting shaft rapidly advance, taking the biopsy. This is the most commonly used type of system.

Some automated systems now allow the operator to select between these two different modes on the same disposable device. Other systems allow the operator to determine the length of the specimen, i.e. the forward throw of the needle – very useful if the biopsy is close to a vital structure. Make sure you familiarize yourself with the systems in your hospital and get the best out of the devices.

**Tip:** Remember that with a fully automatic system, the biopsy is taken from the tissue 10–20 mm in front of the needle tip, depending on the size of the specimen notch.

# Aftercare

There is no fixed regimen for post-biopsy care. The aftercare varies with the site of biopsy, coagulation status and general condition of the patient. Ensure that a written care plan is given to the staff who will care for the patient. If there is no established local protocol, the proforma below can be modified to suit most procedures.

**Sample proforma for patient aftercare**

| Patient name | | ID No. |
|---|---|---|
| Date | Time | |
| Procedure | | |
| Anaesthesia/Sedation | | |
| Needle size | | No. of cores taken |
| Uneventful/Complicated (specify) | | |
| Specimens | In formalin/saline/dry | |
| | Returned with patient/Sent to | |
| Aftercare | | |
| | Flat bedrest for 2 hours | |
| | Pulse and BP | Every 15 minutes for 1 hour |
| | | Every 30 minutes for 1 hour |
| | | Every 60 minutes for 2 hours |
| | | Every 4 hours until discharge |
| | Analgesia as necessary | |
| Other, e.g. fluids only | | |
| Information for discharge | | |

# Draining fluid collections and abscesses

Tapping fluid collections to drain them or to obtain fluid for laboratory investigation is an important and frequently requested procedure. The vast majority of collections can be managed with an appropriately-sized and positioned catheter but success depends on understanding a few key concepts.

## Assessing abscesses

Use the pre-intervention imaging to identify:

- **The exact anatomical location of the collection**. An understanding of the anatomical boundaries will dictate the ideal drain position and approach. Large collections will shrink and to achieve complete drainage, the drain should be placed in the most dependent portion of the collection.
- **The content of the collection**. Ultrasound offers the most useful assessment of the viscosity of the collection and the presence of loculi and septa. Look for the following features, which will influence the type and number of drains required:

| Anechoic collection | Probably clear fluid, e.g. urinoma |
| Few scattered echoes | Turbid fluid, e.g. thin pus |
| Extensive or swirling echoes | Thick fluid, e.g. viscous pus |
| Diffuse echoes with gas | Organized abscess or phlegmon |
| Simple collection | Single drain |
| Loculated collection – thin | Single drain-synechiae |
| Loculated collection – thick | Multiple drains-septae |
| Multiple collections | Multiple drains |

 **Tip:** The ultrasound appearances are not an infallible guide and occasionally will be misleading – always try a diagnostic aspiration.

## Which drain

*Drain size* At the risk of stating the obvious, viscous fluid will not drain through a small-calibre drainage catheter. Use a 6–8Fr catheter for clear fluid, 8–10Fr catheter for thin pus, 10–12Fr catheter for thick pus and a 12–22Fr drain for collections containing debris.

*Drain type* Virtually all drainage catheters are pigtail shaped. The pigtail in some catheters is locked in position to provide anchorage. The mechanism to lock the catheter usually involves tensioning threads between the catheter hub and pigtail. As the locking mechanism varies between individual devices, familiarize yourself with the systems used in your hospital. Failure to unlock the catheter at removal will cause a large exit wound; intense screaming from the patient usually warns the alert operator.

## Diagnostic aspiration

This is also the first step in any drainage procedure.

# Equipment

- 21G needle (of appropriate length).
- 20-mL syringes.
- Specimen pots.

 **Tip:** Ensure that you know which samples are required and how they are to be handled en route to the laboratory. Some specimens must be examined urgently.

# Procedure

Prepare and anaesthetize the skin at the desired puncture site. Aim the needle into the collection and aspirate the desired amount of fluid. If necessary, it is acceptable to traverse bowel with a 21G needle, but this tract cannot be used for drainage. If drainage is anticipated, only take a small sample as this leaves a larger target to aim at.

 **Tip:** Before plunging a needle into a collection, turn on the colour Doppler as this will prevent you from draining an aneurysm!

## Troubleshooting

**Fluid cannot be aspirated** Check that the needle tip is correctly sited within the collection and reposition as necessary. Sometimes the fluid is too thick to aspirate with a 22G needle; try again with an 18G needle. If this is unsuccessful, this is probably a solid mass; consider biopsy.

## Therapeutic drainage

A selection of catheters and guidewires may be needed. A small amount of fluid is usually aspirated as a prelude to drainage; the nature of this specimen helps select which drain will function best.

### Procedure

The precise technique depends on the type of catheter that has been chosen.

Prepare and anaesthetize the skin and the desired puncture site. Make a sufficiently large skin incision to allow passage of the drainage catheter. Pass a needle into the collection, using imaging guidance.

In an **one-step procedure**, the catheter is mounted on a central needle and stylet. A direct puncture technique is used. The central stylet is removed and fluid is aspirated to confirm the tip is within the collection. The needle is held still and the catheter is simply advanced along the needle into the collection. This technique is only advisable for large collections that are easily accessed. Fluoroscopy is not required.

In a **two-step procedure**, fluoroscopy is recommended though the skilled operator can do this under ultrasound alone. A guidewire is passed through the puncture needle into the collection. If a 21G needle was used to puncture the collection, either simply repuncture with an 18G needle or consider using a Neff set to convert to a 0.035-inch wire. The needle is removed over the wire and the track is dilated using fascial dilators to 1–2Fr larger than the drainage catheter.

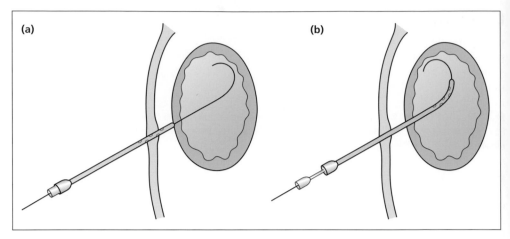

**Fig. 25.4** ■ Catheter stiffener assembly (A) The entire assembly is advanced to the edge of the collection. (B) The Luer lock is loosened and the inner stiffener and the wire are held stationary and the drainage catheter pushed forwards.

Fix the wire securely to ensure that it does not kink and that you do not lose wire position during catheter exchanges.

The catheter stiffener assembly is then passed over the wire into the collection. When you reach either a significant bend or the collection, detach the stiffener, hold the stiffener and the wire fixed in position, and slide the catheter forward over the guidewire (Fig. 25.4). The stiffener and guidewire are removed and the catheter is allowed to form. Most self-retaining catheters are introduced in this way.

 **Tip:** Always insert plenty of guidewire as this allows a degree of latitude if you kink the wire.

Whichever technique is used, ensure that there is free drainage and that you have obtained adequate specimens for laboratory analysis. **When the collection contains pus, aspirate it as completely as possible!** In addition, consider gentle saline irrigation of the cavity as this helps to clear thick pus and other semisolid debris. Make sure that you have a suitable drain bag to attach to the drainage catheter; sometimes special adaptors are needed. Do not wait until pus is running over your shoes to find this out!

Securely attach the catheter to the patient. There are several ways to do this:

- Suturing the catheter to the skin
- Using adhesive anchor systems
- Using adhesive tape – only secure with waterproof tape.

Make sure that the final position will be practical and as comfortable as possible for the patient.

 **Tip:** Don't attach a conventional 3-way tap to a 12Fr drain – you have just reduced the lumen to 6Fr!

# Follow-up

Remember to write in the case notes if you have inserted a locking pigtail drain, just in case they decide to remove the drain.

The volume of fluid drained is charted. Febrile patients usually settle within 24–48 hours if there is adequate drainage. Most simple fluid collections drain quickly, with a steady decrease in the volume of fluid draining. Large inflammatory collections (e.g. pseudocyst, empyema) may take several weeks to resolve.

Thick viscous collections require irrigation and aspiration to ensure effective drainage. It is essential the catheter is aspirated three times a day. Use a 50-mL syringe for maximum suction and then irrigate with 5–10 mL of saline. The drain may need to be repositioned or replaced as the situation evolves.

The drain catheter can be removed when there is minimal drainage (<10 mL/day) and the collection has resolved as documented by CT or ultrasound. Catheters should be promptly removed when they have fulfilled their role so that they do not become a source of infection in their own right.

## Troubleshooting

**The drainage catheter will not advance into the collection** Ensure that the skin incision is large enough.

- Use fluoroscopy to check for wire kinking. If the wire is kinked and there is sufficient wire, pull it until the kink is outside the skin, then insert a dilator and exchange for a stiffer wire.
- Large drains may need to be placed through a peel-away sheath which is positioned over a stiff guidewire.

**The collection is loculated and does not drain freely** Thin loculi can be disrupted by moving the catheter back and forth within the collection.

- If this is not successful, fibrinous bands can be broken down by instilling streptokinase into the collection. This is particularly useful for loculated empyema.
- Some collections require multiple drainage catheters.

**The catheter drains initially but then stops** Hopefully, the collection is completely drained.

- Re-image the patient to assess the catheter position and the size of the collection.
- The drainage bag has been positioned above the collection, e.g. on the patient's locker. Place the bag in a dependent position.
- The catheter is correctly positioned, but there is a kink in it or the drainage tubing. Kinks are almost always external and are often caused by fiddling with the catheter or dressings. Reattaching it appropriately can often salvage the catheter. If there is any doubt, replace the catheter/drainage tube.
- The catheter may need to be repositioned or replaced if the collection has changed size or shape or if the catheter has been displaced.
- The catheter is blocked. Gentle flushing may clear it. If this fails, try using a guidewire to unblock it. An irreversibly blocked catheter must be exchanged. Catheters which have been in place for a week or more usually have a well-established tract. The catheter can be removed and a hydrophilic guidewire passed through the tract into the collection. A new drain is then simply positioned over the wire. An alternative option is to cut the hub off the catheter and then pass a sheath over the outside of the catheter. The catheter is removed and a guidewire passed into the collection through the sheath; the sheath is removed and a new catheter positioned over the wire.

**Fever does not settle after 48 hours** Failure to improve implies incomplete drainage or another source of sepsis. If this occurs, the patient should be re-imaged. Further drainage is often required. This scenario is common in patients with infected pancreatic pseudocysts.

**There is a sudden increase in drainage or a change in the composition of the effluent** This implies that a fistula has developed; an injection of contrast into the drainage catheter will usually demonstrate the problem. Sometimes it is necessary to perform an alternative study if the fistula tract acts as a one-way valve. A fistula will usually resolve if there is an adequate alternative route of drainage, although prolonged drainage may be necessary. Where there is a connection with an obstructed system, this will also need to be drained if the fistula is to resolve.

# Biopsy and drainage of specific areas

## Liver

Liver biopsy is one of the most frequently requested interventional procedures, and it is usually one of the simplest to perform. Biopsies are either targeted to a focal lesion or random cores in diffuse liver disease. Non-targeted biopsies are usually taken from the right lobe. When there are multiple lesions, choose the most accessible. To minimize the risk of haemorrhage when taking a biopsy of peripheral lesions, always make a tract that passes through 2–3 cm of normal liver before hitting the target (Fig. 25.5).

When taking a biopsy of the right lobe of the liver, a lateral approach is usually chosen. The ribs can interfere with access; choose an approach which allows scanning parallel to the line of the ribs. Sometimes the needle has to be angled up or down to accommodate this.

Mild shoulder tip pain is not uncommon after liver biopsy and the patient should be warned that this may occur. The risks of biopsy are increased in the presence of biliary obstruction and ascites. Drainage is recommended before biopsy. In the presence of mildly deranged clotting, consider a plugged biopsy.

### Plugged liver biopsy

The essence of this procedure is to prevent haemorrhage from the liver capsule by embolizing the needle tract, using Gelfoam injected through a sheath in the needle tract. Using a sheath has the potential advantage of allowing more than one needle to pass through the same tract.

**Fig. 25.5** ■ Direct biopsy of peripheral liver lesions (A) increases the risk of extracapsular bleeding. Choose an approach (B) that passes through a cuff of normal liver tissue.

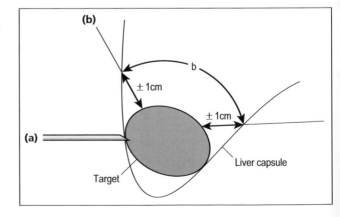

## Equipment

- 18G biopsy needle.
- 18G sheathed needle.
- Gelfoam sheet.

## Procedure

Prepare the Gelfoam in advance by cutting the sheet into 1-mm pledgets and soak them in contrast. Discard the needle from the 18G sheathed needle and fit the sheath over the biopsy needle. The needle and sheath are advanced into the liver as a single unit (Fig. 25.6). The biopsy is performed in the conventional fashion. The needle is withdrawn, leaving the sheath in situ and the adequacy of the specimen is confirmed. The tract is now embolized by injecting 1–2 mL of the Gelfoam pledgets as the sheath is withdrawn. Post-biopsy aftercare is the same as for a standard liver biopsy.

# Transjugular liver biopsy

Transjugular liver biopsy (TJB) is a much more complicated and expensive procedure. It is reserved for patients with diffuse liver disease and deranged coagulation or ascites for whom plugged biopsy would still pose significant risk. The rationale for TJB is that there is no puncture of the liver capsule and therefore any bleeding from the needle tract will be contained within the liver or auto-transfuse into the hepatic vein. TJB is not carte blanche to perform liver biopsy in any patient; as always, attempts should be made to correct the underlying coagulopathy before the procedure.

## Anatomy

The hepatic veins join the IVC just below the right atrium. Biopsy is most safely performed from the right hepatic vein while angling the sheath anteriorly. This ensures the biopsy is taken from the maximum volume of parenchyma and avoids inadvertent capsular perforation. Anterior biopsy from the middle hepatic vein should be avoided.

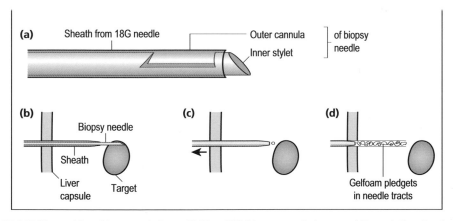

**Fig. 25.6** ■ Plugged liver biopsy technique. (A) The 18G biopsy needle is passed through the sheath of an 18G needle. (B) The needle and sheath are advanced into the liver and the biopsy taken. (C) The biopsy needle is removed and Gelfoam pledgets injected through the sheath as it is withdrawn. (D) The final result is a tract embolized with Gelfoam.

Differentiating the right from the middle hepatic vein can be difficult in the AP projection but is easily done from a lateral projection.

## Equipment

- Basic angiography set.
- 5Fr sheath.
- Cobra II catheter.
- Hydrophilic and Amplatz guidewires. A 1-cm floppy tip Amplatz wire is very useful in small livers.
- Transjugular cutting needle liver biopsy set (Cook UK), which contains a 7Fr 49-cm long sheath, an angled metallic sheath stiffener, a 5Fr straight catheter and a 60-cm long cutting biopsy needle. A metal arrow on the hub of the stiffener indicates the orientation of the curve.

## Procedure

*Access* Ultrasound-guided right IJV puncture.

*Catheterization* Pass the J wire and Cobra catheter into the IVC, taking particular care steering through the right atrium. Rotate the catheter so that its tip points towards the patient's right; slowly withdraw it until the tip engages the RHV. Advance the hydrophilic wire and Cobra catheter into the vein.

*Runs* Hand inject a few millilitres of contrast to ensure that the catheter is not wedged, then perform a hepatic venogram. The RHV is the target vein and typically has a suitably shallow angle that allows the sheath entry. The angled stiffener within the sheath gives excellent torque control but poor cornering ability and will only negotiate suitably angled veins.

*Biopsy* An Amplatz extra-stiff wire is passed into the hepatic vein; take care not to puncture the liver capsule with the guidewire (Fig. 25.7). Exchange the 5F sheath for the reinforced sheath, which is passed 3–4 cm into the hepatic vein. Use the directional indicator on the

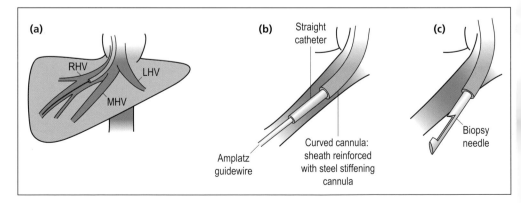

**Fig. 25.7** ■ Transjugular liver biopsy technique. (A) Catheterize the RHV using a Cobra II catheter. Then exchange for an Amplatz super-stiff wire. (B) Advance the curved cannula into the right hepatic vein using a co-axial straight catheter and the Amplatz wire. Remove the catheter and wire to leave the curved cannula in place. (C) Turn the curved cannula anteriorly to abut the vein wall and advance the long biopsy needle into the liver parenchyma to take the biopsy.

hub to direct the sheath anteriorly until it abuts the vein wall. The cutting needle is primed and advanced into the sheath until the needle tip is a few millimetres beyond the end of the sheath in the liver parenchyma. The patient is instructed to breath-hold and the inner stylet is depressed, taking the biopsy.

# Kidney

The kidney is the most vascular organ in the body and biopsy is associated with an increased risk of haemorrhage. Most renal biopsies in native and transplant kidneys are performed to investigate the aetiology of renal failure. These biopsies should be taken from either the upper or the lower pole of the kidney. Avoid biopsy adjacent to the renal pelvis as this greatly increases the risks of urinary and vascular complications. Few biopsies are performed to investigate the nature of renal masses as these are usually dealt with surgically.

# Adrenal glands

The adrenal glands are usually approached posteriorly in the prone or lateral decubitus position; large lesions can be biopsied anteriorly. In most cases, CT is the best imaging guidance. Always measure vanillylmandelic acid levels in patients who have an adrenal mass with no known primary tumour. When phaeochromocytoma is suspected, α-adrenergic blockade is recommended to minimize the risk of hypertensive crisis.

# Pancreas

Pancreatic biopsy is indicated in the investigation of a mass at the head of the pancreas. There is usually associated biliary and pancreatic duct obstruction. If obstructed, the biliary tree should be drained before starting. The pancreatic duct cannot be drained and there is a risk of pancreatitis and pseudocyst formation.

Pancreatic biopsy can usually be performed under ultrasound guidance. The biopsy track may be transgastric but care should be taken to avoid inadvertent biopsy through the transverse colon (Fig. 25.8). Plastic biliary stents are readily seen on ultrasound and can be used to target pancreatic biopsy. As pancreatic biopsy is often painful, sedation and analgesia are recommended.

Peripancreatic abscesses, pseudocysts and phlegmons are common complications of pancreatitis. Infected collections often require drainage. The management of complex pancreatitis is best left to a specialist team but the following guidelines are generally applicable. Collections in the lesser sac can usually be approached anteriorly through the transverse mesocolon between the stomach and transverse colon. Collections in the left paracolic gutter are more difficult to approach and are best done with CT guidance to avoid colonic puncture. Loculated collections may require several drains. As always, frequent review is mandatory. This often entails serial CT scanning. Large pseudocysts, which continue to drain, can be treated by cyst gastrostomy.

 **Alarm:** If you cannot confidently identify the colon, opacify it with contrast. Do not risk a colonic kebab!

# Retroperitoneum

Most retroperitoneal masses are best biopsied on CT unless they are very large. The retroperitoneum can be approached anteriorly if there is a window without bowel. The posterior approach is particularly useful for paraspinal masses.

**Fig. 25.8** ■ Relationship between the stomach, pancreas and transverse colon. Transgastric biopsy is acceptable but take great care to avoid the colon.

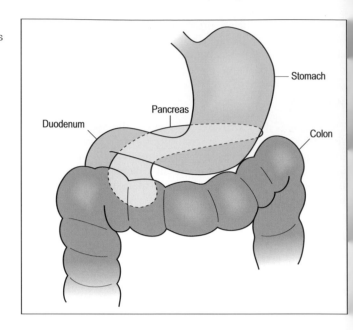

## Pelvis

The commonest difficulty in pelvic biopsy or drainage is identifying a route that does not transgress bowel or bladder. Gravity causes pus to collect in the prerectal space; this is difficult to access from an anterior approach. Alternative options include transrectal, transvaginal and transgluteal approaches.

The posterior transgluteal route traverses the sacrosciatic notch and uses CT guidance (Fig. 25.9). The patient is scanned in the prone position (Fig. 25.10) and the approach is planned in the conventional fashion. **Remember that the sciatic nerve and gluteal vessels pass through the anterior portion of the notch**. To avoid them, the tract should pass as close to the sacrum as possible. Burrowing through this much muscle can be difficult and may be uncomfortable for the patient both during and after the procedure. Pericatheter inflammation can cause sciatica even when the catheter is appropriately placed.

Ultrasound-guided transrectal and transvaginal drainage and biopsy are readily performed and well tolerated. Although these approaches are unfamiliar, the basic principles of biopsy and drainage apply. These routes offer a direct approach to posterior collections, with the advantage of draining well in the supine position. Most suitable probes have needle guides. Use sterile covers over the probe and guide. The collection is punctured under direct visualization. As always, aspirate some fluid; if it is purulent, formal drainage is performed; if not, the collection is aspirated to dryness. Catheter fixation is difficult and self-retaining catheters are preferred. The catheter can be taped to the patient's thigh and drained into a leg bag.

**Transrectal procedures** cause surprisingly little discomfort but this is a 'dirty' route (Fig. 25.11). A cleansing enema is recommended to remove any faecal residue and antibiotic prophylaxis must be given. Contamination of the collection with faecal organisms is a potential pitfall but is thought not to occur because of the positive intra-abdominal pressure during defaecation. The patient is scanned in the lateral decubitus or lithotomy position. Drains up to 12Fr can be used. Catheter displacement during defaecation is common even with self-retaining catheters.

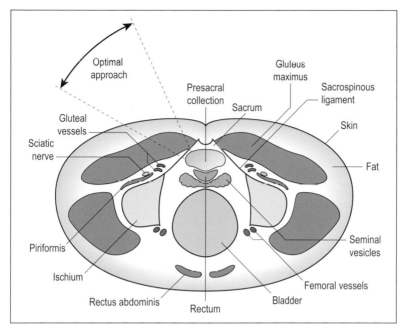

**Fig. 25.9** ■ Approach for transgluteal drainage through the greater sciatic notch. Optimal path is posteromedial to avoid the gluteal vessels and sciatic nerve.

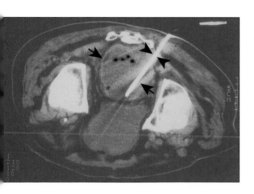

**Fig. 25.10** ■ Transgluteal route for drainage of a presacral abscess (arrows). The catheter (arrowheads) passes close to the sacrum to avoid the sciatic nerve and gluteal vessels that lie anteriorly.

The **transvaginal approach** is performed with the patient in the lithotomy position (Fig. 25.12). Sedation is recommended as the procedure tends to be uncomfortable and the vaginal wall can be difficult to traverse. The vagina and perineum are cleaned with povidone iodine solution. Catheters up to 12Fr can be used but require employing serial fascial dilators over a stiff guidewire.

# Complications of biopsy and drainage

Fortunately, complications following biopsy are rare and the majority of complications are minor. The risks vary between individual patients and differing sites and are discussed in the relevant sections. The most important complications are:

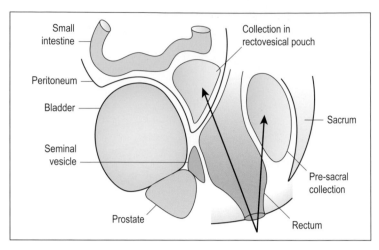

**Fig. 25.11** ■ Sagittal section through male pelvis showing routes for transrectal drainage.

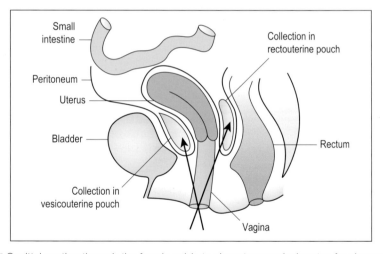

**Fig. 25.12** ■ Sagittal section through the female pelvis to show transvaginal routes for abscess drainage.

*Bleeding* This may occur even in the best hands, particularly in the presence of a vascular lesion or organ. Ensure that the blood clotting and platelets are optimized before starting.

 **Alarm:** The risk of haemorrhage is highest during:
- Biopsy of vascular organs (liver, spleen and kidneys) in the presence of abnormal clotting
- Biopsy adjacent to major blood vessels
- Biopsy of known vascular tumours, particularly when there is no surrounding normal tissue to tamponade bleeding.

In high-risk patients it is wise to group and save or even cross-match blood for the procedure.

*Perforation of a hollow viscus* Bowel can usually be avoided by using an appropriate approach. If the intestine must be traversed, use a fine needle (22G) rather than a cutting needle.

*Pneumothorax* This is common following biopsy of lung or mediastinal masses. Pneumothorax can also occur when the pleural space is traversed during biopsy of upper abdominal lesions. Remember that the pleural space extends much further down posteriorly. This problem can be anticipated and the patient should be warned that it might be necessary to have a chest drain following the procedure.

*Fistula* May occur when performing biopsies in the presence of an obstructed system. For this reason, it is advisable to perform drainage before biopsy. This is particularly important in the presence of biliary obstruction.

*Infection* This is rare if proper aseptic precautions are taken and the intestine is not traversed. When the bowel is traversed, e.g. transrectal biopsy, then prophylactic antibiotics should be given, e.g. gentamicin (80 mg) and metronidazole (500 mg). If the colon is punctured, seek surgical advice. The patient will usually settle on conservative management, nil by mouth and antibiotics.

*Tumour seeding of the biopsy tract* This is rare but can occur with any tumour. The risk can be minimized by passing through a 'normal' section of the target organ or the potential field of resection.

*Death* This is usually due to haemorrhage and is very rare in routine biopsies.

# Suggestions for further reading

Bakal CW, Sacks D, Burke DR, et al. Quality improvement guidelines for adult percutaneous abscess and fluid drainage. J Vasc Interv Radiol 2003;14:S223–S225.

Georgian-Smith D, Shiels WE. Freehand interventional sonography in the breast: basic principles and clinical applications. Radiographics 1996;16:149–161.

Gupta S. New techniques in image guided percutaneous biopsy. Cardiovas Intervent Radiol 2004;27:91–104.

A comprehensive and contemporary overview with useful insights into newer modes of CT guidance and also advanced biopsy techniques.

Livraghi T, Lazzaroni S, Civelli L, et al. Risk conditions and mortality rate of abdominal fine needle biopsy. J Intervent Radiol 1997;12: 57–64.

Includes recommendations to minimize risks; a very worthwhile read.

Spies JB, Berlin L. Complications of percutaneous needle biopsy. AJR Am J Roentgenol 1998;171:13–17.

## Pelvic

Alexander AA, Eschelman DJ, Nazarian LN, et al. Transrectal sonographically guided drainage of deep pelvic abscesses. AJR Am J Roentgenol 1994;162:1227–1230.

Feld R, Eschelman DJ, Sagerman JE, et al. Treatment of pelvic abscesses and other fluid collections: efficacy of transvaginal sonographically guided aspiration and drainage. AJR Am J Roentgenol 1994;163:1141–1145.

## Thoracic

Hubsch P, Bankier AA, Wilding R, et al. Thoracic anatomy relevant to CT interventions. Semin Intervent Radiol 1994;12;211–217.

Moore EH. Technical aspects of needle aspiration lung biopsy: personal perspective. Radiology 1998;208:303–318.

Beautiful article with a wealth of practical information – a must read.

Moulton JS, Moore TP. Coaxial percutaneous biopsy technique with automated biopsy devices: value in improving accuracy and negative predictive value. Radiology 1993;186:515–522.

## Liver

Choh J, Dolmatch B, Safadi R, et al. Transjugular core liver biopsy with a 19 gauge spring loaded

cutting needle. Cardiovasc Intervent Radiol
1998;21:88–90.

Smith TP, McDermott VG, Ayoub DM.
Percutaneous transhepatic liver biopsy with tract
embolization. Radiology 1996;198:769–774.
Good practical description of the technique.

### Renal

Christensen J, Lindequist S, Knudsen DU, et al.
Ultrasound guided renal biopsy with biopsy gun
technique – efficacy and complications. Acta
Radiol 1995;36:276.

### Adrenal

Hussain S. Gantry angulation in CT guided adrenal
biopsy. AJR Am J Roentgenol 1996;166:537–539.

Welch TJ, Sheedy PF II, Stephens DH.
Percutaneous adrenal biopsy; review of a 10 year
experience. Radiology 1994;193:341–344.

### Pancreas

Dodd LG, Mooney EE, Layfield LJ, et al. Fine-
needle aspiration of the pancreas: A cytology
primer for radiologists. Radiology
1997;205:203–209.

VanSonnenberg E, Wittich GR, Chon KS, et al.
Percutaneous radiologic drainage of pancreatic
abscesses. AJR Am J Roentgenol
1997;168:979–984.
The best results achievable with a very aggressive
radiological approach.

# 26

# Percutaneous renal intervention

## Percutaneous nephrostomy

Percutaneous nephrostomy is one of the most frequently performed interventional procedures and is a technique in which every radiologist should feel completely confident. The commonest indication is ureteric obstruction, which leads to gradual progressive renal loss, and nephrostomy is usually an elective procedure. In an infected obstructed system, the resultant rapid renal loss and septicaemia are an indication for urgent drainage.

### Equipment

- Undilated or minimally dilated system: 21G Accustick/Neff co-axial access set.
- Dilated system: 19G sheathed needle.
- Heavy duty 3-mm J guidewire (shorter guidewires, usually about 60 cm length make it easier).
- Fascial dilators to one size greater than the drain size.
- 6–8Fr pigtail nephrostomy drain.
- 5Fr Cobra catheter.
- Angled hydrophilic wire.

### Procedure

The performance of a safe nephrostomy requires an understanding of renal anatomy, good ultrasound guidance and basic catheterization skills.

*Target zone* The renal arteries and renal veins enter the kidney at the renal hilum and divide into larger anterior and smaller posterior divisions passing around the renal collecting system. Much has been made of Brödel's avascular line but in practice the least vascular zone, and therefore the safest area, lies within the arc shown (Fig. 26.1).

Interpolar posterior calyces in the mid and lower pole are the best target and provide the most favourable approach for intervention. Direct puncture of the renal pelvis should be avoided as this increases the risk of major vascular injury and persistent urine leak. Puncture of the upper pole calyces is only necessary for nephrolithotomy and is associated with a significant risk of pneumothorax (Fig. 26.2). Avoid anterior punctures; in addition to providing the least favourable access and causing renal haemorrhage, you may well traverse the colon, liver or spleen.

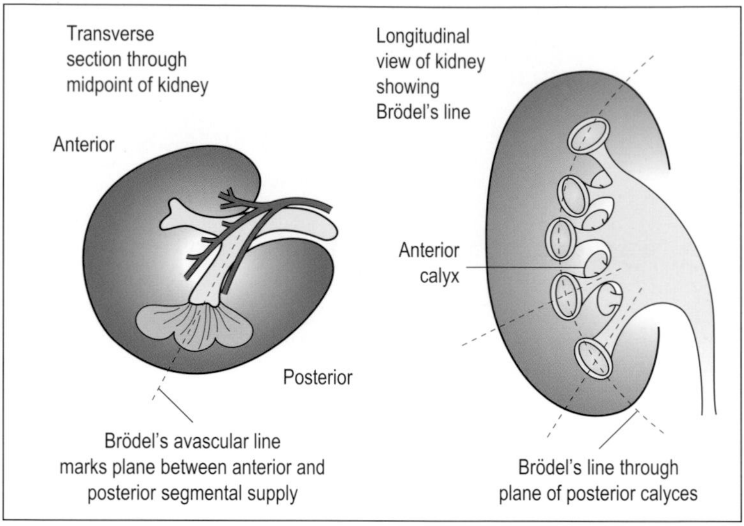

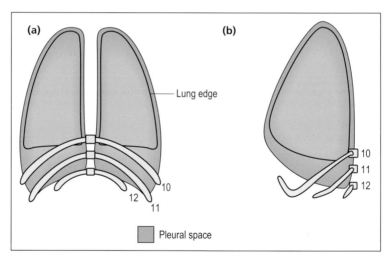

**Fig. 26.1** ■ Optimal approach for nephrostomy – posterior, lower or interpolar calyces along Brödel's avascular line.

**Fig. 26.2** ■ Surface markings of the pleural spaces and the lungs relative to the lower ribs of (A) the posterior and (B) the lateral chest walls.

***Ultrasound-guided puncture*** Ultrasound guidance is by far the easiest and safest technique. It is easy to be anxious to get to the needlework, but take time at the start to get the ultrasound just right. If you have not read the section on ultrasound-guided punctures (Chapter 23, Imaging Guidance for Intervention), then read it now if nothing else!

Scan the patient in either a prone or a prone/oblique position, using a posterolateral approach to aim for a posterior interpolar calyx. Drape the patient, infiltrate local anaesthetic along the needle track and make a 5-mm skin nick with a scalpel. Advance the puncture needle under continuous ultrasound guidance. When the needle tip reaches the calyx, advance it 5–10 mm with a darting motion. There may be a sudden 'give' as the calyx is entered. Apply gentle suction while slowly withdrawing the needle; aspiration of urine indicates entry to the system. Do not completely decompress the system, as it makes subsequent wire and catheter manipulation more difficult.

*Achieving drainage* It seems nothing could be simpler now than to advance the nephrostomy drain into position, but many procedures go astray at this stage and frustrating hours can then be spent trying to puncture a now undilated system. If you are using a co-axial set, initially introduce the 0.018-inch wire, ensuring the soft leading section (the most radio-opaque section on fluoroscopy) is completely within the pelvicalyceal system. The support from the stiffer section of the wire is needed to advance the co-axial dilator system. Exchange the needle for the co-axial dilator system over the guidewire.

Using fluoroscopy, introduce an 0.035-inch J wire, which should advance without resistance. If you are lucky, it will pass down the ureter but often it will pass into an upper pole calyx or coil in the renal pelvis. Ideally, the guidewire should be passed into the ureter; it may be necessary to use a Cobra catheter to direct it. Advance dilators over the guidewire to 1Fr larger than the drain. Leave the dilator in place on the wire to tamponade the track.

In an uninfected system, a 6Fr nephrostomy catheter is adequate, but pus requires at least an 8Fr drain for satisfactory drainage. Advance the nephrostomy drain until the tip is just within the ureter, then withdraw the wire to form the pigtail.

Inject a small amount of contrast to confirm your position but generally, unless you have performed an immaculate puncture, a formal nephrostogram should be left for 24 hours, as blood clot can simulate stones. Never overdistend an obviously infected system with contrast. This is a sure way to give the patient septicaemia. Aspirate the drainage catheter:

- Pus: completely decompress the system
- Blood – rosé coloured: connect to drainage bag
- Blood – claret coloured: lavage with normal saline until it clears to rosé.

Finally, **secure** the catheter in position with either an adhesive dressing or a suture. Make sure that the catheter is firmly attached or you will be replacing it later!

# Troubleshooting

**Difficult visualization** Optimize the ultrasound; spend time looking for a good acoustic window before you start.
- Use a suitable probe: 3.5–5 MHz is best for nephrostomy.
- Use the best ultrasound machine available.

**Aspiration of urine but cannot advance guidewire** The needle sheath is sitting against the wall of the calyx. Do not use force as the calyx can be perforated. Very gently inject a little contrast to outline the position and carefully retract the needle sheath and advance the guidewire.

**Unable to advance dilators/drainage catheter** Check the skin nick. Is it large enough? Is the guidewire kinked? The wire most often kinks either at the skin surface or at the renal cortex. If you have inserted enough wire into the ureter or renal pelvis, it will be possible to withdraw the kink outside the skin. If there is insufficient wire to allow this, it is usually possible to thread a 4Fr dilator over the most kinked wire into the renal pelvis. Insert a stronger wire and this time do not let the wire ride forward during catheter insertion. Rarely, a stronger wire than the heavy duty J wire is needed. Steer a 4Fr catheter into the ureter, then gently insert an Amplatz wire.

**The pelvicalyceal system is undilated** Exceptional for an emergency nephrostomy. Optimize your chances and use the best ultrasound machine. Consider giving 1 L normal saline and furosemide prior to nephrostomy to try to distend the system slightly. A co-axial system is best as it is fairly unlikely you will access a suitable calyx first pass. Some operators will use contrast and puncture using fluoroscopic guidance. For the more advanced, inject carbon dioxide after entering the pelvicalyceal system, and, as this floats, it allows targeting of a suitable calyx.

**Tip:** Do not try to jump too many French sizes but, as a general rule, go up in steps of two. Remember to dilate the tract to 1Fr larger than that of the drainage catheter.

# Renal transplant nephrostomy

The good news about transplant nephrostomy is the target is closer and therefore ultrasound guidance easier. It is essential to avoid the temptation to perform a direct puncture of the renal pelvis. Ensure that the path of the nephrostomy catheter passes through parenchyma. Generally, transplant kidneys have an outer fibrotic capsule and it will require serial dilators to allow passage of the drainage catheter. Remember to insert plenty of wire; if necessary, use a catheter to steer down into the ureter. Finally, transplant kidneys do tend to be a bit more vascular, so do not be alarmed by bleeding during catheter changes as the nephrostomy drain will tamponade the tract.

**Alarm:** Finishing off: remember when documenting the procedure to highlight that this is a locking pigtail catheter. Removal without releasing the locking mechanism is painful and can disrupt the pelvicalyceal system or fracture the catheter. Finally, hopefully this catheter will be removed, and in addition to releasing the lock, make sure that the nylon suture doesn't get left behind when the catheter is withdrawn, as it can act as a nidus for infection or stone formation.

# Antegrade ureteric stent insertion

Antegrade stenting is performed when long-term ureteric drainage is required. It is more comfortable for the patient than having a nephrostomy and has the obvious advantage of not needing any drainage bag. Ureteric stents can be placed retrogradely or antegradely. The antegrade approach is used when:
- There is a nephrostomy in situ.
- The retrograde approach has failed.

## Indications
- Benign or malignant ureteric obstruction; malignant obstruction is by far the commonest indication.
- Ureteric injury, often in combination with nephrostomy drainage.
- Ureteric calculus undergoing lithotripsy.

# Equipment

- Guidewires: 3-mm J, Amplatz, stiff hydrophilic.
- Catheters: Cobra or Torcon blue.
- Peel-away sheath (usually 9Fr).
- Ureteric stent system (Pusher/suture or pusher/plug).
- 8Fr nephrostomy catheter.

# Procedure

1. A percutaneous nephrostomy may already be present. Alternatively, perform a nephrostomy aiming for a middle or lower pole calyx.
2. A shaped catheter, either a Cobra or a Torcon blue (Cook UK) is inserted using a J guidewire for access.
3. Contrast is introduced via the catheter to outline the ureter and the level of obstruction.
4. A hydrophilic wire (Terumo) is inserted into the catheter and directed down the ureter. The catheter is advanced down the ureter until it is just above the stricture.
5. The hydrophilic wire is gently advanced and rotated and will readily pass through the majority of strictures.
6. The catheter is advanced beyond the stricture and into the bladder.
7. It's useful to distend the bladder at this stage with dilute contrast; this creates space for the pigtail of the stent to form and makes the procedure less uncomfortable for the patient.
8. The guidewire is now exchanged for an appropriately stiff wire such as an Amplatz super-stiff wire. Try to create a loop of wire within the bladder, and leave the catheter and wire in situ and prepare/assemble the ureteric stent system.
9. The tract should be dilated to 1Fr greater than the stent being inserted.
10. The ureteric stent system is inserted over the wire and, holding the wire perfectly still, it is advanced until the distal stent marker lies several centimetres within the bladder (Fig. 26.3).
11. The proximal end of the stent is positioned within the renal pelvis and the guidewire is withdrawn.
12. If an inner stiffener catheter is present, carefully withdraw it while keeping forward pressure on the pusher to maintain the stent in position.
13. Usually ureteric stent systems have a variant of one of two methods to allow stent retraction if pushed in too far. Method one is the pusher/suture system: a suture looped through the final sidehole of the stent can be pulled to retract the stent. If the stent is in a satisfactory position, one side of the looped suture is cut close to the skin and the suture carefully removed. This isn't foolproof. For tips on how to avoid and manage suture-related mayhem, see the troubleshooting section below. Method two is the pusher/plug system: this has an inner catheter plugged into the ureteric stent that can be released by pressing a button on the hub that advances a pusher, releasing the stent. Care needs to be taken to ensure that the release button is not accidentally pushed during insertion.
14. A guidewire is inserted through the delivery system and a nephrostomy catheter placed in the renal pelvis. The nephrostomy catheter should be capped off and if the stent functions adequately, it can be removed after 24 hours.

# Troubleshooting

**Unable to negotiate the stricture with a guidewire** It is usually possible to negotiate strictures even if no route through can be seen on ureterograms. It takes skill and patience to negotiate these strictures, not force! Get a ureterogram and advance the catheter so the tip of

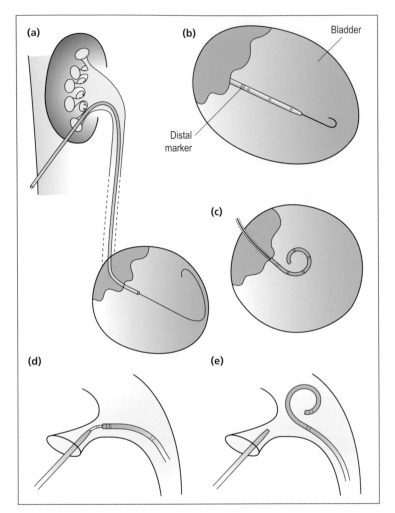

**Fig. 26.3** ■ Ureteric stent insertion. (A) The catheter and guidewire are passed into the bladder. (B) The stent is advanced until the distal marker is in the bladder. (C) The guidewire is withdrawn until a pigtail forms in the bladder. (D) The proximal end of stent is positioned so that pigtail will form in the renal pelvis. The guidewire is pulled back and final adjustments made to the stent position. (E) The central pusher catheter is withdrawn to release the stent.

the catheter is in the apex of the stricture. Use a hydrophilic wire and torque device to gently probe the stricture. This can take some time in the most difficult lesions. If this fails, it is often worth leaving a nephrostomy in and allowing the system to decompress and the ureteric oedema to settle over a few days. If, after several attempts, no route can be found, it may be worth considering extra-anatomic stenting (see Suggestions for further reading).

**Unable to advance the catheter through the stricture** Occasionally, the guidewire can traverse the stricture but the catheter will not follow. Try a 4Fr or hydrophilic catheter and try to rotate the catheter while advancing through the stricture. If this fails, take a deep breath and withdraw the guidewire and insert a 3-mm J guidewire down to the level of the stricture before advancing a 9Fr peel-away sheath into the distal ureter. The increased stability and reduction in friction mean it is now often possible to advance a catheter. Exceptionally, this may fail and it is worth crossing the stricture with a 0.018-inch wire and using a low-profile, small vessel balloon to dilate the stricture.

**Unable to advance the stent through the stricture** Advance a peel away sheath across a stiff wire into the distal ureter or bladder. The reduction in friction means the stent usually passes readily. Remember to take care not to accidentally pull back the stent when peeling the sheath apart.

**The pusher becomes impacted in the stent** With some stent systems, the pusher can become impacted in the stent after the stent has been pushed through. This means when the pusher is withdrawn, the stent comes back with it. Always screen during withdrawal of the pusher and if the stent seems to be coming back with the pusher, rotating the pusher can often separate them.

**The retraction sutures are entangled with the stent** In practice, these sutures are often a cause of problems. Prevention is better than cure and when advancing the stent, always make sure the suture loop is not wrapped round the stent. If, after the loop has been cut, the suture is still pulling back the stent, don't just pull like fury – it is possible to remove the stent, leaving an unsightly exit wound and a failed procedure. An elegant solution is to thread the longest part of the suture loop through a 5Fr dilator; using this as a buttress against the stent, it is usually possible to withdraw the suture.

# Complications of nephrostomy and antegrade ureteric stenting

**Disruption of the renal pelvis/extravasation of contrast** This will settle, providing the urinary system is adequately drained.

**Bleeding** Some degree of haematuria is to be expected, particularly if multiple passes have occurred. Haematuria should clear within 48 hours. A blood clot in the pelvicalyceal system will lyse spontaneously because of the endogenous urokinase.

Renal angiography ± embolization are occasionally required if there is persistent haematuria.

**Inadvertent puncture of adjacent structures** Pneumothorax and colonic, liver and splenic puncture are all possible. These are much less likely to occur under ultrasound guidance.

# Percutaneous nephrolithotomy (PCNL)

This technique uses percutaneous access to the kidney to dilate a tract that permits stone removal via a nephroscope. Practice varies between centres as regards the roles of the radiologist and the urologist, but more and more urologists will perform the access without radiological assistance.

As always, reconnaissance is essential and it is vital that you understand the anatomy of the pelvicalyceal system and the stone-bearing calyces, as this will determine the target calyx. Before the procedure, decide with the urologist which calyx is likely to allow the most stone clearance. Remember that more than one puncture may be required to clear a large complex staghorn.

There are a variety of different techniques to achieve PCNL, but in principle the case should follow the steps described below.

## Accessing the system

1. The urologist will place a retrograde catheter into the ureter.
2. The patient is turned prone and prepped and draped. Fluoroscopy is used to identify the target calyx and an entry point on the skin; generally, this should be inferior and lateral to the calyx; the exact amount will depend on the size of the patient. If you are targeting an upper pole calyx, the puncture will be more vertical. Remember, with upper pole punctures, going through the pleura is not good because it will leave a rather large hole.
3. The urologist can then inject contrast from below to outline the calyx and help distend the system.
4. Usually a 19G sheathed needle is used for access, and this is directed down towards the target calyx. Hitting a stone creates a characteristic feel to the puncture.
5. Now the tricky bit; there isn't much space, as you will have – nine times out of 10 – punctured a stone-bearing calyx. Carefully advance the plastic sheath over the needle until it just enters the PC system. Try to manipulate a stiff hydrophilic wire into the PC system and down into the ureter. If the urologist has put in a retrograde catheter, get them to distend the system a little just prior to puncture, to create some space for your hydrophilic wire.

 **Tip:** If the calyx is full of stone, try to puncture at the calyceal fornix as there is often a tiny amount of space there (Fig. 26.4).

6. Once you have gained access with the hydrophilic wire, place a catheter into the ureter and exchange for an Amplatz super-stiff wire or similar.

## Dilating the tract

Choose between using either balloon dilation (e.g. Nephromax) or serial Amplatz dilators. The serial dilators take more time and involve more X-ray exposure for everyone, although they are a bit cheaper – but don't let us influence your choice. A few units use Alken dilators, which are metallic tubes that telescope over each other. The advantages with these are that they are reusable and have a zero tip, so that you can dilate up to the edge of the stone-bearing calyx, without going into the calyx, which might cause calyceal rupture (Fig. 26.5). Either way, take care to think about what the leading edge of the dilation is doing to the kidney – don't push too much into the pelvis as it can completely disrupt the system. If you are using the balloon, remember to pre-load the final sheath onto the balloon shaft. The balloon is then inflated with a pressure device, and fluoroscopy used to confirm that it has completely inflated. With the balloon inflated, the sheath is advanced over the balloon with a twisting motion. This isn't for the faint-hearted, as a fair amount of (controlled) force is required to take the sheath into the system. Deflate the sheath and hold your breath – **keep the guidewire well down into the ureter**.

## Removing stone

It is not unusual for there to be a bit of bleeding at the point of access, particularly from 'cortical vessels' if the sheath hasn't quite gone in far enough. The urologist usually complains

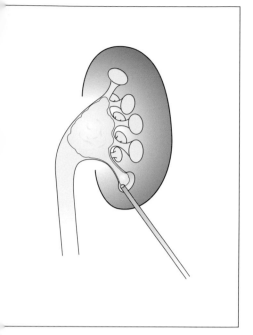

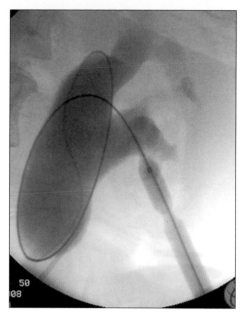

**Fig. 26.5** ■ Balloon dilation of the tract. Note careful positioning of the balloon just at the edge of the calyx.

**Fig. 26.4** ■ In a stone-bearing calyx try to aim for the calyceal fornix as there is potentially more space.

at this point about a variety of aspects of the puncture. This is traditional and resolves once the first stone fragment is visible. If bleeding is genuinely brisk, then simply reinsert the balloon to tamponade the tract.

The stone is then broken up, often by ultrasound and pneumatic drill (Lithoclast) or, less commonly, by laser and extracted via the tract. This bit can take a while, so get comfortable and make sure they aren't pulling out your access wire.

After a while, intermittent fluoroscopy will be used to determine the residual stone burden. It is not always possible to remove all the stone; generally, fragments that are smaller than 4 mm will pass spontaneously.

## Which tube to leave behind?

There has been a progressive move towards reducing the size of the drainage catheter or even completely doing away with it – tubeless PCNL. This element is likely to vary from centre to centre but generally, if you are convinced that there is bleeding during the procedure, most operators will leave a larger catheter, e.g. 20 Fr. An uncomplicated PCNL may well have a smaller 8–10Fr catheter left in situ.

## Complications

The most feared complication is haemorrhage. Immediate management includes clamping the drainage catheter, fluid resuscitation and a low threshold to renal angiography and embolization.

Injury to innocent bystanders during access is a definite risk, and colonic and pleural puncture are the most frequently reported.

# Suggestions for further reading

Barbaric ZL. Percutaneous nephrostomy for urinary tract obstruction. AJR Am J Roentgenol 1984:143;803–809.

Cockburn JF, Borthwick-Clarke A, Hanaghan J, et al. Radiologic insertion of subcutaneous nephrovesical stent for inoperable ureteral obstruction. AJR Am J Roentgenol 1997;169:1588–1590.
An impressive technique only to be performed with a responsible adult in the room.

Dyer RB, Chen MY, Zagoria RJ, et al. Complications of ureteral stent placement. Radiographics 2002;22:1005–1022.

Farrell TA, Hicks ME. A review of radiologically guided percutaneous nephrostomies in 303 patients. J Vasc Interv Radiol 1997;8:769–774.

Ferral H, Stackhouse DJ, Bjarnason H, et al. Complications of percutaneous nephrostomy tube placement. Semin Intervent Radiol 1994;11:198–206.
A contemporary update on an established technique.

Milty HA, Train JS, Dan SJ. Placement of ureteral stents by antegrade and retrograde techniques. Radiol Clin North Am 1986;24:587–600.

Zegel HG, Pollack HM, Banner MP, et al. Percutaneous nephrostomy: comparison of sonographic and fluoroscopic guidance. AJR Am J Roentgenol 1981;137:925–927.
Just in case you are in any doubt about the superiority of ultrasound guidance.

# 27

# Biliary intervention

Biliary intervention mainly involves biliary drainage and stent insertion. Until recently, PTC and endoscopic retrograde cholangiopancreatography (ERCP) were the mainstays of investigating the biliary system. Advances in non-invasive imaging, in particular CT and magnetic resonance cholangiography, have markedly decreased the need for percutaneous transhepatic cholangiography in the investigation of the jaundiced patient. In many centres, MR cholangiography is increasingly used to determine the site and nature of biliary obstruction. MR cholangiography can be invaluable in planning the procedure, particularly for biliary drainage in patients with hilar lesions.

## Percutaneous transhepatic cholangiography

PTC is now rarely used as a primary technique to evaluate the biliary tree. In most patients, the role of PTC has been downgraded to a component stage of biliary drainage. Before embarking on PTC, remember that patients with jaundice often have deranged liver function and abnormal clotting. Check platelets and coagulation before starting (see the section on patient preparation, Chapter 1, Preparing for Successful and Safe Procedures). Correct any underlying coagulation abnormality before proceeding; vitamin K is often all that is required but needs to be given at least a day in advance. In urgent cases, use FFP. Ensure that the patient is adequately hydrated and that antibiotic prophylaxis has been given prior to the procedure

## Equipment

- Chiba needle or Neff/Accustick access set.
- Connecting tube.
- C-arm fluoroscopy and a good ultrasound machine with a suitable probe and biopsy guide.
- IV access.
- Sedatives and analgesics.

## Procedure

*Planning your approach* It is helpful to review any cross-sectional imaging before starting to assess the site of the causative lesion, the distribution of duct dilation and to check for ascites. It almost always pays for you to have a quick look with the ultrasound before starting. Look

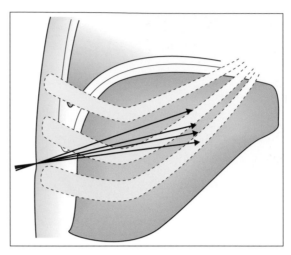

**Fig. 27.1** ■ Pattern of Chiba needle punctures at PTC. Note the pleural reflection extends below the aerated lung.

for dilated ducts and consider whether the ducts are uniformly dilated or there appears to be a segmental pattern of obstruction. Ultrasound guidance is always used for left lobe punctures but is equally valuable to direct right-sided punctures. The patient should be prepared according to the planned approach to the right or left lobe. The procedure is much simpler if the hole in the drape is positioned over the puncture site. Before starting:

- Take a control film of the right upper quadrant to look for calcification
- Make sure intravenous antibiotics (check the local preference) to cover Gram-positive and Gram-negative bacteria have been given.

***Right-sided punctures*** Blind puncture is traditionally made from the right flank below the 10th rib. The point of puncture is in the mid-axillary line. Place sponge forceps at the proposed site of puncture, then fluoroscope to ensure it is over the liver and below the pleural reflection.

**Tip:** If you don't feel comfortable with this approach, use ultrasound to direct operations.

Infiltrate with local anaesthetic down as far as the peritoneum but try to avoid puncturing the liver capsule. The intercostal vessels run along the inferior border of the ribs and therefore it is best to puncture at the top edge of a rib. Make the initial pass with the needle, aiming just cranial to the hilum of the liver. Angulate it about 20° cranially and 20° ventrally (Fig. 27.1).

The needle is advanced 10–15 cm into the liver, the central stylet is removed and the connecting tube attached to the needle. Under fluoroscopy, gently inject full-strength contrast as the needle is withdrawn slowly.

**Tip:** You know you are injecting at the correct rate when the needle tract outlines as a thin line of contrast. Big splurges in the liver parenchyma indicate overinjection.

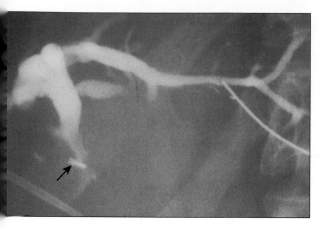

**Fig. 27.2** ■ PTC from a left-sided approach showing a surgical clip (arrow) occluding the common bile duct following laparoscopic cholecystectomy.

Look for filling of bile ducts and blood vessels. As the bile ducts fill, contrast tends to flow towards the hilum; in obstructed ducts, the contrast often swirls as it dilutes. Portal vein and hepatic artery branches flow towards the periphery of the liver, whereas hepatic vein branches flow cranially towards the right atrium. Remember that the biliary radicles course together with portal vein and hepatic arterial branches in the portal triads, so that if you hit one, you are close to the others.

When you hit a bile duct, slowly inject contrast under continuous fluoroscopy. The dependent ducts tend to fill first, so the right posterior duct outlines before the remaining right ducts or the left. The bile ducts have a complex three-dimensional anatomy and AP and both oblique views are required to analyse them. Take spot radiographs of any abnormal areas. Do not overdistend the bile ducts as this is a sure-fire recipe for cholangitis.

If this is the exceptional case, and you were only in the biliary system for diagnostic purposes, then it's the end of the procedure; pull the needle out and put a plaster over the puncture site. You can press on it if you like but it will not stop the liver from bleeding.

*Left-sided punctures* The same principles apply; left-sided punctures are made from a substernal approach with ultrasound guidance (Fig. 27.2). Usually, the target is the S3 duct as it is anterior and inferior; try to puncture it as peripherally as possible. This will give you a bit more space, particularly for wire manipulation around the bend of the left main duct towards the hilum.

# Interpretation

- **Filling defects**: are caused by gallstones, tumour or blood. Gallstones appear as discrete, smooth intraluminal filling defects, sometimes visible on the plain film. Tumour may form mural nodules or strictures. The blood clot appears as extensive serpiginous intraluminal filling defect. Its appearance resembles tramlining seen in DVT (Fig. 27.3).
- **Strictures**: are caused by tumour or sclerosing cholangitis. The distribution of strictures should be noted and recorded.
- **Beading**: due to sclerosing cholangitis.
- **Dilated ducts:** due to downstream blockage.
- **Displaced ducts**: due to adjacent mass.
- **Distension of the gallbladder**: usually the result of downstream obstruction; this is typically caused by pancreatic carcinoma.

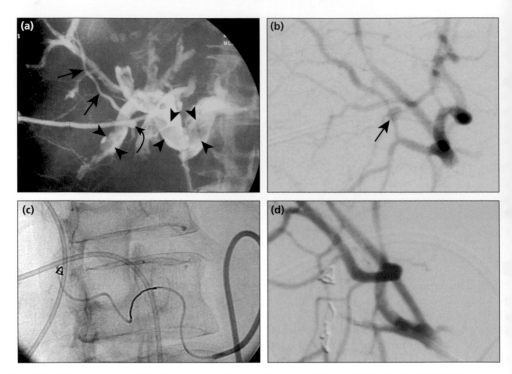

**Fig. 27.3** ▨ Haemorrhage following percutaneous transhepatic drainage. (A) Cholangiogram shows extensive blood clot (arrowheads) within the bile ducts. Note filling of a branch hepatic artery (arrows) and a false aneurysm (curved arrow) adjacent to the biliary drain. (B) Selective hepatic angiogram confirms the false aneurysm (arrow). (C) Coil embolization via a microcatheter. (D) Completion angiogram showing aneurysm exclusion. Adjacent hepatic artery branches are preserved.

## Troubleshooting

**There is ascites** This increases the risk of bleeding from the liver capsule and makes advancing stiff drainage catheters more difficult as the liver moves away from catheter. If there is extensive ascites, it should be drained before PTC. In the presence of a small amount of fluid, you can proceed if the liver abuts the peritoneum at the proposed puncture site. Many operators would choose to perform an ultrasound-guided left lobe puncture in the presence of small volume ascites. Make sure that you only make a single puncture of the liver capsule.

**You do not hit a bile duct at the first attempt** If you do not hit a bile duct on the first pass, angle the needle 5° caudal and dorsal to the initial pass and try again. Do not pull the needle right out of the liver. Stop before you cross the capsule, as fewer punctures = less risk of bleeding. If the patient is not distressed, make up to five attempts and ask the radiographer to alert your boss that you may require assistance.

**Contrast extravasates from the bile duct** Unfortunately, you have lost position or were in a small peripheral branch. This nearly always requires redirecting your puncture. If there is residual contrast in the biliary system, you can aim for this.

**The left ducts do not fill** The right-sided ducts are dependent and fill preferentially; sometimes the left ducts will only fill if the patient is turned right side up. Be careful not to dislodge the needle as you move the patient.

**Extensive intraluminal filling defects are seen** This usually represents haemobilia and is an indication to stop if you are in only for diagnostic purposes. The patient should be closely monitored and resuscitated as necessary. The vast majority of cases of haemobilia will settle with conservative management; however, you should be prepared to perform a hepatic angiogram if bleeding continues (Fig. 27.3).

**The patient has a rigor on the table** The patient has cholangitis and will rapidly deteriorate. Sepsis is more common in patients with benign strictures than those with neoplastic disease. If the biliary system is obstructed, make sure to place a drain and leave this on free drainage. Contact the referring clinician immediately. Aggressive resuscitation is often required.

# Percutaneous biliary drainage

Percutaneous biliary drainage is performed in patients with obstructive jaundice in whom endoscopic drainage is unsuccessful or who have complex hilar lesions. The commonest indications are malignant disease of the bile ducts or pancreas.

 **Tip:** Patients with Roux en Y loops who develop biliary obstruction almost always require percutaneous drainage.

## Equipment

As for cholangiography, plus:

- Co-axial percutaneous access kit.
- Guidewires: stiff 0.018-inch platinum-tipped wire, heavy duty 0.035-inch 3-mm J wire, curved stiff hydrophilic wire, Amplatz wire.
- Catheters: dilators (at least 4–7Fr), 30-cm straight catheter, biliary manipulation catheter, Cobra II, Berenstein.
- Drains: there are many alternatives – pigtail, internal external drain, e.g. Ring catheter, Cope loop.
- Stents: most people use self-expanding metal stents if permanent drainage is required.
- Peel-away sheath.
- Sutures or catheter-retention device.

## Procedure

It is useful to consider the Klatskin classification of hilar cholangiocarcinoma (Table 27.1). In practice, it is only necessary to drain about a sixth of the liver to relieve the jaundice and the accompanying pruritus. This can usually be achieved with a single, judiciously placed drain or stent. The left hepatic duct has a longer course before it divides and so a left-sided approach may offer more effective drainage for type II and type III tumours. For distal obstruction, the right-sided approach is usually chosen as it is technically simpler. Before starting, review the previous imaging to decide the most promising approach. Sometimes one lobe of the liver has atrophied and it is now too late to salvage function in it; use the other lobe!

**Table 27.1** Number of stents required depending on tumour site

| Klatskin type | Site | No. of stents to treat completely |
|---|---|---|
| Type I | Common hepatic duct | 1 |
| Type II | Confluence of left and right hepatic ducts | 2 |
| Type III | Confluence of hepatic ducts and first-order branches | 3+ |

Frequently, with a right-sided approach to hilar tumours, the initial duct entered is not appropriate for drainage, usually as it is too near the hilum. Use the first puncture to opacify the biliary system and fluoroscopically target a more suitable duct with a second Chiba needle.

**Biliary drainage: a step-by-step guide**

1. **Obtain IV access**: give antibiotics, sedation and analgesia – biliary drainage is painful.
2. **Perform a cholangiogram**: use a co-axial set; this allows conversion to a 0.035-inch wire if you hit a suitable duct.
3. **Choose the optimal duct for drainage**: in practice, any duct draining a large part of the liver. Choose a duct with a straight approach to the site of obstruction that can be accessed from the conventional puncture sites.
4. **Puncture the duct**: aim for a point where the duct is large enough to accommodate the catheters and drains that you plan to use, but remember that there are fewer complications the more peripherally you puncture. Guide the puncture with fluoroscopy and rotate the C-arm or the patient to demonstrate the position of the needle relative to the duct. When you are close to the duct, it will start to move when the needle is moved back and forwards. When you reach the duct, it will indent as the needle tip contacts it. There is usually 'a give' when the duct is entered.
5. **Confirm intraduct position**: free backflow of bile indicates that you are in the duct. If this is not forthcoming, either inject a small amount of contrast or try to see if the guidewire will pass along the duct; make sure you put a decent length of the 0.018-inch wire into the duct (certainly all the opaque floppy section).
6. **Exchange the 0.018-inch wire for the 0.035-inch J wire**: using the co-axial set.
7. **Dilate a tract into the duct**: this is usually uncomfortable, so remember to give the patient adequate analgesia/sedation. Use 5Fr or 6Fr dilators, depending on the size of catheter you intend to use.
8. **Introduce the catheter you hope to use to cross the stricture**: most operators use either a Cobra or a biliary manipulation catheter.
9. **Take a sample of bile**: for microbiology ± cytology.
10. **Cross the stricture**: this is often harder than it sounds. We usually start with the curved hydrophilic wire. The process is similar to crossing a stricture or occlusion in a blood vessel (see Chapter 15, Angioplasty and Stenting, p. 163).
11. **Confirm intraluminal position**: always ensure that you are either back in the bile duct or through to the duodenum.
12. **Exchange for the heavy duty J wire or Amplatz super-stiff wire**: an angled approach will need a stronger support wire.
13. **Position the drain catheter/stent**: internal/external drains must have sideholes on each side of the obstruction but not into the liver parenchyma. Stents must completely cover the lesion.
14. **Confirm free drainage**: make sure you do this before you attach the catheter!
15. **Fix the drain catheter to the skin**: there are many options for this; none is foolproof, so either use a suture or a proprietary skin fixation device.

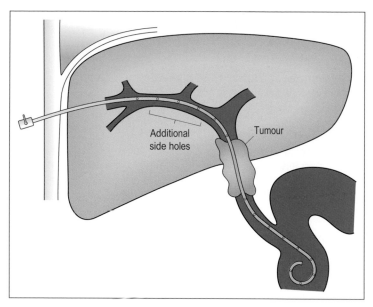

**Fig. 27.4** ■ Internal/external biliary drainage catheter. Note that additional sideholes are often required to drain the proximal biliary tree.

# Which drainage catheter?

There is a bewildering choice of drains available; the choice in biliary drainage depends on the anatomy.

*Straight drain* Only used as a last resort as a temporary measure when it is not possible to negotiate through a stricture into a large enough duct to form a pigtail. Straight catheters are easy to remove, often unintentionally. They should not be trusted and should be exchanged for a 'proper drain' as soon as possible.

*Pigtail drain* Use these when you cannot cross the obstruction but can access a sufficiently central duct. Even pigtail catheters can be inadvertently dislodged, so a self-retaining device, e.g. a locking pigtail loop, is preferable. Pigtail catheters are usually used as a temporary measure until a definitive drainage procedure is performed.

*Internal/external drain* These drains are more secure than straight catheters or pigtails. They have multiple sideholes over a long length of the catheter (Fig. 27.4). When they are placed across the stricture, bile can be drained externally to a bag, or internally to the duodenum. Additional sideholes should be punched along the proximal catheter to permit drainage from the intrahepatic biliary tree. Take care that no sideholes extend proximal to the liver parenchyma as bile may then drain into the peritoneal cavity, particularly in patients with ascites. The position of the most proximal sidehole can be determined by this simple test: before inserting the drain, put a green needle into the most proximal sidehole, then advance a guidewire into the drain. The guidewire will stop at the needle. Bend the guidewire at the hub of the drain. Insert the drain into the patient. Final positioning can be determined by using the previously bent wire to indicate the most proximal sidehole.

Rarely, internal/external drains may be used for long-term drainage. In this case, they should be allowed to drain externally for about a week before converting to internal drainage. The advantages of internal drainage are:

- Bile salts are not lost.
- It allows the patient to be ambulant without a bag.
- Skin excoriation is less common.
- The mature tract allows access for repeat procedures if the drain blocks.

 **Tip:** When punching extra sideholes in drainage catheters, use a proper hole punch rather than a needle as the results are much better. Do not punch holes directly opposite each other or in very close proximity as this will weaken the catheter and may result in catheter fracture.

## Troubleshooting

**Guidewire or catheter reluctant to advance** Bile is an effective lubricant and passage of guidewires and catheters is usually easy. If you experience difficulty, this usually indicates a problem, e.g. you are not in the duct any more. Stop and confirm intraluminal position by aspiration ± contrast injection.

**Initial cholangiogram fades** Either inject more contrast through the initial puncture needle or through the catheter if you used the PTC tract to access the biliary tree.

**Unable to cross the lesion with the guidewire** Do not be despondent; it is often very difficult to cross an occlusion in a very dilated system. Put in a pigtail drain (preferably self-retaining) and leave the catheter on free drainage for 2–3 days. When you try again, the system will be less capacious and less oedematous; frequently, it is now much simpler. If you still cannot succeed, seek an expert opinion. The adviser will help you decide whether to persist or to settle for permanent external drainage.

**Unable to cross the lesion with the catheter** Try a 4Fr hydrophilic catheter or a tapered Van Andel catheter. If this is not successful, try to pre-dilate the lesion with an low profile angioplasty balloon. If the balloon will not cross the entire lesion, try to dilate it in stages. It is sometimes necessary to sacrifice the guidewire position and re-cross the lesion with a 0.018-inch guidewire to allow use of a low-profile angioplasty balloon. These rarely fail to cross the lesion.

**Unable to cross the lesion with the drain or stent** Consider balloon dilatation. If this fails, make sure that you have a stiff guidewire across the lesion and then insert a peel-away sheath. Cross the lesion with this if you can; if not, position it close to the obstruction and try again.

**Biliary bleeding** Stop and put in a drain. Resuscitate the patient as necessary and monitor closely. Try again in 48 hours.

**Drainage stops** Review the patient yourself. Often there is a benign cause, such as kinking or clamping of the drain tube. If this is not the cause, try flushing the drain with saline as this may salvage a blocked catheter. If none of the above is successful, perform a cholangiogram through the drain to determine the problem; usually the catheter has been pulled out.

# Biliary stenting

Plastic and metal stents are available. Metal stents have a longer patency but cannot be removed; they are generally avoided in benign disease or when the patient has a long life-expectancy. Stents can be placed endoscopically, percutaneously or as part of a combined procedure.

## Plastic stents

These stents are cheap but are more likely to occlude than metal stents. Endoscopic stent placement is the first choice in most centres, with the other techniques reserved for those patients in whom endoscopic access has failed. The combined procedure, as its name suggests, involves percutaneous and endoscopic techniques. The radiologist performs a percutaneous drainage and passes a catheter and long guidewire (4.5 m!) into the duodenum. The endoscope is now positioned alongside the catheter and the guidewire is snared. The wire is pulled out through the endoscope and then used to deliver the stent. The radiologist's job is to keep tension on the guidewire and to abut the percutaneous catheter against the stent. The stent and catheter can then be pulled through the stenosis. Plastic stents (Coons stents) can be placed percutaneously but require at least a 10Fr tract compared with the 6/7Fr tract required for a metal stent, and are therefore rarely used now.

## Metal stents

Many units now deploy metal stents for malignant biliary obstruction. This is associated with extra capital costs, but these are offset by:

- Better patency, reducing the cost of re-intervention as they will frequently stay patent for the remainder of the patient's lifetime.
- Ability to treat the patient in a single session in radiology because of the smaller tract size (usually 6Fr or 7Fr).
- The patient is spared the inconvenience of an external tube.
- Smaller tracts are required through the liver.

A variety of metallic stent types are used in the biliary system. The Wallstent has been extensively used to palliate jaundice. It is flexible and comes in sufficiently long lengths to allow most lesions to be treated. The alternative is to use a Nitinol-type self-expanding stent. While there is perhaps less experience with this stent type in the biliary system, it does have the advantage of very predictable shortening and placement.

The majority of biliary stent insertions occur in two stages, with initial decompression achieved preferably with an internal/external drain. Cholangiography is then performed and the pattern of disease assessed. Aim to cover the entire diseased segment with the stent. Hilar tumours often require stenting out to second order ducts to achieve satisfactory drainage.

# Roux loop access

Many patients with benign biliary strictures will have choledochoenterostomy, usually to a proximal jejunal loop. Benign strictures tend to recur and therefore an access loop of bowel is often apposed to the anterior abdominal wall. Roux loop access is preferable to percutaneous transhepatic access to the bile ducts when repeated intervention is required.

## Equipment

As for percutaneous drainage.

## Procedure

*Access* The Roux loop is punctured percutaneously. This sounds straightforward, but the bowel loop in question looks just like any other. Kind surgeons fix the Roux loop to the anterior abdominal wall and place radio-opaque marker clips to identify it, which greatly simplifies the procedure. However, it is more likely that there will be no markers, so either:

- Perform a limited abdominal CT to identify and mark the position of the loop that is anastomosed to the bile duct (see Chapter 23, Imaging guidance for intervention, CT guidance, p. 279).
- Perform a percutaneous cholangiogram using a Chiba needle and then aim for the correct loop.
- Consider using ultrasound, but this is rarely helpful.

*Catheterization* Puncture the loop with a Neff set. Inject contrast to confirm intraluminal position, then introduce the guidewire. Dilate the tract and then place a heavy duty J wire well into the lumen. You can now place a shaped catheter into the loop and use this to negotiate through the loop and into the bile duct. This approach can be used to perform diagnostic cholangiography, and intervention such as angioplasty can be performed through the loop.

# Percutaneous gallbladder drainage (cholecystostomy)

This is generally indicated to drain an infected gallbladder in a critically ill patient or in unexplained sepsis, particularly in intensive care patients. It also provides an alternative option for imaging the biliary tree in patients in whom ERCP and PTC have failed.

An acutely inflamed gallbladder will be thick walled and adherent to the peritoneum and can be drained from an anterior transperitoneal approach. In theory, non-inflamed gallbladders are better punctured transhepatically. In this way, any bile leakage will not cause peritoneal irritation. An additional advantage of transhepatic puncture is that the gallbladder shrinks towards the drainage catheter, whereas with transabdominal puncture the catheter may be displaced when the gallbladder decompresses.

Use ultrasound to guide gallbladder puncture and take particular care to maintain access and insert a self-retaining catheter. Vasovagal reactions are not infrequent and atropine should be readily available. Drainage is usually performed for at least two weeks to allow a mature tract to form. Cholangiography should be performed to confirm cystic duct patency before the tube is removed. If there is obstruction, infection will recur or a biliary fistula will form. Clamp the tube for 48 hours prior to removal to confirm satisfactory internal drainage.

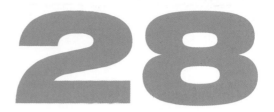

# Percutaneous fluoroscopic gastrostomy

This straightforward procedure is principally used to provide nutritional support for patients with swallowing disorders. There are two variants to the radiological technique: the traditional radiologically inserted gastrostomy (RIG) and a new variant, the peroral image guided gastrostomy (PIG). The traditional fluoroscopic gastrostomy (RIG) technique places a 12–14Fr tube, which can be prone to blockage. PIG delivers the gastrostomy via the oral route, allowing placement of larger-calibre tubes (14–20Fr) that are often easier to manage in the long term.

Feeding via a percutaneous gastrostomy is associated with gastro-oesophageal reflux and aspiration in over a third of patients. To prevent this, some practitioners choose to manipulate the tube around the duodenal loop into the jejunum, i.e. percutaneous gastrojejunostomy. The initial technique is similar for both procedures.

## Equipment

Commercial kits are available for both the PIG and RIG insertions and in practice most departments will use a kit. Essentially this contains:

- RIG insertion:
  - 18G Seldinger needle
  - J guidewire 0.038 inch
  - Fascial dilators to 1Fr greater than the drain
  - A self-retaining catheter.
- PIG insertion:
  - 18G Seldinger needle
  - J guidewire 0.038 inch
  - Headhunter catheter
  - Super-stiff wire
  - A 'push' gastrostomy tube and adaptor.

If percutaneous gastrojejunostomy is necessary, a Cobra catheter, hydrophilic guidewire and gastrojejunostomy tube are needed. Some gastrostomy kits have specific extension catheters for gastrojejunostomy.

## Technique

### RIG

A nasogastric tube is inserted on the ward and any gastric content aspirated. The stomach is insufflated with air to bring it into apposition with the anterior abdominal wall; this can be

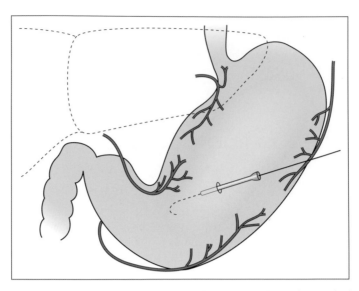

**Fig. 28.1** ■ Puncture site or percutaneous gastrostomy with puncture directed towards the pylorus.

easily confirmed on fluoroscopy. The target is a puncture at the mid/distal body of the stomach, equidistant from the lesser and greater curves to minimize the risk of arterial injury. Avoid puncture through the transverse colon and left lobe of the liver, which are adjacent innocent bystanders (Fig. 28.1).

Infiltrate local anaesthesia, go all the way in with the green needle and make a scalpel incision. Puncture vertically down; avoid punctures directed towards the fundus as these will be tricky to convert later to gastrojejunostomy. The final puncture through the gastric wall requires a short stabbing motion. It is usually possible to see the gastric wall tenting away from the needle when it is necessary to make that final thrust (Fig. 28.2). Confirm entry into the stomach by injecting contrast through the needle, then insert the J guidewire.

T fasteners or anchors can be used to maintain the stomach in apposition with the anterior abdominal wall. Practice is variable, but more practitioners are using T fasteners/anchors even for a straightforward gastrostomy and certainly in the face of an uncooperative patient, ascites or a post-surgical stomach.

**How to use T fasteners/anchors** T fasteners, sometimes called suture anchors, are a short metal bar attached to a suture/needle, that are delivered through a puncture needle into the stomach (Fig. 28.3). An introducer needle is preloaded with the suture anchor and directed into the stomach. Contrast is injected to confirm position and a wire guide is then inserted into the needle, which pushes the anchor out into the stomach cavity. The introducer needle may then be removed and traction applied to the suture to bring the stomach into apposition with the anterior abdominal wall. While maintaining tension, the thread is sutured to the skin surface. The suture is cut after a period of approximately two weeks to permit tract formation.

A variety of other fixation devices are available on the market. We can't describe them all but make sure you absolutely understand the one on your kit, as inadequate fixation can result in significant complications.

The next step is tract dilation. You may have a distant memory of anatomy tutorials and the three muscular layers of the stomach. Practically, this means you need to push hard with the serial dilators. Usually, systems then use a peel-away sheath that allows the self-retaining catheter to be advanced into the stomach. There are a variety of different retention methods

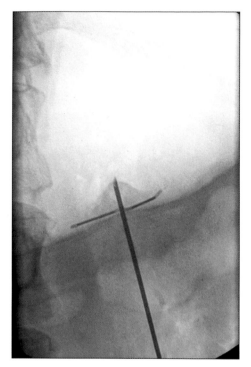

**Fig. 28.2** ■ Characteristic 'tenting' of the stomach wall. Note two suture anchors have been previously deployed.

including the usual pigtail loop catheters and balloons that tamponade against the gastric wall. Inject contrast to confirm satisfactory position, then secure the catheter to the skin.

 **Tip:** Keep the guidewire in until the position is confirmed with contrast. If you have somehow not got the catheter all the way in, you have a rescue option through the same gastric puncture.

If percutaneous gastrojejunostomy is required, the initial steps are identical but a Cobra catheter is used to negotiate around the duodenum; the gastrojejunostomy catheter may then be placed with its distal tip just beyond the ligament of Treitz.

## PIG

The initial technique for percutaneous access to the stomach is similar, but suture anchors are not required with this technique. The gastrostomy tube for this technique is a completely different design and is pulled down through the orophaynx (Fig. 28.4). This technique can pull down oral flora to the gastrostomy site and therefore a single dose of cefuroxime 750 mg is advised.

A 4Fr sheath is placed through the gastrostomy tract and the oesophagus is catheterized retrogradely with a Headhunter catheter and hydrophilic wire. This is more difficult than it sounds and can take 10–15 frustrating minutes. The catheter is advanced up the oesophagus and brought out through the mouth. The guidewire is exchanged for a 260-cm stiff wire. Working at the head end, the gastrostomy tube is then advanced over the wire until the distal extent exits the anterior abdominal wall. The catheter and wire are removed to avoid any risk

**Fig. 28.3** ■ Suture anchors. (A) Basic design. (B) The suture anchor is pushed into the stomach using a guide wire. (C) Traction on the suture anchor brings the stomach against the abdominal wall.

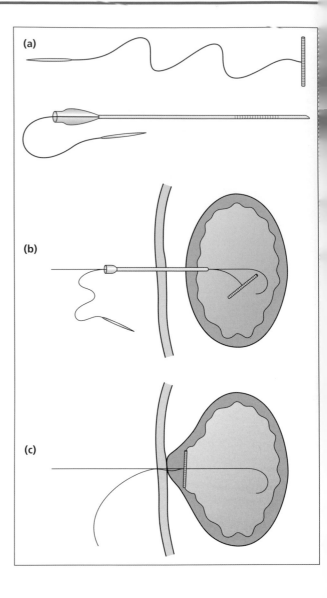

**Fig. 28.4** ■ Peroral gastrostomy tube. Arrows indicate the point of separation of the long dilator from the gastrostomy tube.

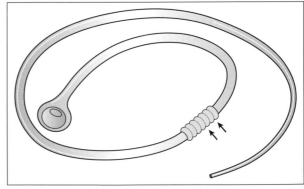

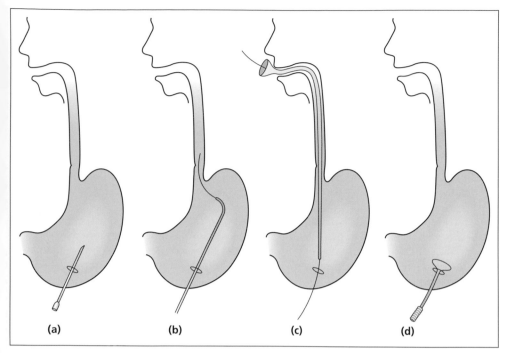

**Fig. 28.5** ■ Technique for PIG. (A) Percutaneous access to the stomach. (B) Retrograde catheterization of the oesophagus. (C) Push gastrostomy os advanced over the wire via the peroral route. (D) Gastrostomy tube is pulled down and the internal fixation collar is pulled against the gastric mucosa.

of 'cheese-wiring' and the gastrostomy tube is pulled down into the stomach. It's a good idea to prepare the patient at this stage for the sensation of the tube crossing the oropharynx; a reasonably quick passage through the oropharynx is a mercy for the patient. The gastrostomy tube can then be fixed in place with the supplied fixation disc (Fig. 28.5).

## Aftercare

The patient should fast for 6 hours post procedure, then if they are okay, start water for 6 hours at ~50 mL/hour. If this is tolerated, commence enteral nutrition.

## Results

Technical success rates are usually in excess of 95% for radiological gastrostomy. Complications occur in approximately 5% of patients and are principally peritonitis or puncture of adjacent viscera.

## Troubleshooting

**Unable to pass a nasogastric tube** It is often possible to negotiate oesophageal strictures using an angiographic catheter and hydrophilic wire using the techniques described in oesophageal stenting.

**Difficult access** If it proves difficult to be certain that you have safe access avoiding other structures, the gastrostomy can often be safely performed under CT guidance.

**Difficulty getting the catheter through the gastric wall** A stiff guidewire and a peel-away sheath can be helpful, particularly if trying to negotiate the duodenum for a gastrojejunostomy. Keeping the stomach air distended can also help.

**Difficulty accessing the oesophagus retrogradely during a PIG procedure** Pass a wire antegradely down the oesophagus via the nasogastric catheter. It is then usually straightforward to snare the wire using the gastric access.

**Access is lost after tract dilation** Not usually possible to rescue this puncture. The patient will get a gastric leak from the hole created by the dilation and may have a stormy few days. Inform the ward and give antibiotics and fast and supportive care. All the more reason to make a real effort to maintain access until satisfactory position is achieved with the final catheter. Repuncture at a later date.

**The gastrostomy tube falls out after insertion** If after less than 7 days, particularly if T fasteners have not been used, there is unlikely to be a track. Start again. If more than 7 days later, a track is likely to be present, and for long-term gastrostomies this can be maintained by the attending clinical team passing a Foley catheter, until a formal gastrostomy catheter can be replaced.

## Suggestions for further reading

Cope C. Suture anchor for visceral drainage. AJR Am J Roentgenol 1980;135:402–403.

Ho CS, Yeung EY. Percutaneous gastrostomy and transgastric jejunostomy. AJR Am J Roentgenol 1992;158:251–257.

Laasch HU, Wilbraham L, Bullen K. Gastrostomy Insertion comparing the options: PEG, RIG or PIG? Clin Radiol 2003;58:398–405.

Excellent description of the PIG technique.

Wollman BD, Agostino HB. Percutaneous radiologic and endoscopic gastrostomy: a 3-year institutional review. AJR Am J Roentgenol 1997;169:1551–1553.

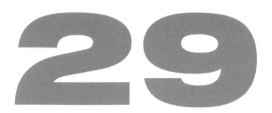

# Gastrointestinal stent insertion

Gastrointestinal stent insertion is being used with increasing frequency at either end of the gastrointestinal tract. In essence, the principles of gastrointestinal stenting are not too different from stenting other systems. The stricture or occlusion is traversed with catheters and guidewires and then a stent deployed to restore 'flow'. The procedures are technically straightforward, provide excellent symptom relief and are well within the capabilities of most radiologists.

## Oesophageal stent insertion

Oesophageal stenting is used to palliate dysphagia, particularly in malignant disease. Oesophageal carcinoma is a common condition, and 50% of patients are irresectable at the time of diagnosis. Traditional palliation of dysphagia with radiotherapy and plastic endoprostheses has a high complication rate and significant insertion-related mortality. Self-expanding metallic endoprostheses allow durable palliation of dysphagia in a single treatment session, with minimal morbidity and mortality. Oesophageal stents come in two main types: covered stents and bare stents. Covered stents have lower rates of occlusion secondary to tumour ingrowth but initial designs had a high rate of migration. Improvements in design have reduced the stent migration rate to less than 10% and most centres will now use covered stents for all patients. A few stents are available that contain a one-way valve to prevent reflux and even have a suture loop to permit repositioning/retrieval. Advances in radiotherapy and chemotherapy mean retrievable stents are an increasingly used option.

Accurate sizing is not important, but using a device that is approximately appropriate in size is required. In reality, few operators measure the true length of the lesion, as the vast majority of these lesions are covered by a single stent. As a guide, the length should be at least 2 cm longer than the lesion at either end. Large diameter stents, i.e. around 30 mm, are best reserved for the dilated oesophagus as they cause considerable pain in a normal-calibre oesophagus.

## Equipment

- Oesophageal stent: 18–25-mm diameter.
- Hydrophilic guidewire, Amplatz super-stiff guidewire: 260 cm.
- Berenstein/vertebral catheter.
- Oesophageal dilation balloons: 10–20 mm.

# Procedure

Perform an initial contrast swallow of the oesophagus with non-ionic contrast, to identify the approximate level of the stricture. The throat is subsequently anaesthetized with lidocaine spray (Xylocaine) and the patient positioned in the prone oblique position. IV sedation is administered and appropriate monitoring commenced.

Using fluoroscopic guidance, the oesophagus is catheterized via the *oral route*; it's tricky to get an oesophageal stent through the nose later in the procedure! It can take a little time to steer past the epiglottis; use a lateral projection and steer posteriorly. Try to avoid putting a guidewire deep into the trachea as this almost certainly will cause a coughing fit. The catheter is advanced to the approximate level of the lesion and a small amount of non-ionic contrast injected to outline the upper extent of the stricture. The catheter is then used to manipulate the hydrophilic guidewire through the stricture, using the techniques outlines in Chapter 15, Angioplasty and Stenting. The lower extent of the stricture can often be identified from the previous contrast injection but, if necessary, the catheter can be pulled back while slowly injecting contrast to define the distal margin. The distal extent of lesions at the gastro-oesophageal junction can usually be outlined by air within the stomach. The position of the stricture can be indicated either by radio-opaque markers or bony landmarks but remember these markers are a considerable distance from the oesophagus and even minor patient movement may be significant. The Amplatz guidewire is inserted into the stomach and the stent is then carefully advanced over the Amplatz wire and deployed in position (Fig. 29.1). Deployment mechanisms vary between devices, but most devices are deployed by progressive retraction of a sheath (see Chapter 15, Angioplasty and Stenting). Unless the stent is very narrow, most operators will not post dilate and prefer to wait for the stent to expand itself (Fig. 29.1).

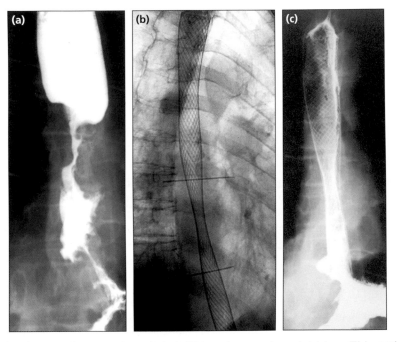

**Fig. 29.1** ■ Deployment of an oesophageal stent. (A) Irregular oesophageal stricture. (B) Immediately after deployment the stent was narrow but was not post dilated. (C) The stent was fully open at 24 hours.

**Tip:** If the markers move or there is difficulty being sure of the length and position, use a long angiographic sheath over the wire to depict the proximal and distal extent of the stricture without losing wire position.

# Aftercare

Clear fluids are permitted 4 hours after the procedure. If this proceeds uneventfully, a light diet may be commenced. It is not essential to perform a routine follow-up oesophageal study, but some centres will re-study at 24 hours. All patients should be advised to cut food into small pieces and encouraged to drink fizzy drinks, particularly cola, as they tend to prevent the stent from progressive sludging with food. If the stent extends over the cardia, the patient should be commenced on a proton-pump inhibitor to alleviate oesophageal reflux.

# Retrievable stents

Most of the available retrievable stents have a suture loop that will collapse down the stent when pulled taut. This is generally easiest under direct visualization at endoscopy, but it can be undertaken by the skilled interventionalist using a short reverse curve catheter to go through the loop and a long wire which can be directed retrogradely back up the oesophagus and captured in the mouth. Both ends of the wire are then put through a sheath (12–14Fr will do) and the sheath gently advanced to just above the stent. The guidewire is pulled tight, and the proximal extent of the stent will just about collapse into the sheath, and the entire ensemble can be withdrawn.

# Results

Primary technical success is achieved in 95–100% of patients, with significant relief of dysphagia in most series. Complications consist of migration <10%, haemorrhage ~3% and fistula/perforation 2–3%.

# Troubleshooting

**The stent migrates through the cardia** Stent migration is more common with a stent that extends across the cardia and *slightly* more common with covered stents. If this is partial at the time of insertion, then it may be possible to anchor the stent by inserting an overlapping stent. More often, this occurs some time after the initial insertion and the stent is within the stomach. Most stents are left in situ within the stomach, but if the patient is symptomatic, the stent can be retrieved (but not reused!) at endoscopy, using an overtube.

**The stent occludes** An acute occlusion usually indicates a food obstruction. Perform a contrast study of the oesophagus; if contrast is still percolating through, then try some cola! If this fails, the stent can usually be readily cleared at endoscopy.

More insidious onset of dysphagia indicates the stent has become occluded secondary to tumour overgrowth or tumour ingrowth. If tumour overgrowth has occurred, then often a second stent will resolve this. If the problem is tumour ingrowth, then either a covered stent or laser therapy should be considered.

**The lesion is high in the oesophagus** The majority of lesions are in the lower third but high lesions in the upper third of the oesophagus need particularly critical positioning to avoid stenting open the vocal cords! Endoscopy during stent placement to identify the position of the cricopharyngeus muscle can be very useful. For the very brave, an alternative is a 1-mL submucosal injection of Lipiodol at endoscopy to pinpoint the upper extent of the lesion. The Ultraflex oesophageal stent comes in a proximal release variant, and this permits more accurate proximal placement. It is generally better to use smaller devices in the upper oesophagus and the Ultraflex stent, which has less radial force, may prove more comfortable for the patient.

**The patient develops chest pain post deployment** This often occurs and is secondary to the expansile force of the stent. The sensation almost always resolves spontaneously.

# Oesophageal fistulae and perforations

There is increasing experience in the use of covered stents in the treatment of oesophageal perforations and fistulae. Malignant fistulae are readily treated by accurate placement of a covered oesophageal stent. Benign perforations are technically fairly straightforward but long-term results may be less favourable due to overgrowth of granulation tissue at the stent margins. In this group of patients, most operators would place a temporary/retrievable covered oesophageal stent; the only significant technical difference is definitely avoiding pre/post dilation as this would expand the oesophageal defect.

# Gastric oulet/duodenal stent placement

Gastric outlet obstruction secondary to either intrinsic or extrinsic tumour involvement can be readily treated by gastrointestinal stent placement. The technique is essentially the same as for oesophageal placement. Make sure the stomach has been emptied by a nasogastric tube prior to intervention, as an empty stomach is a shorter and easier route. Even with this help, it can be difficult to advance the stent round the greater curve of the stomach and the use of a long sheath can be invaluable. In a few patients, it is impossible to advance the stent from an oral route and the procedure can be performed by creating a gastrostomy (see Chapter 28, Percutaneous Fluoroscopic Gastrostomy) to allow a much more direct route. It is usual to leave the gastrostomy in situ for a few weeks rather than removing immediately, as a leak may occur.

# Colorectal stent placement

Acute left-sided colonic obstruction is a common surgical emergency. Frequently, the patient is dehydrated, frail and has not had sufficient time for accurate staging of malignant disease. Emergency surgery and primary colonic anastomosis is associated with a high surgical morbidity and mortality, and colorectal stenting is an increasingly frequent treatment method for this group of patients.

## Equipment

- Vertebral/Berenstein catheter.
- Stiff hydrophilic guidewire.
- Amplatz super-stiff wire.
- Large calibre sheath: 10–12Fr, 60 cm long.
- Colonic stents: an ever-increasing variety of these devices are available. Most are simple to deploy and we can only suggest that you familiarize yourself with the devices available in your own department. Typically, colorectal stents are between 20 mm and 30 mm diameter and approximately 100 mm long.

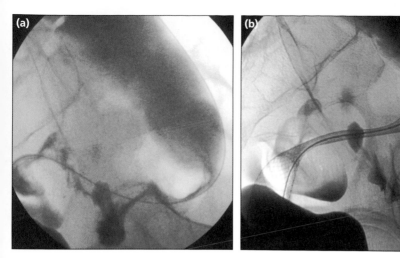

**Fig. 29.2** ■ (A) Gastrografin enema showing rectosigmoid tumour. (B) Post deployment the position is satisfactory, but note that the stent remains narrowed.

**Tip:** It's easy to find yourself with too short a wire in this procedure, particularly if you 'borrow' an endoscopic stent. Always think about the length of the stent deployment system.

# Technique

Rectosigmoid lesions can be negotiated with fluoroscopic guidance alone; however, lesions higher in the colon usually need the company of an endoscopist. Place the patient in the left lateral position and administer conscious sedation. Introduce a small amount of water-soluble contrast to outline the stricture. It is often best at this stage to turn the patient prone or prone-oblique to profile the stricture. Advance the catheter and guidewire combination and carefully negotiate the stricture. This is often harder than it would appear, as the capacious colon offers little in the way of support for the catheter and it can be useful to insert a sheath to provide additional support. Once through the stricture, carefully insert the stiff guidewire. Advance the stent over the wire; this can be difficult if following a tortuous colon and, again, a large calibre sheath may be invaluable. Centre the stent over the lesion and deploy (Fig. 29.2). Regardless of how tight the stent looks, *don't* post dilate. This greatly increases the risks of perforation and misadventure. A successful stent is usually indicated by an escape of gas/faecal fluid, in most cases from the patient!

Finally arrange for a plain film of the abdomen the next day to assess stent expansion, and check the stent position to make sure it has not migrated.

# Results

Most stents are inserted for malignant obstruction and the overall success rate should be around 90%. Complications occur in 10% of patients and consist of perforation, migration and sepsis. Palliation is achieved in over 80% of patients and ~20% of patients will have recurrent symptoms secondary to either tumour ingrowth or overgrowth; most can be treated by additional stent insertion. Colorectal stents have been placed for a variety of benign indications, including diverticulitis, anastomotic stricture and colonic fistula, but tend to have a rather more complicated clinical course. Overall, they are best avoided in benign disease, except in exceptional circumstances.

## Troubleshooting

**Can't negotiate the stricture** Is the colon below the stricture empty? If the colon below the stricture is full of faecal material, then arrange for a bowel washout. Generally, endoscopic assistance helps identify the stricture and the use of a sheath to 'prevent the catheter flopping about' in the colon is helpful.

**Oops, I've perforated the bowel** Catheter or guidewire perforation is usually without clinical consequence, and it is appropriate to persevere and complete the procedure. Perforation secondary to either balloon dilation or stent expansion is more serious and may lead to surgical intervention.

**The stent has migrated** Management depends on the clinical situation. If the stent was placed for temporary relief of acute obstruction, then often there is no need to replace the stent. If a palliative case, the original stent can usually be readily retrieved and another stent placed over the stricture.

# Suggestions for further reading

Camurez F, Echenagusia A, Gonzalo S, et al. Malignant colorectal obstruction treated by means of self expanding metallic stents: effectiveness before surgery and in palliation. Radiology 2000;216:492–497.

Conio M, Caroli_Bosc F, Demarquay JF, et al. Self-expanding metal stents in the palliation of neoplasms of the cervical oesophagus. Hepatogastroenterology 1999;46:272–277.

A good series in a tricky area.

Morgan R, Adam A. Use of metallic stents and balloons in the esophagus and gastrointestinal tract. J Vasc Interv Radiol 2001;12:283–297.

If you have only time to read one article on gastrointestinal, this is the one.

Morgan RA, Ellul JPM, Denton ERE, et al. Malignant oesophageal fistulas and perforations: management with plastic-covered metallic endoprostheses. Radiology 1997;204:527–532.

O'Sullivan CJ, Grundy A. Palliation of malignant dysphagia with expanding metallic stents. J Vasc Interv Radiol 1999;10:346–351.

Sabharwal T, Hamady MS, Chui S, et al. A randomised and prospective comparison of the Flamingo Wallstent and Ultraflex stent for the palliation of dysphagia associated with lower third oesophageal carcinoma. Gut 2003;52:922–926.

Well-conducted study; turns out there's not much to choose between them.

Wojciech C, Tranberg K-C, Cwikiel W, et al. Malignant dysphagia: palliation with oesophageal stents – long-term results in 100 patients. Radiology 1998;207:513–518.

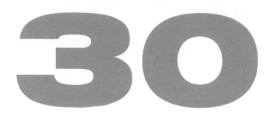

# Tumour ablation

Minimally invasive thermal ablation techniques use alterations in tissue temperature to kill tumour cells. The objectives of tumour ablation are to increase patient survival and sometimes to palliate local symptoms and painful tumours. There are several techniques which cause either tissue heating (radiofrequency (RF), microwave, laser, focused ultrasound) or freezing (cryotherapy). Advantages over surgical tumour resection are due to the minimally invasive nature of these therapies, which allows a wider spectrum of patients to be treated and reduces morbidity and mortality. Some treatments are performed on an outpatient /day case basis, with potential to decrease costs.

## Radiofrequency ablation

RF ablation (RFA) is the most widely used minimally invasive image-guided tumour ablation technique and is used for treating a wide variety of focal primary or secondary tumours in many organs, particularly the liver, lung, bone and kidneys.

**General principles of RFA**
- Tumour size should be less than 5 cm if a complete cure is the aim, regardless of the site of origin.
- Curative tumour ablation treatment must include a 0.5–1-cm margin of healthy tissue around the target lesion in order to obliterate any microscopic satellite foci and avoid early local recurrence.
- Multiple overlapping spheres (Fig. 30.1) or cylinders of necrosis may be needed to have adequate ablation of tumour, and systems that are based on co-axial guidance can be advantageous for larger lesions.
- For tumours larger than 5 cm, the main role of RFA is to debulk the lesion prior to chemotherapy or for pain relief.

There are a variety of different systems available for RFA, but the core principles and science behind RFA remain the same. In essence, RFA applicators are introduced percutaneously under CT or ultrasonographic guidance into the target tumour. The applicators have straight or expandable electrodes (Fig. 30.2). A high-frequency alternating current (460–500 kHz) is delivered through the lesion, which causes agitation of the tissue ionic molecules producing frictional heating (Fig. 30.3). The applied electrical current exits the body through grounding pads attached at the thighs (Fig. 30.4). Local tissue temperatures between 60°C and 100°C produce protein denaturation, immediate cell death and coagulative necrosis of the tumour.

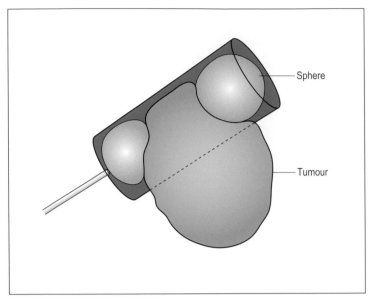

**Fig. 30.1** ■ Multiple spheres may be needed for complete tumour ablation.

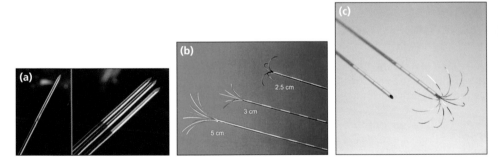

**Fig. 30.2** ■ (A–C) Common electrode types.

 **Tip:** The end point of ablation is assessed either by a change in electrical impedance or by measurement of the temperature at the electrode tip. Check that you are familiar with the parameters of the equipment you are using.

# RFA systems

There are three major systems currently in use, which differ in the power of the generator, size of needles and electrical parameters, and, most importantly, the electrode technique to maximize treatment volumes. Although temperature and impedance are measured in several of the systems, each one uses one parameter to maximize treatment diameter, and each system has a specific algorithm for treatment, which requires varying degrees of operator input. Both temperature and impedance are very interrelated and reflect tissue cooking or overcooking in a similar fashion. Temperature information at the periphery of the thermal

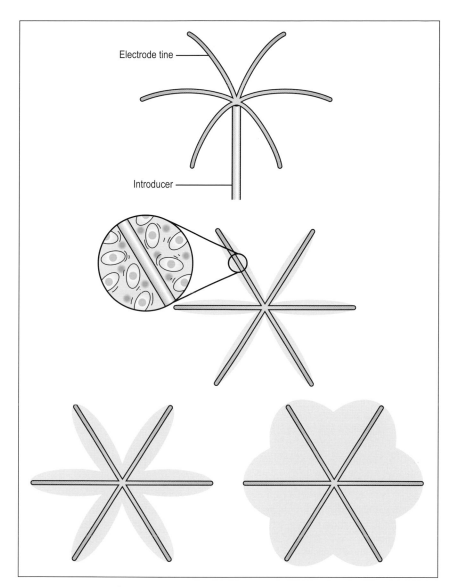

**Fig. 30.3** ■ Stages of RFA.

lesion (from thermocouples on the RFA probes or external thermocouples) may help to assess skip areas next to vessels from the heat sink. The three systems are:

 **Tip:** RF electrodes have a 'bare' metal area at the active portion to allow current to pass. The remainder of the electrode is covered in an electrically insulated coating to prevent non-target heating. The bare area is not always at the electrode tip!

1. Covidien (formerly Tyco Healthcare Valleylab): monopolar single straight or cluster electrodes that internally circulate chilled water to cool adjacent tissue. This decreases charring and vaporization, and thus increases ablation volume and shortens ablation

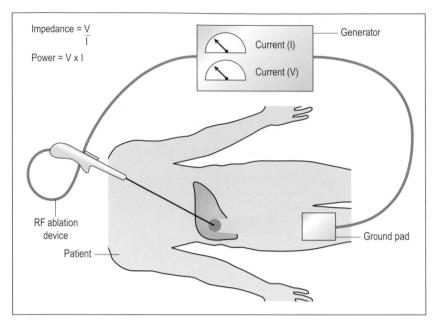

**Fig. 30.4** ■ Patient with generator and grounding pads. The RFA probe acts as the cathode of an electrical circuit that is closed by the application of dispersing pads on the patient's thighs.

time. The bare portion of the needle is some millimetres away from the tip (Fig. 30.1), hence the electrode tip should be passed slightly beyond the distal margin of the lesion. The system automatically monitors tissue impedance, which is used to determine when to stop ablation

**Tip:** Tract ablation is possible with the depression of the tract ablate button on the generator, coupled with a slow withdrawal of the electrode.

2. Boston Scientific: impedance-based, monopolar LeVeen electrode with an umbrella configuration. This has a co-axial introducer system which is positioned before the electrode is inserted. This simplifies pre-RFA biopsy, multiple needle placement for treatment and CT scanning to check needle position before inserting the electrodes. Tines are usually initially deployed along the periphery of the deep aspect of the tumour. All electrode probe tips are active. The end point of ablation is a large increase in impedance (termed 'roll-off').
3. Rita Medical Systems: multiple tines that take a Christmas tree-like configuration. Once the needle is in position, treatments are made with the tines extended by different amounts to maximize ablation volume (think of the multiple trails made by one of those fireworks that makes you go 'ooooooooohhh' and you will have the idea!). Ideally, the probes should be placed at the proximal portion of the target lesion, and then gradually extended until they reach the deep aspect of the tumour. The tips of the RITA hooks have thermocouples that report real-time temperature at the treatment volume margin. This is used to regulate current and automatically maximizes treatment volume set for the target temperature.

## Cookbook

**Covidien** Place needle tip to far end of desired thermal lesion. Turn on generator and then the water pump, after verifying temperature rise. Start with low current (100–800 mA) for a minute before increasing. In pulsing mode, the current max will take care of itself, based on tissue impedance. Peak currents should be sustained for >10 seconds. Treat for 12 minutes. Turn off generator and pump simultaneously and wait 30 seconds for maximum temperature (60–90°C). If less than 70°C, a repeat treatment in a slightly different area is needed since this temperature achievement is unlikely to have a sufficient tumour ablation and could have been a result of a neighbouring vessel (heat sink effect).

For 0–2-cm tumours, a single electrode will suffice; when tackling 2–5-cm lesions, the triple cluster with multiple ablations (spheres) is required.

**Boston Scientific** LeVeen probes come in a range of sizes (2–5 cm); choose a probe 0.5–1 cm larger than lesion size. Deploy probe tines fully once the probe tip is in the centre of the lesion. Verify position of tines on imaging. Push start on generator; check the manufacturer's recommended starting power for probe size and generally increase wattage by increments of 10 W/min. When impedance 'roll-off' is reached, the generator will stop. Wait 30 seconds, and restart second burn at 70% of last maximum power reached. For large lesions, reposition probe and restart algorithm. Finally, consider tract ablation by retracting tines to almost full retraction, select generator to 30 W, and pull probe back slowly.

**Rita** If using the Intelliflow Pump system in the Starburst Xli and Talon with adjuvant saline perfusion, the peristaltic pump must be primed and tested prior to probe insertion. Follow the manufacturer's guidelines. Under image guidance, the probe is placed within lesion. Ensure safe full deployment; verify with imaging. Deploy tines, in stages to incremental size and temperature targets – 2, 3, 4, 5 … cm marks, with power set to 50, 70,90, 110 … watts, and target temperatures at 80, 105, 110°C … and treat for time intervals or until target temperature is reached. If target temperature is not reached at any stage in 3 minutes, increase power by 20 Ws. If target temperature is not reached, rotate the probe as it may be close to the vessel.

 **Alarm:** Tumour ablation must be performed using sustained progressive heating. It is essential that you are familiar with the indications for the endpoints of the system you are using.

# Imaging guidance for RFA

Fluoroscopy, ultrasound, CT and MRI are the modalities used, with ultrasound and CT being the most useful and practical. Imaging has five distinct purposes:

**Planning**: ultrasound, CT, MRI and more recently, positron emission tomography (PET) are used for planning/assessing suitability.

**Targeting**: ideal qualities of a targeting technique include clear delineation of the tumour(s), treatment electrodes and the surrounding anatomy, coupled with real-time imaging and multiplanar and interactive capabilities (Fig. 30.5).

**Monitoring**: important aspects of monitoring include how well the tumour and/or target is being covered by the ablation zone and whether any adjacent normal structures are being affected at the same time.

**Controlling**: MRi is currently the only modality with real-time temperature monitoring. When using cryotherapy, CT clearly delineates formation of the iceball.

**Assessing treatment response**: post procedural imaging:

- Size of lesion – increase in size is normal during the first 1–4 weeks due to reactive changes after ablation. At 3 months, the lesion should be equal to or smaller than the pre-procedural size. Considerable reduction in the size is expected at 6 months and thereafter.

**Fig. 30.5** ■ (A) Exophytic renal tumour. (B) Tined electrode opened within tumour.
(C) Confirmation of electrode coverage in different planes.
(D) Post-procedure image showing satisfactory ablation.

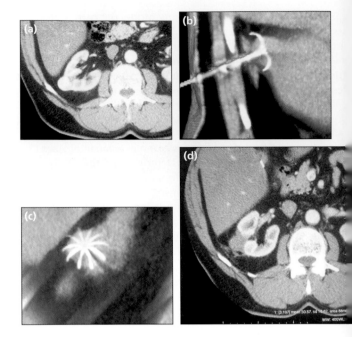

- Contrast enhancement – no central or peripheral enhancement is expected at any time after ablation.

Another important follow-up tool is tumour markers – elevation in organ-specific tumour markers points to recurrence or new lesions.

**Tip:** If using ultrasound guidance, start with the deeper portions of the tumour to prevent microbubbles produced during ablation of the superficial parts blocking your view!

When using CT, utilize the multiplanar images and reconstructions for better evaluation of probe and electrode tips.

**RFA key procedural steps:** The key to complete and successful ablation is the precise placement of the electrode relative to the tumour.
- Review all pertinent cross-sectional images, including MPR.
- Note the size and number of tumours, anatomical relationship of the tumour to vital structures.
- Plan the point of entry, a safe trajectory, and the end position of the needle; understanding image guidance is essential. See Chapter 23, Imaging guidance for intervention for useful tips.
- Ensure ground pads are secure and be familiar with the electrode/generator and regimen for heating.
- Ensure strict sterility is used.
- Ensure adequate analgesia and sedation for during and after the procedure; some treatments will require general anaesthesia.
- Inject local anaesthetic from the skin to the surface of the target organ (expect for lung lesions).
- Advance the electrode towards the tumour along anaesthetised tract and deploy.
- At the end of the procedure, perform scan to check for any immediate complications.

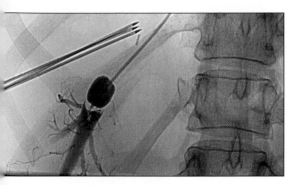

**Fig. 30.6** ▪ Occlusion balloon within hepatic vein to reduce heat sink effect.

## itfalls/limitations/suboptimal treatment

Tissue vaporization/charring – temperatures above 100°C vaporize water and carbonize the tissue adjacent to the electrode, both of which degrade the electrical conductance and result in suboptimal treatment effect. Vigilant intralesional temperature monitoring helps avoid this scenario.

- Heat sink phenomenon – if the target lesion abuts a blood vessel 3 mm or larger, the flowing blood carries heat away from the adjacent tumour, reducing effectiveness. Heat sink effect can be minimized by reducing blood flow using an occlusion balloon (Fig. 30.6), embolization or pharmacological modulation of blood flow.
- Size of lesion – see discussion above.

## Adjunctive techniques

These are used to increase the safety and applicability of RFA and other ablation techniques and have resulted in some ingenious solutions.

*Minimizing collateral damage* Protecting adjacent viscera from thermal injury is an important consideration. Other organs and viscera can be displaced away from the intended ablation zone. Several techniques are described.

- **Fluid displacement (hydrodissection)**: sterile water or similar isotonic solution (e.g. dextrose) is used to separate the tumour and the organ deemed at risk by injection through a fine needle inserted between them.
- **Balloon displacement**: the use of fluid-filled balloons positioned between the kidney and adjacent viscera has also been described.
- **Gas displacement**: instillation of carbon dioxide or air to form an insulating thermal cushion is another successful technique.
- Retrograde or percutaneous antegrade infusion of chilled water during RFA of the kidney protects the adjacent collecting system from thermal injury during ablation of central tumours (Fig. 30.7).

*Improving access* An improved window can sometimes be created to improve the path to the tumour.

- **Intentional pneumothorax**: an iatrogenic pneumothorax is created by instilling air into the pleural surface without producing injury to the lung surface. This can be performed for the treatment of upper-pole renal cell carcinoma with RFA or for central lung tumours.

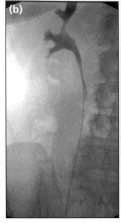
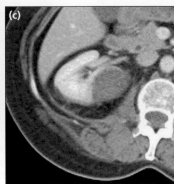

Fig. 30.7 ■ (A) CT scan of central renal tumour. RFA of this was likely to cause ureteric heat injury. (B) Internal ureteric cooling with cold irrigation via catheter to reduce heat injury. (C) Post ablation scan demonstrated no hydronephrosis and no ureteric stricture.

# Complications of RFA

New techniques bring new complications and essentially the potential complications can be divided into three categories.

## Complications of electrode placement

- **Bleeding** – depends on tumour location and character of the underlying parenchyma.
- **Infection** – strict sterility; risk factors are diabetes and biliary enteric communication (for liver RFA).
- **Tumour seeding** – commoner in superficially located, poorly differentiated hepatocellular carcinoma. Meticulous technique is required for initial placement of the electrode, with care taken to ensure optimal positioning on the first pass. Use co-axial needle, with the advancement of the inner electrode only through the tumour. 'Hot withdrawal' technique to coagulate tract site may reduce tumour seeding and also reduce bleeding rate.
- **Pneumothorax** – similar to lung biopsy; traversing fissures or long transpleural tracts increases the risk.

## Complications of thermal therapy

- **Post-ablation syndrome**: this is one of the commonest complications of RFA and presents with constitutional symptoms such as fever (low grade) and arthralgia. Seen more commonly when large tumour volume is treated. Supportive treatment with pain medication and rest is all that is required. Strict adherence to aseptic technique and eradication of pre-existing infection prior to the procedure help avoid post-ablation syndrome.

    **Alarm:** Persistent fever after 2–3 weeks should raise suspicion for infection.

**Non-target damage**: bile duct strictures, cholecystitis and perforated bowel have all been recorded. Colon is at higher risk than small bowel (more mobile) or stomach (thicker wall and fewer adhesions).

**Grounding pad burns**: The grounding pads heat up during RFA; if you feel the leading edge of the pad, this is all too evident during the treatment. Grounding pad burns are well recognized and largely avoidable.

### Avoiding grounding pad burns

- Use larger grounding pads and orientate to maximize the leading edge of the grounding pad (electric current concentrates at the leading edge of the pad).
- Place the grounding pads far away from the leading electrode.
- Shave excessive hair before applying the pad and make regular checks to ensure that sweat has not caused the pads to peel away from the skin.
- Temperatures beneath the grounding pad surface are not uniform, with the greatest heating at the edges of the pad and in pads closest to the electrodes. For this reason, care should be taken to ensure that the grounding pads are equidistant from the electrode.
- Electric burns can also occur when current between the RF electrode and the dispersive pads returns via an alternative route of arm-fingers-thigh. This is more so with RFA of lung lesions. Blankets/insulating material should be positioned between the arms and the body and legs to reduce this risk.
- For prolonged ablation, place ice packs over ground pads.

## Organ-specific complications

- These are covered in the sections on specific applications.

## Metal implants

RFA in patients with cardiac pacemakers may require temporary deactivation of the device during ablation as the RF wave generation could potentially interfere with pacemaker function (automatic implantable cardioverter-defibrillator – inactivate the ventricular arrhythmia sensor).

- Metal jewellery and cosmetic body piercing should be checked for.
- Large implants (hip, knees) are safe to treat.
- Small implants, such as cochlear implants, represent an unknown risk.

## Specific RFA applications

We can't cover every possible application for RFA but have focused on the commonest scenarios.

## Liver

The liver remains the organ with the greatest number of patients eligible for treatment with RFA, given the large number of patients with primary or secondary hepatic malignancies and the low number eligible for surgical resection.

Central (near the hilum) lesions should be avoided because of the risk of central bile duct and vascular injury. Consider the use of co-axial access needles to allow for easy repositioning of probes in larger lesions, as image guidance may become obscured. This is particularly common with ultrasound. Tract ablation is advisable in the liver to reduce tumour tract seeding and bleeding.

Difficult lesion sites, such as near the dome of diaphragm or pericardium, can be mitigated with general anaesthesia for respiratory control, injection of Lipiodol oil for lesion identification for echo-poor lesions, or prior coil insertion for fluoroscopic CT guidance and the use of single electrodes (no tines).

Caution should be used when treating patients with significant liver impairment, e.g. Child's grade C, as they are more likely to have coagulation disorders or liver failure post treatment. Similarly, bleeding complications are more common with concurrent systemic chemotherapy – particularly biological therapies such as bevacizumab (Avastin). Liver abscess is more common in patients with a compromised sphincter of Oddi (after biliary reconstruction).

Bleeding is usually minimal, and bleeding adjacent to an ablated lesion usually stops by itself. It is useful to coagulate the tract and apply direct pressure in this scenario. Follow-up CT is essential in patients who have had intra-procedural bleeding or significant ongoing pain.

**Tip:** Prevention of bleeding: coagulation factor correction is essential. Real-time imaging with colour Doppler ultrasound/CT fluoroscopy helps to avoid injury to blood vessels.

## Kidney

Indications remain limited to patients who are not ideal surgical candidates or those with limited foci of metastatic disease. Small and exophytic tumours are best suited for treatment with RFA, but selected patients with larger or central tumours may be successfully treated.

The single blood supply makes the kidney prone to infarction injury. Treatment of a central lesion increases the risk of haematoma, infarction, urinoma, cutaneous fistula and ureteral stricture. Bladder outlet obstruction has been described secondary to large blood clots after treatment of a renal lesion.

Thermal damage to the psoas muscle or nearby nerves may cause transient intercostal, groin or leg numbness or hip flexion weakness.

**Tip:** Whenever possible, avoid a posterior approach through the anterior surface of the psoas muscle, where nerves reside.

## Adrenals

RFA may be used to treat primary malignant tumours, metastases or hormonally active tumours. If adrenal insufficiency is a risk, adrenocorticoid and mineralocorticoid replacement therapy may help avoid an adrenal crisis.

For hormonally active tumour metastases (phaeochromocytoma, aldosteronoma, insulinoma), administration of appropriate drugs and continuous monitoring are essential (e.g. nitroprusside drip and complete α- and β-blockade with arterial pressure monitoring for phaeochromocytoma, glucose drip and frequent glucose level determinations for insulinoma). However, even with protective measures, these procedures entail high risk: the sudden release of metabolically active hormones (e.g. insulin, catecholamines) may cause hypoglycaemia or a hypertensive episode.

Hypertensive crisis is possible even in the absence of phaeochromocytoma. Use of general anaesthesia with blood pressure monitoring is prudent.

# Bone tumours

In the case of palliative ablation of bone metastases, the principal aim of RF is to ablate the bone–tumour interface, which is the primary source of pain. Large ablation volumes are generally avoided near the spine and sacrum, to avoid nerve injury. A passive thermocouple may be inserted alongside the RF electrode to monitor temperature rise at the level of the foramina.

**Alarm:** When performing RF ablation of osteolytic vertebral lesions, the presence of an intact posterior cortex to shield the spinal canal cannot be overstressed.

Ablation of sclerotic lesions is possible with reduced power to avoid early impedance increase. Newly developed bipolar RF electrodes are of special interest in spinal and paraspinal applications. In bipolar arrays, the current flows from the tip of one electrode to the other and no grounding pads are used. In this way, heat is generated around the tip of the active and grounding probe and mainly limited between them. This allows improved protection of surrounding tissues. RFA can be performed in conjunction with vertebroplasty. Ensure that there is a time gap when the ablated zone has had time to cool down before injecting the cement.

Bone tumours consolidated with osteosynthesis should be avoided, particularly when the electrode is close to metallic structures.

- The coaxial technique using a bone biopsy needle should be handled with care.
- The bone needles are not insulated and the active part of the electrode should not be in contact with these needles to avoid loss of energy and coagulation of the needle tract.

Plasma-mediated RF ablation is a recently engineered technique that causes tissue dissolution at low temperatures and achieves tumour debulking before cementoplasty in patients with advanced metastases compromising the spinal canal.

*Osteoid osteoma* The nidus must be identified on cross-sectional imaging and targeted during placement of the RF electrode. An insulating guiding needle, probably of 13G size or larger, which can be trephined or hammered (with a mallet) precisely into the lesion, is required. Once in position, the electrode is coaxially passed through the guiding needle into the nidus and the ablation is performed.

# Lung

- Indications include stage 1 small volume non-small cell lung cancers in inoperable patients, small limited metastases, and palliation of chest wall pain refractory to other therapies.
- CT guidance is best, as MR and ultrasound have poor resolution.
- Position the patient to allow the shortest and safest route, avoiding fissures.
- During positioning of the arm, care must be taken to avoid brachial plexus traction injury. Access should be planned to:
  - Pass over the superior aspect of a rib to reduce the risk of injuring an intercostal artery
  - Avoid passing through an interlobar fissure or bulla.
- To reduce migration of electrode tip during CT scanning, consider:

- Introducing the coaxial needle as close to vertical as possible – this reduces downward gravitational torque
- Using the coaxial technique and only placing the electrode when the needle tip is in position
- Using a multiple tine electrode.
- Lesions surrounded by lung parenchyma can be ablated with minimal discomfort. Treating lesions of the pleural surface/ribs can be painful and occasionally may require general anaesthesia.
- Commonest complication is pneumothorax. It is treated by aspiration or a chest drain.
- Normal coagulation profile must be established prior to lung RFA. Pulmonary haemorrhage in a patient with already compromised pulmonary function can have disastrous consequences.
- Electric impedance of lung tissue is high relative to other tissues; thus for small tumours surrounded by air-filled lung, RF power delivery at levels appropriate for tumours located within the lung parenchyma would likely lead to premature charring and incomplete ablation. Therefore, power delivery for small tumours that do not abut the pleura should be started at a lower power level and increased more slowly than with a large tumour or tumours that are pleural based.
- Pleural reaction tends to be worse at day 6–7 – warn the patient in advance, just as with post-ablation syndrome.
- Peripheral or complete tract ablation is not advisable in the lung as this may lead to risk of delayed pneumothorax.
- CT imaging immediately after RFA will show a halo of ground-glass opacity, which is a marker of thermal changes within the lung.

# Microwave (MW) ablation

MW radiation is at the higher frequency part of the RF spectrum. MW radiation excites molecules farther away from the source than RF and therefore the ablation zone is larger for MW ablation (MWA) and far less dependent on tissue thermal conductivity. Other advantages of MWA over RFA include less pain, reduced tissue charring and heat sink effect, faster ablation and lack of need for ground pads.

MWA is a newer technology than RFA, hence there are fewer clinical results.

# Cryoablation

Cryotherapy is the application of extreme cold to freeze and destroy tumours. Percutaneous cryoablation has been shown to be an effective treatment modality for primary malignancies of the kidney, liver, lung, and prostate, as well as for metastatic lesions of bone.

As compressed argon gas passes through the cryoablation needle, the tip is cooled, forming an iceball that engulfs and destroys the tumour.

The basic features of cryosurgical ablation have been established as rapid freezing, slow thawing, and repetition of the freeze–thaw cycle. At subzero temperatures, ice crystals first form outside the cell, causing shrinkage and damage. As the temperature continues to fall, intracellular ice forms, causing additional injury to the cell. During the thaw cycle, the ice melts and water enters the cell, causing expansion and further disruption to the cell. All the parts of the freeze–thaw cycle contribute to tissue injury.

Cryotherapy ablation begins with a freeze cycle lasting approximately 10 minutes. This is followed by several minutes of thawing, whereby the cryoablation needle is warmed, resulting

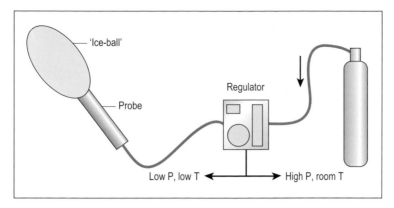

**Fig. 30.8** ■ Argon gas stored at high pressure is supplied to the probe via a regulator. The sudden drop in pressure results in a temperature drop. This is transmitted to the tissues surrounding the uninsulated portion of the probe, resulting in an 'ice-ball' visible under US, MRI or CT imaging. P, pressure; T, temperature.

in a thawing of the target tissue. Thawing is a prime factor in the destruction of cancer cells. The freeze–thaw cycle is then repeated, as it is known to be an important factor in effective ablation treatment.

The current generation of cryotherapy probes are available as thin as 1.7 mm in diameter.

Place cryoprobes before obtaining biopsy, since bleeding due to biopsy can obscure the tumour, making subsequent cryoprobe placement difficult, if not impossible (Fig. 30.8).

## Advantages of cryoablation over RFA and MWA

• Ablated zone is visible during the procedure, thus allowing for real-time feedback.
• The procedure is less painful and, therefore, conscious sedation is adequate.

## Disadvantage of cryoablation

There is a higher risk of bleeding as there is no tract ablation or coagulation of injured blood vessels with cryoablation.

## Suggestions for further reading

Carl T, Millward SF, Gervais DA, et al. Reporting standards for percutaneous thermal ablation of renal cell carcinoma. J Vasc Interv Radiol 2009;20:S409–S416.

Gervais D, Goldberg SN, Brown DB, et al. Society of Interventional Radiology Position Statement on Percutaneous radiofrequency ablation for the treatment of liver tumours. J Vasc Interv Radiol 2009;20:S342–S347.

Goldberg SN, Grassi CJ, Cardella JF, et al. Image guided tumour ablation: standardization of terminology and reporting criteria. J Vasc Interv Radiol 2009;20:S377–S390.

Mauro M, Murphy K, Thomson K, et al. Image-guided interventions, Volume 11. Saunders Elsevier, Edinburgh, 2008.

Rhim H, Dodd GD, Chintapalli KN, et al. Radiofrequency thermal ablation of abdominal tumours: lessons learned from complications. Radiographics 2004;24:41–52.

Rose SC, Thistlethwaite PA, Sewell PE, et al. Lung cancer and radiofrequency ablation. J Vasc Interv Radiol 2006;17:927–951.

Rose S, Dupuy DE, Gervais DA, et al. Research reporting standards for percutaneous thermal ablation of lung neoplasms. J Vasc Interv Radiol 2009;20:S474–S485.

Sabharwal T, Katsanos K, Buy X, et al. Image-guided ablation therapy of bone tumours. Semin Ultrasound CT MR 2009;30:78–90.

# Respiratory system

## Biopsy of pulmonary and pleural masses

Most central endobronchial lesions are biopsied bronchoscopically. Inaccessible lesions are usually biopsied under CT guidance. Large parenchymal lesions can be biopsied under fluoroscopic guidance, which is certainly faster. Ultrasound is useful for lesions abutting the pleural surface.

### Planning

Planning the procedure with review of previous imaging is essential. The majority of this type of biopsy will be undertaken with CT guidance. Plan a route that, if possible, does not transgress aerated lung, as this minimizes the risk of pneumothorax. Many parenchymal lesions will need a pleural puncture. The route chosen should puncture the pleural surface perpendicularly and particularly avoid puncture of bullae and fissures, as these usually cause a substantial air leak. Always puncture just above the rib, since the neurovascular bundle travels along the inferior margin. Patient cooperation is essential and breathing instructions should be explained and practised. It is best to get the patient to breath-hold in early inspiration. The patient must be warned of the risks of pneumothorax (around 20%; about 2–5% require formal drainage), haemoptysis and air embolism. It is mandatory to have oxygen monitoring, and equipment for chest drainage should be immediately available.

## Aspiration versus cutting biopsies

In suspected malignant disease, FNA biopsy will produce satisfactory results. Limiting the number of pleural punctures reduces the risk of pneumothorax and if a number of passes are anticipated, then the use of a co-axial needle technique is strongly recommended. Cutting needle biopsy is generally used where previous FNA has been negative or when benign disease or lymphoma is suspected.

### Post-procedural care

Most complications occur either immediately at biopsy or within a few hours. Immediately after biopsy, the patient should be positioned puncture side down as there is evidence this minimizes the size of pneumothorax. Expiratory erect chest films should be obtained 1 hour and 3 hours after biopsy. The patient may be discharged if clinically stable and the 3-hour chest X-ray is satisfactory. The patient should be given instructions to rest and avoid lifting, straining or any other manoeuvres likely to cause a Valsalva. Minor blood streaking in the sputum is acceptable, but the patient must return to hospital if there is more significant blood loss.

## Complications

Pneumothorax is the commonest complication and is more frequent if there is emphysema or obstructive airways disease. There are no absolute guidelines as to which patients require chest drainage. Symptomatic pneumothorax, a pneumothorax >30% or a progressively expanding air leak are all likely candidates. Some patients can be simply managed by aspiration of the pneumothorax. Haemoptysis occurs in 5–10% of patients and is more likely with cutting needle biopsy. If there is a significant haemoptysis, withdraw the biopsy needle immediately and place the patient biopsy side down to avoid aspiration into the other lung. If bleeding persists, consider bronchoscopic tamponade or pulmonary or bronchial artery embolization. Air embolism is a rare but potentially catastrophic complication that occurs when there is a bronchovenous communication. Needle withdrawal, 100% oxygen and Trendelenburg positioning to prevent cerebral air embolism are recommended.

## Pleural effusions

Ultrasound guidance is ideal for diagnostic and therapeutic thoracocentesis. Diagnostic thoracocentesis can be performed with a 21G needle. Specimens are obtained for microbiology, biochemistry and, in appropriate patients, cytology.

Prompt drainage of complicated parapneumonic effusions (pH < 7.0, glucose <40 mg/dL, lactate dehydrogenase >1000 IU/L or positive Gram stain) will reduce the risk of empyema.

## Thoracocentesis

The technique for thoracocentesis is straightforward:

- Position the patient seated leaning forward with the back facing the radiologist. Cross the patient's arms and support this position with pillows if necessary.
- A small diagnostic aspirate can be readily obtained with a 21G needle attached to a 50-mL syringe.
- Small effusions can be aspirated through a hypodermic needle. Larger collections are more effectively treated with a drain.
- Formal drainage of non-viscous pleural fluid requires only 6F–8Fr drains; infected pleural collections can usually be managed with 16Fr catheters.
- Therapeutic thoracocentesis is performed either with a Seldinger technique or, for large effusions, with a one-step technique. Blunt dissection of the soft tissues with forceps will aid the passage of larger-calibre catheters through the chest wall.
- Connect the chest drain to a closed system or an underwater seal drain.
- Arrange a post-procedural erect chest X-ray.

Some infected effusions will not drain because of the presence of multiple loculi, and intrapleural fibrinolysis can be useful. Streptokinase is the most commonly used agent and typically is given as a 250 000 U dose in 100 mL normal saline once daily. The tube is clamped for 1–2 hours, then returned to suction. Several doses are usually required, with success judged by clinical and radiological resolution of the effusion. Complications are rare.

# Bronchial artery embolization

Bronchial artery embolization is a technically demanding but potentially life-saving intervention. Embolization is most frequently performed in patients with chronic inflammatory lung disease, such as cystic fibrosis, tuberculosis or bronchiectasis, who have developed hypertrophied, fragile bronchial arteries.

Embolization is usually reserved for patients who have sustained massive haemoptysis. The conventional definition is haemoptysis in excess of 300 mL in 24 hours. In reality, the operator will usually only get a vague approximation of the volume loss but it is usually obvious the patient needs intervention. Continued haemoptysis usually leads to aspiration and hypoxia, and therefore prompt treatment is essential. Embolization does not cure the chronic lung disease, and therefore, typically, patients require repeated embolization sessions, with each treatment becoming more difficult as smaller vessels are involved.

Preintervention assessment must include chest radiography. Opinions on the value of fibreoptic bronchoscopy vary; occasionally, it will lateralize the source of bleeding but in many patients with massive haemoptysis blood will be present in both right and left bronchi. Contrast-enhanced CT can be valuable, as modern scanners will visualize bronchial and non-bronchial systemic feeder vessels and visualize the abnormal parenchyma, allowing the embolization to be directed to the most appropriate area.

*Anatomy* The bronchial arteries usually arise from the descending aorta between T4 and T6; however, both the number of vessels and the exact site of origin are variable. The most frequent pattern is a common intercostobronchial trunk on the right side and a single bronchial artery on the left side, although there are many variations (Fig. 31.1). Infrequently, bronchial arteries can arise directly from an extra-aortic vessel such as the internal mammary, inferior phrenic or subclavian artery.

Patients with chronic lung disease, particularly if this involves pleural surfaces, may have a collateral bronchial supply from a variety of systemic arteries including the subclavian vessels, inferior phrenic, internal mammary artery and thyrocervical trunk. The chest film will usually help identify which of these vessels is most likely to be a significant supply.

*Technique – CFA access* Start with a descending thoracic aortogram using a pigtail catheter positioned just beyond the left subclavian artery. Give at least 30 mL at 15 mL/s with a film rate of 3 FPS. In most patients, particularly those with chronic lung disease, careful scrutiny of

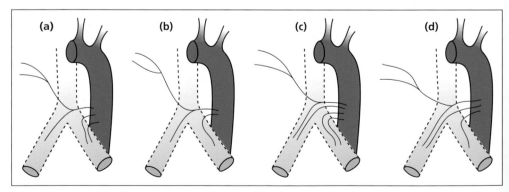

**Fig. 31.1** ■ Bronchial artery anatomy. (A) 41% – two bronchial arteries on the left and an intercostobronchial trunk on the right. (B) 21% – one bronchial artery on the left and one on the right. (C) 21% – two bronchial arteries on the left and two on the right. (D) 10% – one bronchial artery on the left and two on the right.

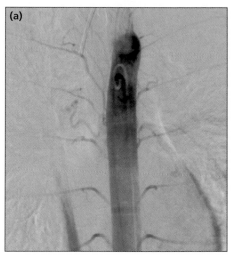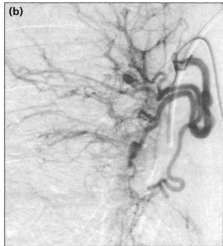

**Fig. 31.2** ■ (A) Descending thoracic aortogram; the bronchial origins can be seen. (B) Selective right bronchial arteriogram showing marked hypertrophy of the bronchial artery.

the run will reveal the origin of the bronchial arteries. If the origins are not visualized, choose a selective catheter and muster all your patience to start systematically hunting for the bronchial arteries between T4 and T6. Catheter choice is very much personal preference for this procedure but a reasonable start is to use a Cobra or Headhunter. If you fail with these catheters, try again with a reverse curve catheter such as a Sos Omni.

 **Tip:** 90% of bronchial arteries are located within the lucency formed by the left main bronchus.

## Interpretation

Hypertrophied bronchial arteries have a very characteristic appearance, with a tortuous course extending from the hila to areas of abnormal lung parenchyma (Fig. 31.2). Shunting to the pulmonary arteries or pulmonary veins is fairly common. Extravasation is very rarely seen in bronchial arterial bleeding. Embolization is definitely indicated when hypertrophied bronchial arteries are seen, particularly when clearly extending to areas of abnormal lung parenchyma. Many operators will embolize morphologically normal bronchial arteries in the face of massive bleeding.

## Embolization

Selective catheterization deep enough to permit embolization may require the use of microcatheters. Obtain good-quality angiograms to exclude an anastomosis with the artery of Adamkiewicz (anterior spinal artery supply), as embolization of this vessel could lead to tetraplegia. PVA particles (355–500 μm) are the most appropriate agent for embolization. Avoid the use of coils, as this simply makes subsequent embolization for patients with chronic lung disease more difficult.

## Complications

There is a long list of potential complications related to bronchial embolization, but these should be balanced against the fairly dismal outcome of uncontrolled massive haemoptysis. The headline complication is undoubtedly paraplegia secondary to inadvertent embolization of the artery of Adamkiewicz, which, rarely, can even occur with catheterization of the artery. Very careful scrutiny of the angiograms for the characteristic hairpin appearance of a spinal artery is mandatory. In addition, repeat angiograms during the embolization are advised, as the spinal artery may not be seen on the initial angiogram due to preferential flow into the hypertrophied bronchial artery. Other rare complications include oesophageal necrosis, bronchial necrosis and pulmonary infarction.

 **Alarm:** If you have catheterized both the bronchial arteries and the potential systemic collaterals and remain unconvinced that the source of bleeding has been identified, perform a pulmonary angiogram. Pulmonary artery pseudoaneurysms, called Rasmussen aneurysms by the cognoscenti, occur in association with chronic infection and are treatable with embolization.

# Tracheobronchial stenting

Tracheobronchial stenting is a useful and simple technique for the palliation of stridor secondary to airways compression by tumours within the upper mediastinum. The technique is usually restricted to the trachea and main bronchi and best reserved for extrinsic tumours. Intrinsic tumours rapidly grow through the open stent mesh usually used in the airway. Generally, self-expanding stents are used, as they do not require occlusion of the airway by a balloon for deployment.

## Preparation

These patients are usually breathless, with reduced oxygen saturations, and appropriate monitoring by skilled personnel is essential. With luck, the patient will have recently had a CT to assess the mediastinum and it is usually possible to measure the size of the affected airway from this examination. As a rough guide, 10-mm self-expanding stents are suitable for the main bronchi and a minimum of 14 mm diameter for the trachea.

## Technique

It is possible to perform this technique without the aid of a bronchoscopist, but why make life hard for yourself? The bronchoscopist will get through the cords easier and may even be able to get beyond the tumour. In addition, they will anaesthetize the airway more thoroughly than a radiologist can, and this may mean that you are not trying to deploy a stent during a coughing fit.

The throat should be thoroughly anaesthetized with lidocaine spray and conscious sedation may be required. The bronchoscopist can usually identify the area of compression, and external radio-opaque markers can be used to indicate the target area. Pass a suitably long wire (260 cm) through the instrument channel of the scope. Take care manipulating the wire in the bronchi as it is still possible to start a paroxysm of coughing. Carefully remove the bronchoscope. If you are already through the tumour and confident that you know the site of the stenosis, now is the time to load on the stent. Occasionally, it is necessary to inject contrast to outline the stenosis. It is nearly impossible to see non-ionic contrast, as it is coughed up so quickly; it is better to use 10 mL of the more viscous Lipiodol. Once you have markers applied to the target lesion, it is usually straightforward to deploy the stent over the target. The only potential difficulty is the cough. Be patient and wait for it to subside before deployment. The bronchoscopist can then go back down (carefully) and directly visualize the stent to admire your work. Often it is obvious from the oxygen saturation monitor that you have done the patient some good.

## Suggestions for further reading

Cameron RJ, Davies HR. Intra-pleural fibrinolytic therapy versus conservative management in the treatment of adult parapneumonic effusions and empyema. Cochrane Database Syst Rev 2008, Issue 2. Art. No.: CD002312. DOI: 10.1002/14651858.

McKusick MA, Andrews JC, Stanson A, et al. Bronchial artery embolization. Chest 2002;121:789–795.

W Yoon, JK Kim, YH Kim, et al. Bronchial and nonbronchial systemic artery embolization for life-threatening hemoptysis: a comprehensive review. Radiographics 2002;22:1395–1409.

# Index